Echinoderms Metabolites: Structure, Functions and Biomedical Perspectives

Echinoderms Metabolites: Structure, Functions and Biomedical Perspectives

Editor

Vladimir I. Kalinin

MDPI • Basel • Beijing • Wuhan • Barcelona • Belgrade • Manchester • Tokyo • Cluj • Tianjin

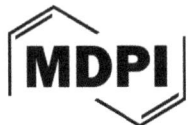

Editor
Vladimir I. Kalinin
Laboratory of Marine Natural
Products Chemistry
G.B. Elyakov Pacific Institute of
Bioorganic Chemistry of the Far
East Branch of the Russian
Academy of Sciences
Vladivostok
Russia

Editorial Office
MDPI
St. Alban-Anlage 66
4052 Basel, Switzerland

This is a reprint of articles from the Special Issue published online in the open access journal *Marine Drugs* (ISSN 1660-3397) (available at: www.mdpi.com/journal/marinedrugs/special_issues/Echinoderms_Metabolites).

For citation purposes, cite each article independently as indicated on the article page online and as indicated below:

LastName, A.A.; LastName, B.B.; LastName, C.C. Article Title. *Journal Name* **Year**, *Volume Number*, Page Range.

ISBN 978-3-0365-1594-6 (Hbk)
ISBN 978-3-0365-1593-9 (PDF)

© 2021 by the authors. Articles in this book are Open Access and distributed under the Creative Commons Attribution (CC BY) license, which allows users to download, copy and build upon published articles, as long as the author and publisher are properly credited, which ensures maximum dissemination and a wider impact of our publications.

The book as a whole is distributed by MDPI under the terms and conditions of the Creative Commons license CC BY-NC-ND.

Contents

About the Editor vii

Preface to "Echinoderms Metabolites: Structure, Functions and Biomedical Perspectives" . . . ix

Vladimir I. Kalinin
Echinoderms Metabolites: Structure, Functions, and Biomedical Perspectives
Reprinted from: *Marine Drugs* **2021**, *19*, 125, doi:10.3390/md19030125 1

Natalia P. Mishchenko, Natalia V. Krylova, Olga V. Iunikhina, Elena A. Vasileva, Galina N. Likhatskaya, Evgeny A. Pislyagin, Darya V. Tarbeeva, Pavel S. Dmitrenok and Sergey A. Fedoreyev
Antiviral Potential of Sea Urchin Aminated Spinochromes against Herpes Simplex Virus Type 1
Reprinted from: *Marine Drugs* **2020**, *18*, 550, doi:10.3390/md18110550 5

Sergey A. Dyshlovoy, Dmitry N. Pelageev, Jessica Hauschild, Yurii E. Sabutskii, Ekaterina A. Khmelevskaya, Christoph Krisp, Moritz Kaune, Simone Venz, Ksenia L. Borisova, Tobias Busenbender, Vladimir A. Denisenko, Hartmut Schlüter, Carsten Bokemeyer, Markus Graefen, Sergey G. Polonik, Victor Ph. Anufriev and Gunhild von Amsberg
Inspired by Sea Urchins: Warburg Effect Mediated Selectivity of Novel Synthetic Non-Glycoside 1,4-Naphthoquinone-6S-Glucose Conjugates in Prostate Cancer
Reprinted from: *Marine Drugs* **2020**, *18*, 251, doi:10.3390/md18050251 21

Sergey Polonik, Galina Likhatskaya, Yuri Sabutski, Dmitry Pelageev, Vladimir Denisenko, Evgeny Pislyagin, Ekaterina Chingizova, Ekaterina Menchinskaya and Dmitry Aminin
Synthesis, Cytotoxic Activity Evaluation and Quantitative Structure-ActivityAnalysis of Substituted 5,8-Dihydroxy-1,4-naphthoquinones and Their *O*- and *S*-Glycoside Derivatives Tested against Neuro-2a Cancer Cells
Reprinted from: *Marine Drugs* **2020**, *18*, 602, doi:10.3390/md18120602 53

Alexandra S. Silchenko, Anatoly I. Kalinovsky, Sergey A. Avilov, Pelageya V. Andrijaschenko, Roman S. Popov, Pavel S. Dmitrenok, Ekaterina A. Chingizova, Svetlana P. Ermakova, Olesya S. Malyarenko, Salim Sh. Dautov and Vladimir I. Kalinin
Structures and Bioactivities of Quadrangularisosides A, A_1, B, B_1, B_2, C, C_1, D, D_1–D_4, and E from the Sea Cucumber *Colochirus quadrangularis*: The First Discovery of the Glycosides, Sulfated by C-4 of the Terminal 3-*O*-Methylglucose Residue. Synergetic Effect on Colony Formation of Tumor HT-29 Cells of these Glycosides with Radioactive Irradiation
Reprinted from: *Marine Drugs* **2020**, *18*, 394, doi:10.3390/md18080394 83

Alexandra S. Silchenko, Anatoly I. Kalinovsky, Sergey A. Avilov, Pelageya V. Andrijaschenko, Roman S. Popov, Pavel S. Dmitrenok, Ekaterina A. Chingizova and Vladimir I. Kalinin
Kurilosides A_1, A_2, C_1, D, E and F—Triterpene Glycosides from the Far Eastern Sea Cucumber *Thyonidium* (= *Duasmodactyla*) *kurilensis* (Levin): Structures with Unusual Non-Holostane Aglycones and Cytotoxicities
Reprinted from: *Marine Drugs* **2020**, *18*, 551, doi:10.3390/md18110551 119

Timofey V. Malyarenko, Alla A. Kicha, Olesya S. Malyarenko, Viktor M. Zakharenko, Ivan P. Kotlyarov, Anatoly I. Kalinovsky, Roman S. Popov, Vasily I. Svetashev and Natalia V. Ivanchina
New Conjugates of Polyhydroxysteroids with Long-Chain Fatty Acids from the Deep-Water Far Eastern Starfish *Ceramaster patagonicus* and Their Anticancer Activity
Reprinted from: *Marine Drugs* **2020**, *18*, 260, doi:10.3390/md18050260 . . . . **141**

Laura Carreón-Palau, Nurgül Şen Özdemir, Christopher C. Parrish and Camilla Parzanini
Sterol Composition of Sponges, Cnidarians, Arthropods, Mollusks, and Echinoderms from the Deep Northwest Atlantic: A Comparison with Shallow Coastal Gulf of Mexico
Reprinted from: *Marine Drugs* **2020**, *18*, 598, doi:10.3390/md18120598 . . . . **155**

Nadezhda E. Ustyuzhanina, Maria I. Bilan, Andrey S. Dmitrenok, Alexandra S. Silchenko, Boris B. Grebnev, Valentin A. Stonik, Nikolay E. Nifantiev and Anatolii I. Usov
Fucosylated Chondroitin Sulfates from the Sea Cucumbers *Paracaudina chilensis* and *Holothuria hilla*: Structures and Anticoagulant Activity
Reprinted from: *Marine Drugs* **2020**, *18*, 540, doi:10.3390/md18110540 . . . . **175**

About the Editor

Vladimir I. Kalinin

Vladimir I. Kalinin (PhD in chemistry and Dr. Sc. in biology (biochemistry)), from 1979 to now has worked at G.B. Elyakov Pacific Institute of Bioorganic Chemistry of the Far Eastern Branch of the Russian Academy of Sciences (Vladivostok, Russia), and from 1998 to now has been the leading scientist. His scientific interests: structure, biological activities, taxonomical distribution, chemotaxonomy significance and evolution of sea cucumber triterpene glycosides. The author and co-author of more than 80 book chapters and scientific articles. Associate Editor of the Natural Product Communications, Member of Marine Drugs Editorial Board, Guest Editor of the SIs of *Marine Drugs* "Marine Glycoconjugates, Trends and Perspectives", "Echinoderms metabolites: structure, function and biomedical perspectives" and "Echinoderms metabolites: structure, function and biomedical perspectives II". Participant of expeditions on r/v "Professor Bogorov" and "Akademik Oparin" in Indian and the Pacific Ocean.

Preface to "Echinoderms Metabolites: Structure, Functions and Biomedical Perspectives"

Echinoderms are unique sources of different metabolites having a wide spectrum of biological activities. All echinoderms possess a unique mechanism of decreasing the lever of free 5,6-unsaturated sterols in their cell membranes –sulfation of these food sterols. Moreover, sea cucumbers and starfish transform these 5,6-unsaturated sterols into stanols or 7,8-unsaturated sterols that allow them to synthesize and keep their own 5,6-sterol-depending membranolytic toxins, namely triterpene oligoglycosides for sea cucumbers and steroid olygoglycosides for starfish, which have protective significance for the producers. Starfish and brittle stars have numerous polyhydoxysteroids and their sulfated and glycosylated derivatives, using them as food emulgators. All echinoderms contain carotenoids and naphthoquinone pigments. The latter are widely presented in sea urchins. The lipid composition of echinoderms is also uncommon and very interesting. For example, they contain cerebrosides and gangliosides characteristic of other deuterostomes, including Chordata, Hemichordata, and Tunicata, relatives of echinoderms. Echinoderms contain lectins, glycan-specific glycoproteins with immunity functions for the producers, and glycoseaminoglycans. Microorganisms associated with some echninoderms and adopted into their toxins may also produce very uncommon metabolites, such as diterpene glycosides synthesized by some fungi associated with sea cucumbers. All the listed as well as other classes of echinoderm metabolites possess significant biomedical potential revealing cytotoxic, antitumor, antifungal, immunomodulatory, antioxidant activity, anti-arthritic, and anti-diabetic action and may also be used as a food supplement for nutrition. The main goal of this Special Issue, "Echinoderm Metabolites: Structure, Functions, and Biomedical Perspectives", is to provide a convenient platform for discussion of all possible scientific aspects concerning low molecular weight and biopolymer metabolites from echinoderms and the microorganisms associated with them, including their isolation and chemical structures, taxonomical distribution and participation in food chains, methods of analysis, biological activities, biosynthesis and evolution, biological functions, and chemical syntheses, including the obtaining of semi-synthetic derivatives of biologically active natural products.

Vladimir I. Kalinin
Editor

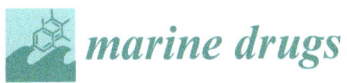

Editorial

Echinoderms Metabolites: Structure, Functions, and Biomedical Perspectives

Vladimir I. Kalinin

G.B. Elyakov Pacific Institute of Bioorganic Chemistry, Far Eastern Branch of the Russian Academy of Sciences, Pr. 100-letya Vladivostoka 159, 690022 Vladivostok, Russia; kalininv@piboc.dvo.ru; Tel.: +7-914-705-08-45

Citation: Kalinin, V.I. Echinoderms Metabolites: Structure, Functions, and Biomedical Perspectives. *Mar. Drugs* 2021, *19*, 125. https://doi.org/10.3390/md19030125

Received: 19 February 2021
Accepted: 25 February 2021
Published: 26 February 2021

Publisher's Note: MDPI stays neutral with regard to jurisdictional claims in published maps and institutional affiliations.

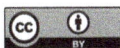

Copyright: © 2021 by the author. Licensee MDPI, Basel, Switzerland. This article is an open access article distributed under the terms and conditions of the Creative Commons Attribution (CC BY) license (https://creativecommons.org/licenses/by/4.0/).

Echinoderms are marine invertebrates belonging to the phylum Echinodermata (from the Ancient Greek words "echinos" (hedgehog) and "derma" (skin)). They have radial symmetry, a unique water vascular (ambulacral) system, and a limestone skeleton, and they include the classes Asteroidea (starfish), Ophiuroidea (brittle stars), Echinoidea (sea urchins), Holothuroidea (sea cucumbers), and Crinoidea (sea lilies). The skeleton of sea cucumbers is reduced by ossicles. Echinoderms have no freshwater or terrestrial representatives and are habitants of all ocean depths. The phylum contains more than 7000 living species [1]. Echinoderms are unique sources of different metabolites having a wide spectrum of biological activities [2]. All echinoderms possess a unique mechanism of decreasing the level of free 5,6-unsaturated sterols in their cell membranes—sulfation of these food sterols [3]. Moreover, sea cucumbers and starfish transform these 5,6-unsaturated sterols into stanols or 7,8-unsaturated sterols, which allows them to synthesize and keep their own 5,6-sterol-dependent membranolytic toxins, namely, triterpene oligoglycosides for sea cucumbers and steroid oligoglycosides for starfish, which have protective significance for the producers [4,5]. Starfish and brittle stars have numerous polyhydroxysteroids and their sulfated and glycosylated derivatives, using them as food emulgators [6]. All echinoderms contain carotenoids [7] and naphthoquinone pigments [8]. The latter are widely presented in sea urchins [9]. The lipid composition of echinoderms is also uncommon and very interesting. For example, they contain cerebrosides [10] and gangliosides [11], which are characteristic of other deuterostomes, including Chordata, Hemichordata, and Tunicata, relatives of echinoderms [12]. Echinoderms contain lectins, glycan-specific glycoproteins with immunity functions for the producers [13], and glycosaminoglycans [14].

In this Special Issue, the echinoderms naphthoquinoids and their analogs are discussed in three articles. The article by Mishchenko et al. concerns the ability of sea urchin pigments (spinochromes)—echinochrome A and its aminated analogues, echinamines A and B—to inhibit different stages of HSV-1 infection in Vero cells and to decrease the virus-induced production of reactive oxygen species. The author found that spinochromes were maximally effective when HSV-1 was pretreated with the tested compounds, revealing the direct effect of spinochromes on the virus particles [15]. Dyshlovoy et al. designed, synthesized, and analyzed a series of 6-S-(1,4-naphthoquinone-2-yl)-D-glucose chimera molecules—novel sugar conjugates of 1,4-naphthoquinone analogs of the sea urchin pigments spinochromes, which were previously known to have anticancer properties. These compounds prevented potential hydrolysis by human glycoside-unspecific enzymes and blocked the Warburg effect—the consumption of sugars by cancer cells that mediates selectivity of their activity against human prostate cancer cells. These substances permeabilize mitochondria membranes, followed by ROS upregulation and release of cytotoxic mitochondrial proteins (AIF and cytochrome C) to the cytoplasm. This leads to the consequent caspase-9 and -3 activation, PARP cleavage, and apoptosis-like cell death [16]. Polonik et al., on the basis of 6,7-substituted 2,5,8-trihydroxy-1,4-naphtoquinone derived from sea urchins, synthesized five new acetyl-O-glucosides of the naphthoquinones. They also synthesized 28 new thiomethylglycosides of 2-hydroxy and 2-methoxy-1,4-naphtoquinones and investigated the cytotoxic activity of 1,4-naphtoquinones (13 compounds) and their O- and

S-glycoside derivatives (37 compounds using the MTT method against Neuro-2a mouse neuroblastoma cells). A quantitative structure–activity relationship (QSAR) model of cytotoxic activity of 22 1,4-naphtoquinone derivatives was constructed and tested. The QSAR model was well appropriated for prediction of the activity of 1,4-naphtoquinone derivatives [17]. Hence, the naphthoquinone metabolites and their analogs and derivatives from echinoderms have good medical perspectives as anticancer and antiviral preparations.

Two articles present isolation, structural elucidation, and biosynthetic interpretation of triterpene glycosides from sea cucumbers. The first one concerns the isolation and structural elucidation of thirteen new mono-, di-, and tri-sulfated triterpene glycosides, quadrangularisosides A, A_1, B, B_1, B_2, C, C_1, D, D_1–D_4 and E from the sea cucumber *Colochirus quadrangularis* from Vietnamese shallow waters. The structures of these glycosides were established by 2D NMR spectroscopy and HR-ESI mass spectrometry. The novel carbohydrate moieties of quadrangularisosides D–D_4, belonging to the group D, and quadrangularisoside E contain three sulfate groups, including one of them occupying an unusual position at C(4) of terminal 3-O-methylglucose residue. Quadrangularisosides A and D_3 as well as quadrangularisosides A_1 and D_4 are characterized by the new aglycones with 25-hydroperoxyl or 24-hydroperoxyl groups in their side chains, respectively. The cytotoxic activities of the isolated compounds were studied. All the compounds were rather strong cytotoxins, but the presence of hydroperoxide groups decreased the activities. Quadrangularisosides A_1, C, C_1, and E possessed strong inhibitory activity on colony formation in HT-29 cells. Due to the synergic effects of these glycosides (0.02 µM) and radioactive irradiation (1 Gy), a decreasing number of colonies was detected [18]. The second article concerns the isolation and structural elucidation of six new monosulfated triterpene tetra-, penta- and hexa-osides, namely, kurilosides A_1, A_2, C_1, D, E, and F, as well as the known earlier kuriloside A, with unusual non-holostane aglycones without lactone, from the sea cucumber *Thyonidium* (= *Duasmodactyla*) *kurilensis* (Levin) (Cucumariidae, Dendrochirotida), collected in the Sea of Okhotsk near Onekotan Island from a depth of 100 m. Structures of the glycosides were elucidated by 2D NMR spectroscopy and HR-ESI mass spectrometry. The cytotoxicity of the isolated compounds was studied. The substances have moderate or low activities [19].

The article by Malyarenko et al. concerns the isolation and structural elucidation of four new conjugates, esters of polyhydroxysteroids with long-chain fatty acids from the deep-water Far Eastern starfish *Ceramaster patagonicus*. The structures of the conjugates were elucidated by NMR and ESIMS and all necessary chemical transformations. Very unusual isolated natural products contain 5α-cholestane-3β,6β,15α,16β,26-pentahydroxysteroidal core and differ from each other in terms of the following fatty acid residues: 5'Z,11'Z-octadecadienoic, 11'Z-octadecenoic, 5'Z,11'Z-eicosadienoic, and 7'Z-eicosenoic acids. Only one similar steroid conjugate with a fatty acid was previously isolated from starfish. The action against cancer cells has been studied. Most of the conjugates are moderately cytotoxic, and one conjugate suppressed colony formation and migration of human breast cancer MDA-MB-231 cells and colorectal carcinoma HCT 116 cells [20].

Another article on steroids concerns the use of free sterols as food markers for deep sea sponges, cnidarians, mollusks, crustaceans, and echinoderms. The authors selected echinoids as their model object because the composition of free sterols in sea cucumber and starfish is deviated by their own cytotoxins and dietary sterols significantly transformed by these classes of echinoderms. The identification of sterols was carried out using the GC–MS method. The authors compared the sterol composition of the representatives of three different phyla, namely, Porifera, Cnidaria, and Echinodermata, collected from a deep- and cold-water region on the one hand, and from a shallow tropical area on the other. They found that shallow tropical sponges and cnidarians had plant and zooxanthellae sterols in their tissues, while their deep-sea counterparts displayed phytoplankton and zooplankton sterols. In contrast, echinoids, a class of echinoderms, the most complex phylum along with hemichordates and chordates (deuterostomes), did not show significant differences in their sterol profiles, suggesting that cholesterol synthesis is present in deuterostomes other than protostomes [21].

The final article covers the polymeric metabolites of echinoderms, namely fucosylated chondroitin sulfates (FCSs), PC and HH isolated from the sea cucumbers *Paracaudina chilensis* and *Holothuria hilla*, respectively. The structural characterization of these polysaccharides was performed by chemical transformations and using advanced NMR spectroscopic methods. Both polysaccharides contain a chondroitin core [→3)-β-D-GalNAc (N-acetyl galactosamine)-(1→4)-β-D-GlcA (glucuronic acid)-(1→]$_n$, bearing sulfated fucosyl branches at O-3 of every GlcA residue in the chain. These fucosyl residues were different in terms of their character of sulfation: PC contained Fuc2S4S and Fuc4S in a ratio of 2:1, whereas HH possessed Fuc2S4S, Fuc3S4S, and Fuc4S in a ratio of 1.5:1:1. It was also observed that some GalNAc residues in HH contain an unusual disaccharide branch of Fuc4S-(1→2)-Fuc3S4S-(1→ at O-6. Sulfated GalNAc4S6S and GalNAc4S units were found in a ratio of 3:2 for PC and 2:1 for HH, respectively. The polysaccharides revealed significant anticoagulant activity in a clotting time assay, which was caused by the ability of these FCSs to induce the inhibition of thrombin and factor Xa in the presence of anti-thrombin III (ATIII) and with the direct inhibition of thrombin in the absence of any cofactors [22].

The materials published in the Special Issue reflect the real diversity of echinoderm metabolites and cover most of their specific classes and biomedical potential as antioxidant, antiviral, anticancer, and even anticoagulant preparations.

Funding: This research received no external funding.

Conflicts of Interest: The authors declare no conflict of interest.

References

1. Wray, G.A. 1999. Echinodermata. Spiny-Skinned Animals: Sea Urchins, Starfish, and Their Allies. Version 14 December 1999 (Under Construction). Available online: http://tolweb.org/Echinodermata/2497/1999.12.14 (accessed on 26 February 2021).
2. Gomes, A.R.; Freitas, A.C.; Rocha-Santos, T.A.P.; Duarte, A.C. Bioactive compounds derived from echinoderms. *RSC Adv.* **2014**, *4*, 29365–29382. [CrossRef]
3. Goodfellow, E.R.M.; Goad, L.J. The steryl sulfate content of echinoderms and some marine invertebrates. *Comp. Biochem. Physiol.* **1983**, *76B*, 575–578.
4. Claereboudt, E.J.S.; Eeckhaut, I.; Lins, L.; Deleu, M. How different sterols contribute to saponin tolerant plasma membranes in sea cucumbers. *Sci. Rep.* **2018**, *8*, 10845. [CrossRef] [PubMed]
5. Goad, L.J.; Rubinstein, I.; Smith, A.G. The sterols of echinoderms. *Comp. Biochem. Physiol.* **1972**, *180B*, 223–246.
6. Stonik, V.A.; Ivanchina, N.V.; Kicha, A.A. New polar steroids from starfish. *Nat. Prod. Commun.* **2008**, *3*, 1587–1610. [CrossRef]
7. Pereira, D.M.; Andrade, P.B.; Pires, R.A.; Reis, R.L. Chemical ecology of echinoderms: Impact of environment and diet in metabolomic profile. In *Ecology, Habitants and Reproductive Biology*; Whitmore, E., Ed.; Nova Science Publisher: Hauppauge, NY, USA, 2014; pp. 58–76.
8. Hou, Y.; Vasileva, E.A.; Carne, A.; McConnell, M.; El-Din, A.; Bekhitaan, A.; Mishchenko, N.P. Naphthoquinones of the spinochrome class: Occurrence, isolation, biosynthesis and biomedical applications. *RSC Adv.* **2018**, *8*, 32637–32650. [CrossRef]
9. Shikov, A.N.; Pozharitskaya, O.N.; Krishtopina, A.S.; Makarov, V.G. Naphthoquinone pigments from sea urchins: Chemistry and pharmacology. *Phytochem. Rev.* **2018**, *17*, 509–534. [CrossRef]
10. Tan, R.X.; Chen, J.H. The cerebrosides. *Nat. Prod. Rep.* **2003**, *20*, 509–534. [CrossRef] [PubMed]
11. Higuchi, R.; Inagaki, M.; Yamada, K.; Miyamoto, Y. Biologically active gangliosides from echinoderms. *J. Nat. Med.* **2007**, *61*, 367–370. [CrossRef]
12. Careaga, V.; Majer, M. Cerebrosides from marine organisms. In *Studies in Natural Product Chemistry*; Atta-ur-Rahman, Ed.; Elsevier B.V.: Amsterdam, The Netherlands, 2014; Volume 42, pp. 59–81.
13. Hasan, I.; Gerdol, M.; Fujii, Y.; Ozeki, Y. Functional characterization of OXYL, a SghC1qDC LacNAc-specific lectin from the crinoid feather star *Anneissia japonica*. *Mar. Drugs* **2019**, *17*, 136. [CrossRef] [PubMed]
14. Chen, Y.; Wang, Y.; Yang, S.; Yu, M.; Jiang, T.; Lv, Z. Glycosaminoglycan from *Apostichopus japonicus* improves glucose metabolism in the liver of insulin resistant mice. *Mar. Drugs* **2020**, *18*, 1. [CrossRef] [PubMed]
15. Mishchenko, N.P.; Krylova, N.V.; Iunikhina, O.V.; Vasileva, E.A.; Likhatskaya, G.N.; Pislyagin, E.A.; Tarbeeva, D.V.; Dmitrenok, P.S.; Fedoreyev, S.A. Antiviral potential of sea urchin aminated spinochromes against herpes simplex virus type 1. *Mar. Drugs* **2020**, *18*, 550. [CrossRef] [PubMed]

16. Dyshlovoy, S.A.; Pelageev, D.N.; Hauschild, J.; Sabutskii, Y.E.; Khmelevskaya, E.A.; Krisp, C.; Kaune, M.; Venz, S.; Borisova, K.L.; Busenbender, T.; et al. Inspired by sea urchins: Warburg effect mediated selectivity of novel synthetic non-glycoside 1,4-naphthoquinone-6S-glucose conjugates in prostate cancer. *Mar. Drugs* **2020**, *18*, 251. [CrossRef] [PubMed]
17. Polonik, S.; Likhatskaya, G.; Sabutski, Y.; Pelageev, D.; Denisenko, V.; Pislyagin, E.; Chingizova, E.; Menchinskaya, E.; Aminin, D. Synthesis, cytotoxic activity evaluation and quantitative structure-activity analysis of substituted 5,8-dihydroxy-1,4-naphthoquinones and their O- and S-glycoside derivatives tested against Neuro-2a cancer cells. *Mar. Drugs* **2020**, *18*, 602. [CrossRef] [PubMed]
18. Silchenko, A.S.; Kalinovsky, A.I.; Avilov, S.A.; Andrijaschenko, P.V.; Popov, R.S.; Dmitrenok, P.S.; Chingizova, E.A.; Ermakova, S.P.; Malyarenko, O.S.; Dautov, S.S.; et al. Structures and bioactivities of quadrangularisosides A, A_1, B, B_1, B_2, C, C_1, D, D_1–D_4, and E from the sea cucumber *Colochirus quadrangularis*: The first discovery of the glycosides, sulfated by C-4 of the terminal 3-O-methylglucose residue. Synergetic effect on colony formation of tumor HT-29 cells of these glycosides with radioactive irradiation. *Mar. Drugs* **2020**, *18*, 394.
19. Silchenko, A.S.; Kalinovsky, A.I.; Avilov, S.A.; Andrijaschenko, P.V.; Popov, R.S.; Dmitrenok, P.S.; Chingizova, E.A.; Kalinin, V.I. Kurilosides A_1, A_2, C_1, D, E and F-triterpene glycosides from the Far Eastern sea cucumber *Thyonidium* (= *Duasmodactyla*) *kurilensis* (Levin): Structures with unusual non-holostane aglycones and cytotoxicities. *Mar. Drugs* **2020**, *18*, 551. [CrossRef] [PubMed]
20. Malyarenko, T.V.; Kicha, A.A.; Malyarenko, O.S.; Zakharenko, V.M.; Kotlyarov, I.P.; Kalinovsky, A.I.; Popov, R.S.; Svetashev, V.I.; Ivanchina, N.V. New conjugates of polyhydroxysteroids with long-chain fatty acids from the deep-water far eastern starfish *Ceramaster patagonicus* and their anticancer activity. *Mar. Drugs* **2020**, *18*, 260. [CrossRef] [PubMed]
21. Carreón-Palau, L.; Özdemir, N.S.; Parrish, C.C.; Parzanini, C. Sterol composition of sponges, cnidarians, arthropods, mollusks, and echinoderms from the deep northwest Atlantic: A comparison with shallow coastal Gulf of Mexico. *Mar. Drugs* **2020**, *18*, 598. [CrossRef] [PubMed]
22. Ustyuzhanina, N.E.; Bilan, M.I.; Dmitrenok, A.S.; Silchenko, A.S.; Grebnev, B.B.; Stonik, V.A.; Nifantiev, N.E.; Usov, A.I. Fucosylated chondroitin sulfates from the sea cucumbers *Paracaudina chilensis* and *Holothuria hilla*: Structures and anticoagulant activity. *Mar. Drugs* **2020**, *18*, 540. [CrossRef] [PubMed]

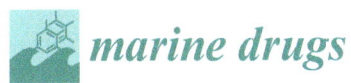

Article

Antiviral Potential of Sea Urchin Aminated Spinochromes against Herpes Simplex Virus Type 1

Natalia P. Mishchenko [1,*,†], Natalia V. Krylova [2,†], Olga V. Iunikhina [2], Elena A. Vasileva [1], Galina N. Likhatskaya [1], Evgeny A. Pislyagin [1], Darya V. Tarbeeva [1], Pavel S. Dmitrenok [1] and Sergey A. Fedoreyev [1]

1. G.B. Elyakov Pacific Institute of Bioorganic Chemistry, Far-Eastern Branch of the Russian Academy of Sciences, 690022 Vladivostok, Russia; vasilieva_el_an@mail.ru (E.A.V.); galinlik@piboc.dvo.ru (G.N.L.); pislyagin@hotmail.com (E.A.P.); tarbeeva1988@mail.ru (D.V.T.); paveldmitrenok@mail.ru (P.S.D.); fedoreev-s@mail.ru (S.A.F.)
2. G.P. Somov Institute of Epidemiology and Microbiology, Far-Eastern Branch of the Russian Academy of Sciences, 690087 Vladivostok, Russia; krylovanatalya@gmail.com (N.V.K.); olga_iun@inbox.ru (O.V.I.)
* Correspondence: mischenkonp@mail.ru; Tel.: +79-084542965
† N.P.M. and N.V.K. contributed equally to this manuscript.

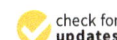

Received: 14 October 2020; Accepted: 2 November 2020; Published: 5 November 2020

Abstract: Herpes simplex virus type 1 (HSV-1) is one of the most prevalent pathogens worldwide requiring the search for new candidates for the creation of antiherpetic drugs. The ability of sea urchin spinochromes—echinochrome A (EchA) and its aminated analogues, echinamines A (EamA) and B (EamB)—to inhibit different stages of HSV-1 infection in Vero cells and to reduce the virus-induced production of reactive oxygen species (ROS) was studied. We found that spinochromes exhibited maximum antiviral activity when HSV-1 was pretreated with these compounds, which indicated the direct effect of spinochromes on HSV-1 particles. EamB and EamA both showed the highest virucidal activity by inhibiting the HSV-1 plaque formation, with a selectivity index (SI) of 80.6 and 50.3, respectively, and a reduction in HSV-1 attachment to cells (SI of 8.5 and 5.8, respectively). EamA and EamB considerably suppressed the early induction of ROS due to the virus infection. The ability of the tested compounds to directly bind to the surface glycoprotein, gD, of HSV-1 was established in silico. The dock score of EchA, EamA, and EamB was −4.75, −5.09, and −5.19 kcal/mol, respectively, which correlated with the SI of the virucidal action of these compounds and explained their ability to suppress the attachment and penetration of the virus into the cells.

Keywords: echinochrome A; echinamine A; echinamine B; herpes simplex virus type 1; Vero cells; glycoprotein gD; molecular docking

---

1. Introduction

According to the World Health Organization, herpes simplex virus (HSV) infections are the second most common viral disease in humans after influenza [1]. HSV type 1 (HSV-1) is a neurotropic virus that can persist in human sensory neurons for life, replicate in epithelial cells during primary infection and reactivation, and cause diseases with a variety of clinical manifestations, from labial herpes to meningitis and encephalitis [2]. Recently, the number of reports on the resistance of HSV-1 against many drugs based on nucleoside analogues, which are acyclovir and its derivatives, has increased [3–5]. Therefore, the search for new antiviral drugs, specifically anti-HSV drugs, remains an important problem.

Many of the cytopathic effects observed during HSV-1 infection are not only due to viral replication but also to oxidative stress caused by the virus, leading to cell damage [6–8]. Therefore, using exogenous antioxidants capable of counteracting the destructive effect of virus-induced oxidative stress on cells is considered a promising strategy [9]. Currently, many laboratories around the world are actively studying antioxidants with different chemical structures as potential therapeutic agents for herpes infection treatment. The largest number of studies on the antiherpetic activity of natural antioxidants is associated with the study of polyphenolic compounds from terrestrial and marine plants [10,11]. In this regard, a class of marine natural polyphenolic compounds found in representatives of Echinodermata, such as sea urchins, sea stars, and ophiurs, is promising [12]. This class is called spinochromes and has been known for over 100 years; nevertheless, extensive investigations of the biological activities of these compounds began only in the last decade [13,14].

Recently, our group discovered the antiviral properties of the most abundant and well-known spinochrome, echinochrome A (EchA), as well as an antioxidant composition consisting of EchA in combination with ascorbic acid and α-tocopherol. It was found that EchA and the composition effectively inhibit the cytopathogenic effect of HSV-1 and tick-borne encephalitis virus [15]. EchA and the antioxidant composition have shown a considerable protective effect on the mouse model of genital HSV type 2 (HSV-2) infection. Both intraperitoneal and oral administration of EchA and the composition significantly improved the survival rate and reduced the vaginal virus load of HSV-2-infected mice [16]. The potential affinity of sea urchin pigments to bind the main protease (Mpro) and the spike protein (S) of SARS-CoV-2 was evaluated in silico [17,18]. EchA showed high affinity to both targets, which indicated its potential as an antiviral drug against SARS-CoV-2 and encouraged further in vitro and in vivo analysis to expand its therapeutic uses.

The first spinochromes containing a primary amino group, echinamines A (EamA) and B (EamB), which are aminated derivatives of EchA, were isolated in 2005 from the flat sea urchin *Scaphechinus mirabilis* [19]. Nowadays, amino derivative of spinochrome E—spinamine E [20] has also been isolated from various species of sea urchins, and the new aminated quinonoid pigment acetylaminotrihydroxynaphthoquinone [21] was detected in the sea urchin *Strongylocentrotus nudus* using UPLC-DAD-MS (ultra performance liquid chromatography-diode array detector-mass spectrometry). The natural origin of these spinochromes is beyond doubt; they were found in both the regular sea urchins *Strongylocentrotus nudus, S. pallidus,* and *S. polyacanthus* and the irregular sea urchins *Echinarachnius parma* and *Scaphechinus mirabilis*, which inhabit the southern and northern seas at different depths up to 200 m [20–23]. The simultaneous presence of three aminated spinochromes—EamA, EamB, and spinamine E—was found in the commercial sea urchin *Evechinus chloroticus* from New Zealand, also known as kina [23].

A number of investigations have reported that spinochromes are strong antioxidants that can block a number of free radical reactions, inhibit lipid peroxidation, and reduce and chelate metal ions [21,24–27]. Recently, using 2,2-diphenyl-1-picrylhydrazyl radical (DPPH) and lipid autooxidation assays, it has been shown that aminated spinochromes EamA and EamB and spinamine E are more potent antioxidants than their hydroxylated analogues [20].

Thus, the aim of this study was to evaluate the anti-HSV-1 activity of EamA and EamB in vitro and in silico as well as their effect on the HSV-1-induced production of reactive oxygen species (ROS) in Vero cells, in comparison with EchA.

2. Results and Discussion

2.1. Physico-Chemical Properties of Aminated Spinochromes

Spinochromes of the sea urchin *Echinarachnius parma* were isolated using a previously described standard procedure [20]: shells were treated with ethanol containing 10% sulfuric acid, and the sum of the pigments was extracted with chloroform and ethyl acetate and then fractionated using repeated column chromatography on Toyopearl HW-40 gel (TOYO SODA, Tokyo, Japan). As a result, EchA, EamA, and EamB were isolated (Figure 1A). According to HPLC-MS (high performance liquid chromatography mass spectrometry) data, *E. parma* extracts also contained spinochromes D and E and three binaphthoquinones [22], which were not used in this study.

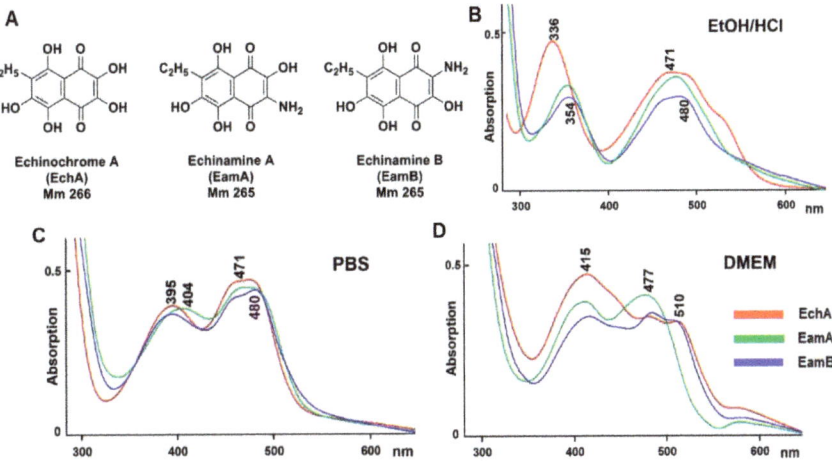

Figure 1. (**A**) Structural formulae of the studied spinochromes. Absorption spectra of the studied spinochromes (0.02 mg/mL) in (**B**) acidified ethanol (pH 1.0), (**C**) phosphate buffered saline (PBS); 0.01 M, pH 7.2, and (**D**) Dulbecco's Modified Eagle's Medium (DMEM) (pH 7.2). Compound spectra were recorded in comparison to the corresponding solvent.

The content of aminated spinochromes in *E. parma* was not higher than 3% of the total amount of quinonoid pigments, which was not enough for biological activity investigations. Recently, several simple and effective synthesis schemes of EamA and EamB have been described [28–32]. However, the most promising method developed by us for obtaining EamA and EamB is the amination of EchA with aqueous ammonia [29]. This reaction led to the formation of a mixture of EamA and EamB in nearly quantitative overall yield, which was successfully separated by column chromatography on a Sephadex LH-20. The HPLC-MS and NMR characteristics of the obtained EamA and EamB coincided with the data of natural echinamines (Supplementary Materials, page 3, Figure S1).

Earlier, we described two specific differences of the aminated spinochromes from their hydroxylated analogues. They have one unit less molecular weight compared to the corresponding hydroxylated spinochrome, and the quinoid electron transfer band in the absorption spectrum of the aminated spinochromes is usually 10–15 nm bathochromically shifted compared with that of their hydroxylated analogues [20]. As seen from in Figure 1B, this is true for both EamA and EamB.

It is known that small-molecule drug substances are ionisable under physiological conditions, forming a number of protomers [33]. Under physiological conditions, for example, in phosphate buffer PBS pH 7.2, all studied spinochromes become ionisable, reflecting a shift in the quinoid absorption band to about 400 nm (Figure 1C). The possible protomeric structures of each spinochrome in the aqueous phase with physiological pH were calculated using MOE 2019.01 software (Figure S2). Under these conditions, echinochrome A forms the largest number of protomers, in which the quinoid fragment of the molecule is presented in the form of triketone, and the negative charge is delocalised in the benzene fragment. The smallest number of protomers was obtained for EamB, one of which takes 77% of the possible structures. Knowledge of the structures of protomers is important for predicting their properties since they determine the binding with biological molecules [34,35]. The absorption spectra of spinochromes in Dulbecco's Modified Eagle's Medium (DMEM) containing glucose, vitamins, salts, L-glutamine, and other amino acids, differed significantly (Figure 1D), possibly due to the presence of different protomeric forms of these compounds in solution, which define the binding with the components of the DMEM.

2.2. Cytotoxicity and Anti-HSV-1 Activity of the Tested Compounds

The cytotoxicity of the spinochromes and acyclovir (ACV) as a positive control against Vero cells was evaluated before testing their antiviral activity. Cells were treated with concentrations of spinochromes from 1 to 200 µg/mL and of ACV from 1 to 1000 µg/mL for 72 h, and cell viability was assessed using the MTT (methylthiazolyltetrazolium bromide) assay. There was no significant difference ($p > 0.05$) between the 50% cytotoxic concentrations (CC_{50}) of the studied spinochromes; their mean CC_{50} values were ~140 µg/mL, while the CC_{50} of ACV was above 1000 µg/mL (Table 1). Therefore, the antiviral activity of the tested compounds against HSV-1 was determined at concentrations below 100 µg/mL.

Table 1. Effects of the tested compounds at different stages of herpes simplex virus type 1 (HSV-1) infection.

Compounds	CC_{50}	IC_{50} (SI)					
		Pretreatment of the Virus	Pretreatment of Cells	Attachment	Penetration	Simultaneous Treatment	Post-Infection Treatment
EchA	142 ± 6	4.1 ± 0.6 (34.6)	83 ± 14 (1.7)	33 ± 6 (4.3)	59 ± 9 (2.4)	35 ± 6 (4.1)	95 ± 18 (1.5)
EamA	146 ± 7	2.9 ± 0.4 (50.3) *	96 ± 16 (1.5)	25 ± 4 (5.8)	56 ± 8 (2.6)	34 ± 6 (4.3)	113 ± 23 (1.3)
EamB	137 ± 6	1.7 ± 0.2 (80.6) *	92 ± 14 (1.5)	16 ± 3 (8.5) *	54 ± 7 (2.5)	30 ± 5 (4.6)	80 ± 14 (1.7)
ACV	>1000	NA	NA	NA	NA	2.1 ± 0.4 (476)	0.1 ± 0.02 (10,000)

Values are presented as the means ± standard deviations. CC_{50} (µg/mL), 50% cytotoxic concentration; IC_{50} (µg/mL), concentration that inhibited 50% of HSV-1 plaque formation; SI, selectivity index (CC_{50}/IC_{50}); NA, no activity. * Statistically significant differences between values of EchA and the echinamines ($p \leq 0.05$).

The inhibitory effect of the tested compounds on different stages of HSV-1 infection was studied by a plaque reduction assay. We used the following treatment schemes [36]: pretreatment of the virus (compounds were added directly to the virus suspension); pretreatment of the cells (cells were treated with compounds for 1 h before infection); attachment (cells were co-treated with the virus and compounds at 4 °C); penetration (cells were infected with the virus at 4 °C and then treated with the compounds at 37 °C); and simultaneous and post-infection treatment (cells were treated with the compounds at the same time as infection or 1 h after infection). The antiviral effect of the tested compounds was compared to that of the untreated virus after 72 h of incubation, and the obtained results were used for calculations of the concentration yielding a 50% reduction in plaque formation (IC_{50}) and the selectivity index (SI) as the ratio of CC_{50} to IC_{50} for each of the compounds.

The pretreatment of HSV-1 (100 plaque-forming units (PFU)/mL) with different concentrations (0.2 to 25 µg/mL) of the tested spinochromes and ACV showed that the spinochromes significantly inhibited HSV-1-induced plaque formation, with IC_{50} values of less than 5 µg/mL (Table 1, Figure S3). Among the three tested compounds, EamB was found to have the highest SI value (80.6) against HSV-1. In comparison, ACV did not show antiviral activity, even when tested up to a concentration of 100 µg/mL. These results indicate the direct effect of spinochromes on HSV-1 particles, with the virucidal activity of EamA and EamB being significantly higher ($p \leq 0.05$) than that of EchA.

The treatment of Vero cells with the tested compounds before infection (pretreatment of cells) had no effect on HSV-1 plaque formation. Post-infection treatment of cells with spinochromes was also ineffective in contrast to ACV (SI of ~1.5 vs. 10,000), which is known to block viral replication [37]. Next, the tested compounds and HSV-1 were added to Vero cells simultaneously to investigate their influence on the early stages of viral infection. In this assay, spinochromes displayed moderate inhibitory activity against HSV-1 ($IC_{50} > 30$ µg/mL; SI of ~4.3) (Table 1).

Thus, the results of HSV-1 pretreatment with spinochromes and the results of simultaneous treatment of cells with HSV-1 and spinochromes revealed that these compounds affect the very early stages of the HSV-1 life cycle, which are the attachment and penetration stages.

The attachment and penetration stages were analysed by shifting the temperature during the infection. It is known that for many enveloped viruses, including HSV-1, a temperature of 4 °C allows for virus attachment to host cells, but not cell penetration, whereas a temperature of 37 °C facilitates virus penetration into the cells [38–40]. In the attachment assay, during which Vero cells were co-treated with HSV-1 and tested compounds at 4 °C, EamA and EchA displayed a moderate inhibitory effect on the binding of the virus to cells (Table 1). At the same time, EamB significantly reduced ($p \leq 0.05$) the HSV-1 attachment to cells (SI = 8.5) compared to EchA (SI = 4.3). For the penetration assay, cells were infected with HSV-1 at 4 °C and then treated with test compounds at 37 °C to facilitate virus entry into the cells. The results showed that the effect of spinochromes on viral entry was not significant (SI of ~2.5). ACV did not affect the attachment and penetration stages of HSV-1 infection when tested up to a concentration of 100 µg/mL.

Thus, it was shown that the tested spinochromes (EamA, EamB, and EchA) exert significant anti-HSV-1 activity, mainly due to their direct virucidal properties, but they also inhibit the attachment of the virus to cells and, to a lesser extent, virus penetration into cells.

2.3. Effect of Spinochromes on HSV-1-Induced Intracellular ROS Production

To determine whether HSV-1 infection induced ROS production, Vero cells were infected with HSV-1 at 100 PFU/mL. At different time points after infection (1, 2, 3, and 4 h), the cells were loaded with the fluorogenic marker (DCF-DA (2′,7′-dichlorofluorescein diacetate)), and ROS production was assessed by changes in the mean fluorescence intensity in the control (uninfected cells) versus the infected cells. The results reported in Figure 2A show that HSV-1 infection of Vero cells induced a significant increase in ROS production at 1 and 2 h post-infection ($p \leq 0.05$), but at 3 and 4 h post-infection the levels of ROS production in the infected cells did not differ from those in the control. These results indicated that HSV-1 was able to induce a high level of ROS at a very early stage of infection, which has also been confirmed by other authors [8,41].

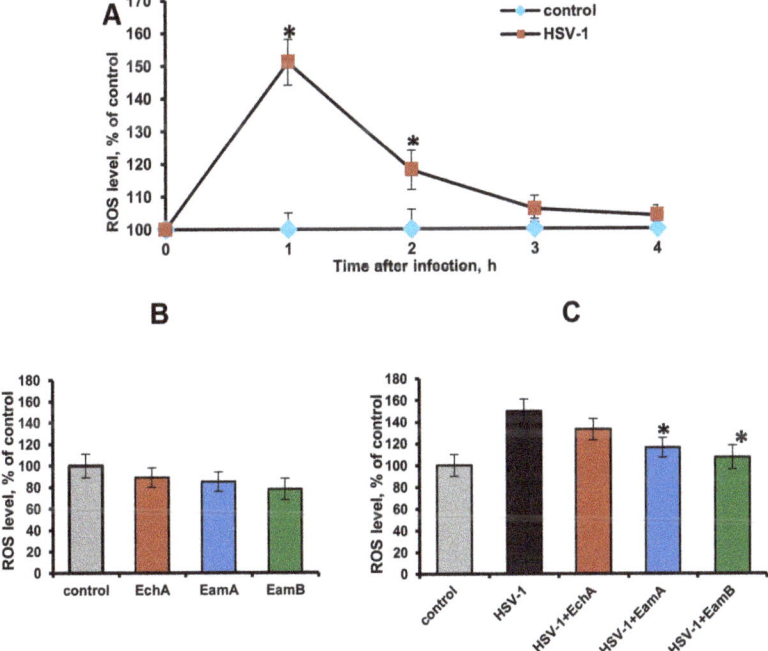

Figure 2. Effects of HSV-1 and spinochromes on reactive oxygen species (ROS) levels in Vero cells. The DCF-DA (2′,7′-dichlorofluorescein diacetate) assay was used to measure the cellular ROS. (**A**) Dynamics

of HSV-1-induced intracellular ROS levels compared to uninfected cells (control). Data are presented as the mean ± SD of three independent experiments. * $p \leq 0.05$ compared with the control. (**B**) Effects of the studied spinochromes (5 µg/mL) on the ROS levels in uninfected cells. (**C**) Effects of HSV-1 (100 PFU/mL) on ROS levels after incubation for 1 h with spinochromes (5 µg/mL). The results include data from three experiments (mean ± SD). * $p \leq 0.05$ compared with HSV-1-infected cells.

The next task was to find out whether the spinochromes could affect the HSV-1-induced ROS production in Vero cells. Since the tested compounds exhibited significant anti-HSV-1 activity, mainly due to direct inactivation of viral particles, as noted above, to study their effect on virus-induced ROS production, HSV-1 was pre-incubated with these compounds. In these experiments, spinochromes were used at a concentration of 5 µg/mL, which is approximately equal to the IC$_{50}$ concentration calculated for them in the virucidal assay. At first, it was found that the tested compounds themselves, when added to Vero cells for 2 h, did not cause a significant decrease in ROS production compared to the cell control ($p > 0.05$) (Figure 2B). At the same time, pretreatment of HSV-1 (100 PFU/mL) with EamA and EamB followed by the 1 h exposure of these mixtures on Vero cells significantly inhibited the early induction of ROS formation by the virus compared with untreated HSV-1-infected cells ($p \leq 0.05$) (Figure 2C).

2.4. Molecular Docking

HSV-1 surface glycoproteins are involved in the processes of adhesion and fusion of the virus with the cell membrane. The HSV-1 glycoprotein gD is involved in the interaction of the virus with the cellular receptors nectin-1, HSEA/M, and 3-O-sulphated heparan sulphate (3-OS HS) [42,43]. The interaction of the gD protein with the receptors triggers the adhesion of the virus to the cell and fusion with the cell membrane. This protein can be used as a target protein to search for compounds that inhibit the initial stages of HSV-1 infection. It was shown with molecular docking that flavonoid myricetin can block HSV infection by directly interacting with the viral gD protein and interfering with virus adsorption [44].

In this work, the interaction of spinochromes with the HSV-1 surface glycoprotein, gD, was studied using molecular docking methods, and it was shown that the studied compounds can directly bind to gD, competing for binding sites of this protein with cellular receptors (nectin-1 and 3-OS HS), thereby preventing the adsorption of the virus to cells.

The search for binding sites for the gD glycoprotein showed that one of the sites overlaps with the site for gD binding to the nectin-1 cellular receptor (Figure S4). Molecular docking of spinochromes into this site showed that spinochromes have two subsites on gD (Figure 3). Analysis of the contacts of the spinochromes with gD showed that the compounds under study form hydrogen bonds with amino acid residues of gD, including the arginine (Arg) 222 residue, which is important for binding to the nectin-1 receptor (Figure 4).

Apparently, the interaction of spinochromes with Arg 222 inhibits the binding of gD to the cellular receptor, nectin-1. The dock score of EchA, EamA, and EamB in Subsite 1 with gD was −4.75, −5.09, and −5.19 kcal/mol, respectively, and correlated with the SI values obtained in the virucidal and attachment analysis (Table 1).

The interaction of gD and 3-OS HS is a key step for triggering the fusion of the virus and cells [43]. Calculation of the electrostatic potential of the molecular surface of the gD protein showed that there are positively charged sites on the surface of the viral protein that can potentially interact with 3-OS HS. The interactions of the 3-OS HS tetrasaccharide and the spinochromes with the glycoprotein, gD, at a positively charged site were tested. It was shown by molecular docking that the 3-OS HS tetrasaccharide and the spinochromes compete for interaction with Arg 67 and Arg 64 residues of the gD protein (Figures 5 and 6). The in silico results allowed for a better understanding and clarification of the mechanism underlying the in vitro anti-HSV-1 action of the spinochromes. The ability of the tested compounds to directly bind to the gD surface of the HSV-1 virus, to compete with the cellular receptors for binding sites on this glycoprotein, and to suppress the attachment and penetration of the virus into the cells was established. Blocking the early stages of HSV-1 infection may be an attractive therapeutic strategy, the advantage of which is that it can prevent the spread of the virus without killing virus-infected cells, as occurs with acyclovir.

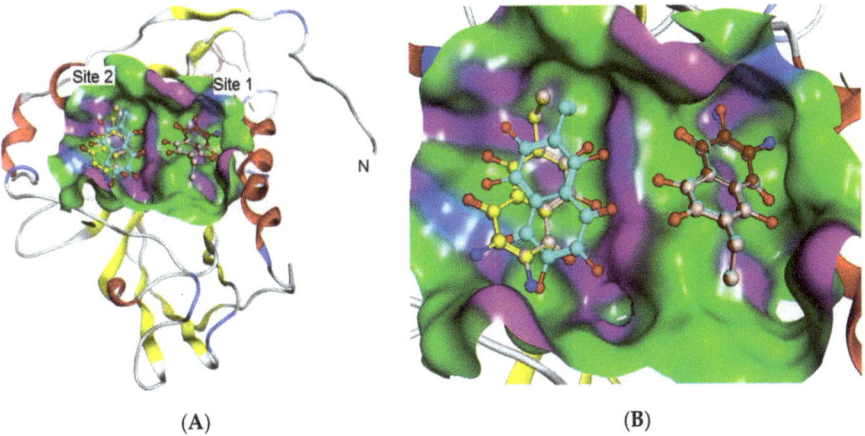

Figure 3. Molecular docking of spinochromes with gD. (**A**) Subsites 1 and 2 of binding of spinochromes to gD. Spinochrome structures are shown in colour as balls and sticks. The gD molecule is shown as a ribbon. (**B**) Molecular surface of gD in the binding sites of the spinochromes. Site 1: EchA (turquoise), EamA (beige), EamB (brown); Site 2: EchA (turquoise), EamA (beige), EamB (yellow). The colour shows the molecular surface of gD: H-bonding (pink), hydrophobic (green), and mild polar (blue).

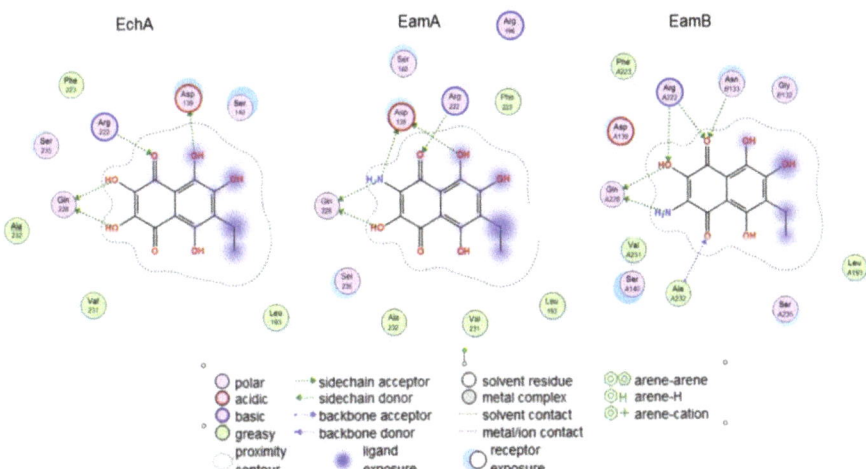

Figure 4. 2D diagrams of EchA, EamA, and EamB contacts with the HSV-1 glycoprotein gD. Abbreviations of aminoacids: alanine (Ala); arginine (Arg); aspartic acid (Asp); asparagine (Asn); glutamine (Gln); glycine (Gly); leucine (Leu); phenylalanine (Phe); serine (Ser); valine (Val).

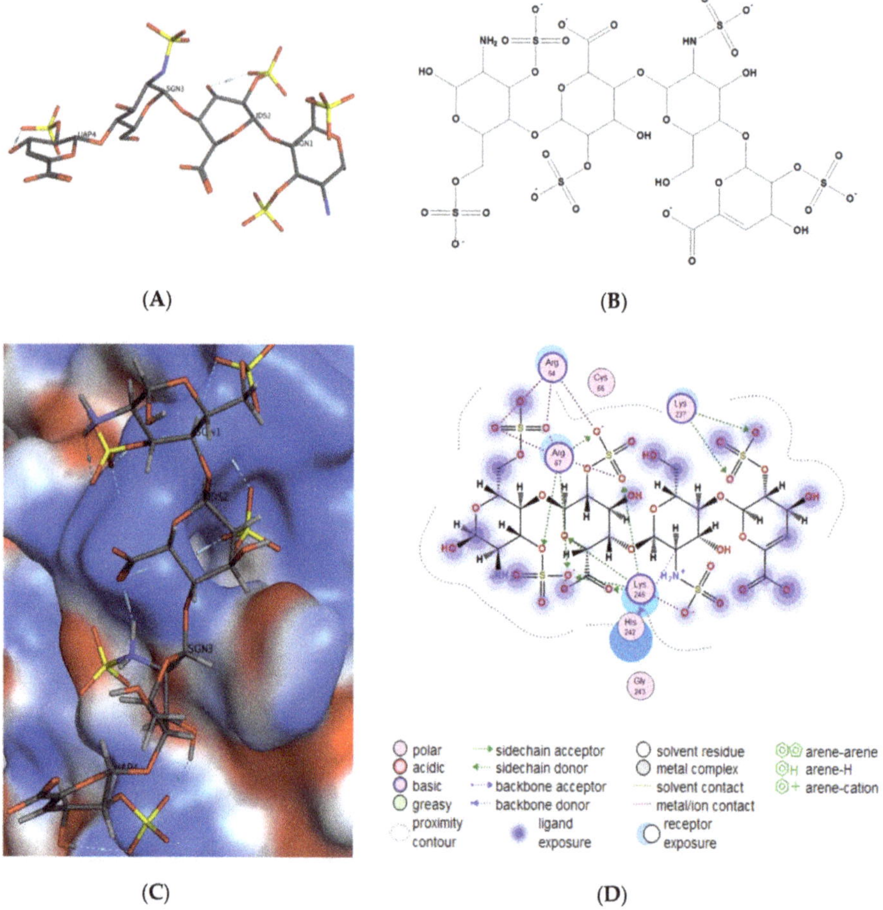

Figure 5. Molecular docking of the 3-*O*-sulphated heparan sulphate (3-OS HS) tetrasaccharide and the herpes simplex virus type 1 (HSV-1) gD membrane glycoprotein. (**A**) 3D structure and (**B**) 2D structure of 3-OS HS obtained using the MOE program. (**C**) The putative binding site of 3-OS HS and gD HSV-1. (**D**) 2D diagram of the contacts of 3-OS HS with gD.

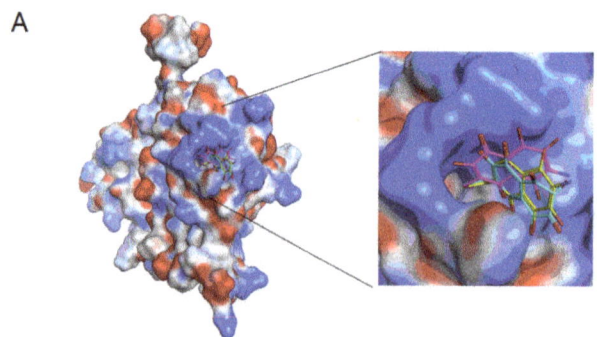

Figure 6. *Cont.*

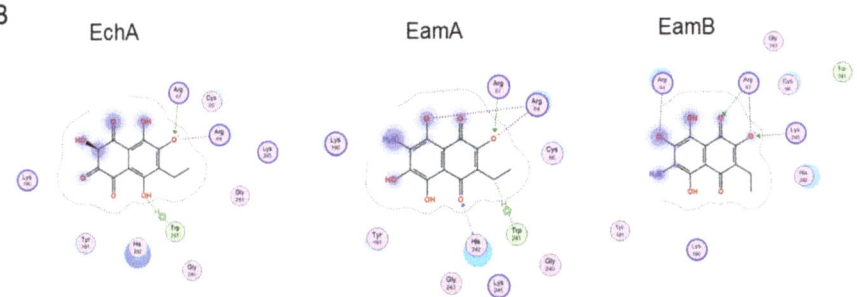

Figure 6. (**A**) Molecular docking of spinochromes into a potential binding site of the 3-OS HS tetrasaccharide and the HSV-1 gD membrane glycoprotein. The electrostatic potential of the gD molecular surface was calculated using the MOE 2019.01 program. The spinochrome structures are shown as sticks. (**B**) 2D diagram of contacts of EchA, EamA, and EamB protomers with gD.

3. Materials and Methods

3.1. Reagents

DMEM (Biolot, St. Petersburg, Russia), fetal bovine serum (FBS, Biolot, Saint Petersburg, Russia), gentamycin (Dalkhimprom, Khabarovsk, Russia), Acyclovir® (ACV; freeze-dried powder for injections; GlaxoSmithKline Pharmaceuticals S.A., Poznan, Poland), dimethylsulfoxide (DMSO; Sigma, Saint-Louis, MO, USA), methylthiazolyltetrazolium bromide (MTT; Sigma, Saint-Louis, MO, USA), 2′,7′-dichlorofluorescein diacetate (DCF-DA; Sigma, Saint-Louis, MO, USA), carboxymethyl cellulose (CMC; MP Biomedicals, Inc., Aurora, OH, USA), crystal violet (Sigma, Saint Louis, MO, USA), and phosphate buffered saline (PBS, Sigma, Saint-Louis, MO, USA) were used.

3.2. Viruses and Cell Cultures

HSV-1 strain L2 was obtained from N.F. Gamaleya Federal Research Centre for Epidemiology and Microbiology, Moscow, Russia. HSV-1 was grown in African green monkey kidney (Vero) cells using DMEM supplemented with 10% FBS and 100 U/mL of gentamycin at 37 °C in a CO_2 incubator. In the maintenance medium, the FBS concentration was decreased to 1%.

3.3. Spinochromes Isolation

The sea urchin *Echinarachnius parma* (Lamarck, 1816) was collected by dredging during the 47th (July 2015) scientific cruise of R/V Academic Oparin, near Iturup Island (45°38′9″ N, 148°22′6″ E; depth of 54 m). EchA was isolated from the sea urchin *E. parma* according to previous work [19]. The purity of EchA was >99% according to the HPLC-MS data (Shimadzu LCMS-2020, Kyoto, Japan).

For EamA and EamB synthesis, 20 mg of echinochrome A was dissolved in 10 mL of ethanol. Then, 5 mL of 25% aqueous ammonia was added, and the mixture was stirred at room temperature. The reaction time was complete in 5 min and acidified to a pH of 1 with 12% hydrochloric acid. The reaction products were extracted with ethyl acetate, the solution was dried with sodium sulphate, and the solvent was removed in vacuo. The residue was chromatographed on a column (1.1 × 40 cm) with Sephadex LH-20 (GE Healthcare Bio-Sciences AB, Uppsala, Sweden) using $CHCl_3$–MeOH (8:1) as the eluent. As a result, 8 mg of echinamine A and 8 mg of echinamine B were obtained. Each compound was fully characterised by NMR and HPLC-DAD-MS data in comparison with the authentic samples isolated from *Scaphechinus mirabilis* ([19]; see Supplementary Materials). According to the HPLC-MS data, the purity of echinamines A and B was more than 98% (Shimadzu LCMS-2020, Kyoto, Japan).

The spinochromes were dissolved in DMSO (Sigma, Saint-Louis, MO, USA) at a concentration 10 mg/mL and stored at −20 °C. For cytotoxicity and anti-HSV-1 activity determination, the stock solutions were diluted with DMEM so that the final concentration of DMSO was 0.5%.

For spectrophotometric studies, 3 mL of either EtOH/HCl (pH 2.0), PBS buffer (pH 7.2), or DMEM (pH 7.2) was first placed in the UV cuvette (10 mm), and then a 20 µL aliquot of the 5 mg/mL methanolic solution of the spinochromes was added. The absorbance was recorded in comparison to the corresponding solvent using a UV 1800 spectrophotometer (Shimadzu USA Manufacturing Inc. Canby, OR, USA).

3.4. Cytotoxicity of the Tested Compounds

The cytotoxicity evaluation of the studied compounds was performed using the MTT assay, as previously described [45]. In brief, confluent Vero cells in 96-well microplates were incubated with two-fold serial dilutions of the tested compounds (1–1000 µg/mL) at 37 °C for 72 h (5% CO_2). Untreated cells were used as controls. Then MTT solution (5 mg/mL) was added, and the cells were incubated at 37 °C for 2 h. After dissolution of formazan crystals, optical densities were read at 540 nm (Labsystems Multiskan RC, Vantaa, Finland). The 50% cytotoxic concentrations (CC_{50}) of the tested compounds able to reduce cell viability by 50% were calculated using regression analysis-generated data from three independent experiments [46].

3.5. Anti-HSV-1 Activity of the Tested Compounds

The inhibitory effects of the tested compounds on HSV-1 replication cycle stages in Vero cells were evaluated by the plaque reduction assay [47,48]. Vero cell monolayers grown in 24-well plates (1×10^5 cells/well) were infected with 100 PFU/mL of HSV-1. The tested compounds and Acyclovir® were used at concentrations from 0.1 to 100 µg/mL.

- *Virucidal assay* (the pretreatment of the HSV-1 with compounds). HSV-1 suspension was pre-incubated with an equal volume of DMEM or various concentrations of tested compounds for 1 h at 37 °C, then the mixture was used to infect cellular monolayers. After viral adsorption for 1 h at 37 °C, the plates were washed, covered with the maintenance medium (DMEM) containing 1% CMC for 72 h at 37 °C (5% CO_2) until plaques formed.
- *Time-of-addition assay*. The tested compounds, at various concentrations, were added to cells at 1 h before viral infection (pretreatment of cells), at the same time with infection (simultaneous treatment) or 1 h after infection (post-treatment). To study a preventive effect, the cells were pretreated with compounds for 1 h, then infected with HSV-1 for 1 h after removal of compounds by washing and overlaid with DMEM with 1% CMC. To study the effect on virus adsorption, cells were treated with compounds and simultaneously infected with HSV-1, then overlaid with DMEM with 1% CMC after removal of the compounds and unbound virus by washing at 1 h after adsorption. To study the effect on the early stage of virus replication, the cells were infected with the HSV-1 for 1 h, and then overlaid with DMEM with 1% CMC containing different concentrations of the studied compounds after removal of virus by washing. Within all procedures, the cells were incubated for 72 h at 37 °C (5% CO_2) until plaques formed.

The attachment and penetration assays were performed as described previously [48,49].

- *The attachment assay*. Pre-chilled at 4 °C for 1 h Vero cells were infected with the virus (100 PFU/mL), and incubated for 3 h at 4 °C with different concentrations of the studied compounds. Then, the compounds and unbound viruses were washed away with cold PBS. The cells were supplied with DMEM containing 1% CMC and incubated for 72 h at 37 °C (5% CO_2) until plaques formed.
- *The penetration assay*. Pre-chilled at 4 °C for 1 h Vero cells were infected with the virus (100 PFU/mL), and incubated for 3 h at 4 °C. The unbound viruses were removed with cold PBS, the cells were treated with medium containing different concentrations of the compounds, and then incubated for 1 h at 37 °C. Viruses that did not enter cells were inactivated with citrate buffer (pH 3.0). Then, the cells were washed with PBS, supplied with DMEM containing 1% CMC, and incubated for 72 h at 37 °C (5% CO_2) until plaques formed.

In all assays, after 72 h of incubation, the cells were fixed with cold ethanol for 20 min, stained with solution of 0.5% crystal violet in 20% ethanol, and the viral plaques were then counted. The plaque formation inhibition rate was calculated according to the following formula [36]: plaque inhibition (%) = 100 − [(P_T/P_C) × 100], where P_T and P_C refer to the number of plaques in the compound-treated cells and the virus-infected cells, respectively. The IC_{50} of each compound was determined as the concentration that inhibited 50% of viral plaque formation, compared to virus-infected cells, and was calculated using a regression analysis of the dose–response curve [46]. The SI was calculated as the ratio of CC_{50} to IC_{50} for each compound.

3.6. Measurement of the ROS Level

The ROS level was measured in the control, the HSV-1-treated cells, and in the same cells with the presence of EchA, EamA, and EamB using the ROS indicator DCF-DA according to prior work [8] with some changes. Treated cells were incubated with 10 µM of DCF-DA for 30 min at 37 °C in the dark. After washing twice with PBS, the intensity of DCF fluorescence of the cells was measured at an λ_{ex} of 485 nm/λ_{em} 520 nm using the PHERAstar FS plate reader (BMG Labtech, Offenburg, Germany).

For all experiments, a monolayer of Vero cells was prepared. Vero cells were seeded in 96-well plates (1 × 10^4 cells/well) and cultured for 24 h at 37 °C in 5% CO_2. The following experiments were performed; each was carried out in three independent replicates.

- *ROS production in HSV-1-infected cells*: Cells were treated with HSV-1 (100 PFU/mL) and cultured at 37 °C. After 1, 2, 3, and 4 h, the cells were washed with PBS and the ROS level was measured in infected (HSV-1) and uninfected cells (control).
- *ROS production in control cells with the presence of spinochromes*: The monolayer of cells treated with the tested spinochromes (5 µg/mL, 100 µL/well) and incubated for 2 h at 37 °C. After washing with PBS, the ROS level was measured. Untreated cells were used as the control.
- *ROS production in control and HSV-1-infected cells with the presence of spinochromes*: HSV-1 (100 PFU/mL) was mixed with the tested spinochromes (5 µg/mL) in a 1:1 (v/v) ratio and incubated for 1 h at 37 °C. Then, the mixture and HSV-1 (100 PFU/mL) were applied to a monolayer of Vero cells. After 1 h of incubation at 37 °C, the cells were washed with PBS and the ROS level was measured. Uninfected and HSV-1-infected cells were used as the control.

3.7. Molecular Docking

We used the crystal structure of echinochrome A (CCDC ID NERLUS code) [50,51]. The structures of Eam A and Eam B were obtained using the molecular editor of the MOE 2019.01 [52] program. The structures of the spinochromes were optimised with the forcefield MMFF94, and the structures of the protomers in the aqueous phase were calculated using MOE 2019.01 software. The crystal structures of the complexes of the HSV-1 gD glycoprotein with the nectin-1 receptor (PDB ID 3UKS) and the HSEA/M receptor (PDB ID 1JMA) were used as a target protein. The structure of the HS tetrasaccharide was obtained from the PDB database (PDB ID 1T8U) and used to obtain 3-O-S HS using the molecular editor MOE 2019.01. For molecular docking, a 3-O-S HS was used, which was solvated in the aqueous phase and optimised with the forcefield Amber10:EHT. The calculation of the electrostatic potential of the molecular surface of glycoprotein gD was carried out using the MOE 2019.01 program. Molecular docking of glycoprotein gD with the spinochromes and 3-OS HS was performed using the Dock module of the MOE 2019.01 software. The structures of 30 complexes were calculated with Score London dG, and the 10 most energetically advantageous complexes were optimised with Score GBVI/WSA dG. Contact analysis was carried out using the Ligand Interaction module of the MOE program.

3.8. Statistical Analysis

Statistica 10.0 software was used for statistical analysis of the experimental data. The results are given as the mean ± standard deviation (SD). Wilcoxon test was used for estimating the differences significant at $p \leq 0.05$ between means of the control and experimental groups.

4. Conclusions

Thus, we found that spinochromes of the sea urchin *Echinarachnius parma* collected at a depth of more than 50 m exhibited significant anti-HSV-1 activity, mainly due to their direct virucidal properties, and their activity increased in the following order: EchA < EamA < EamB. They also inhibited the attachment of the virus to cells and, to a lesser extent, the entry of the virus into cells. One of the mechanisms of anti-HSV-1 activity of spinochromes is due to the fact that the compounds under study can directly bind to gD, competing with cellular receptors for the binding sites of this protein, thereby preventing the adsorption of HSV-1 on cells. Another mechanism of the antiviral action of the spinochromes, which have pronounced antioxidant properties, is due to a decrease in the HSV-1-induced ROS level in the cells.

Echinochrome A sodium salt is a Histochrome drug permitted for clinical application in Russia for the treatment of myocardial infarction and ophthalmological diseases. The ability of EchA to overcome the blood–brain barrier and to inactivate neurotropic viruses such as HSV-1 and tick-borne encephalitis virus makes it a prospective agent for new therapeutic use [15]. Echinamines A and B are the closest structural analogues of EchA. Their low molecular weight, comparable to EchA cytotoxicity, variety of their synthesis pathways with high yield, and more significant antiherpetic activity reported here, open perspectives to investigate their potential for clinical application.

Supplementary Materials: The following are available online at http://www.mdpi.com/1660-3397/18/11/550/s1, Figure S1: HPLC of products of echinochrome A amination reaction. Figure S2: The structures of echinochrome A, echinamine A and echinamine B protomers in the aqueous phase (pH 7) were calculated using the MOE 2019.01 software. Figure S3: Anti-HSV-1 activity of tested compounds in virucidal assay. Figure S4: The gD binding site, defined by the Site Finder module, that overlaps with the gD binding site for the nectin-1 cellular receptor (PDB ID 3SKU).

Author Contributions: Formal analysis, E.A.V. and D.V.T.; funding acquisition, P.S.D.; investigation, N.P.M., N.V.K., O.V.I., E.A.V. and S.A.F.; methodology, N.V.K., O.V.I., G.N.L. and E.A.P.; software, G.N.L.; supervision, N.P.M. and S.A.F.; visualization, G.N.L. and D.V.T.; writing—original draft, N.P.M., N.V.K., E.A.V. and G.N.L.; writing—review and editing, P.S.D. and S.A.F. All authors have read and agreed to the published version of the manuscript.

Funding: This research was funded by the Ministry of Science and Higher Education of Russian Federation, grant number 13.1902.21.0012 (075-15-2020-796) «Fundamental Problems of Study and Conservation of Deep-Sea Ecosystems in Potentially Ore-Bearing Areas of the Northwestern Pacific».

Conflicts of Interest: The authors declare no conflict of interest.

References

1. WHO. Herpes Simplex Virus. News Bulletin. 2016. Available online: https://www.who.int/news-room/fact-sheets/detail/herpes-simplex-virus (accessed on 22 October 2020).
2. Banerjee, A.; Kulkarni, S.; Mukherjee, A. Herpes Simplex Virus: The Hostile Guest That Takes Over Your Home. *Front. Microbiol.* **2020**, *11*, 1–18. [CrossRef]
3. Piret, J.; Boivin, G. Resistance of Herpes Simplex Viruses to Nucleoside Analogues: Mechanisms, Prevalence, and Management. *Antimicrob. Agents Chemother.* **2011**, *55*, 459–472. [CrossRef]
4. Turner, L.D.; Beckingsale, P. Acyclovir-resistant herpetic keratitis in a solid-organ transplant recipient on systemic immunosuppression. *Clin. Ophthalmol.* **2013**, *7*, 229–232. [CrossRef]
5. Pan, D.; Kaye, S.B.; Hopkins, M.; Kirwan, R.; Hart, I.J.; Coen, D.M. Common and new acyclovir resistant herpes simplex virus-1 mutants causing bilateral recurrent herpetic keratitis in an immunocompetent patient. *J. Infect. Dis.* **2014**, *209*, 345–349. [CrossRef]

6. Santana, S.; Sastre, I.; Recuero, M.; Bullido, M.J.; Aldudo, J. Oxidative stress enhances neurodegeneration markers induced by herpes simplex virus type 1 infection in human neuroblastoma cells. *PLoS ONE* **2013**, *8*, e75842. [CrossRef]
7. Georgieva, A.; Vilhelmova, N.; Muckova, L.; Tzvetanova, E.; Alexandrova, A.; Milevaet, M. Alterations in Oxidative Stress Parameters in MDBK Cells, Infected by Herpes Simplex Virus-1. *Compt. Rend. Acad. Bulg. Sci.* **2017**, *70*, 731–738.
8. Marino-Merlo, F.; Papaianni, E.; Frezza, C.; Pedatella, S.; De Nisco, M.; Macchi, B.; Grelli, S.; Mastino, A. NF-κB-Dependent Production of ROS and Restriction of HSV-1 Infection in U937 Monocytic Cells. *Viruses* **2019**, *11*, 428. [CrossRef]
9. Firuzi, O.; Miri, R.; Tavakkoli, M.; Saso, L. Antioxidant therapy: Current status and future prospects. *Curr. Med. Chem.* **2011**, *18*, 3871–3888. [CrossRef]
10. Balakrishnan, D.; Kandasamy, D.; Nithyanand, P. A review on antioxidant activity of marine organisms. *Int. J. Chem. Tech. Res.* **2014**, *6*, 3431–3436.
11. Torky, Z.A.; Hossain, M.M. Pharmacological evaluation of the hibiscus herbal extract against herpes simplex virus-type 1 as an antiviral drug in vitro. *Int. J. Virol.* **2017**, *13*, 68–79. [CrossRef]
12. Thomson, R.H. *Naturally Occurring Quinones*, 2nd ed.; Academic Press: London, UK; New York, NY, USA, 1971; 734p.
13. Hou, Y.; Vasileva, E.A.; Carne, A.; McConnell, M.; Bekhit, A.E.D.A.; Mishchenko, N.P. Naphthoquinones of the spinochrome class: Occurrence, isolation, biosynthesis and biomedical applications. *RSC Adv.* **2018**, *8*, 32637–32650. [CrossRef]
14. Shikov, A.N.; Pozharitskaya, O.N.; Krishtopina, A.S.; Makarov, V.G. Naphthoquinone pigments from sea urchins: Chemistry and pharmacology. *Phytochem. Rev.* **2018**, *17*, 509–534. [CrossRef]
15. Fedoreyev, S.A.; Krylova, N.V.; Mishchenko, N.P.; Vasileva, E.A.; Pislyagin, E.A.; Iunikhina, O.V.; Lavrov, V.F.; Svitich, O.A.; Ebralidze, L.K.; Leonova, G.N. Antiviral and antioxidant properties of echinochrome A. *Mar. Drugs* **2018**, *16*, 509. [CrossRef]
16. Krylova, N.V.; Leneva, I.A.; Fedoreev, S.A.; Ebralidze, L.K.; Mishchenko, N.P.; Vasileva, E.A.; Falynskova, I.N.; Iunikhina, O.V.; Lavrov, V.F.; Svitich, O.A. Activity of compounds containing echinochrome A against herpes simplex virus type 2 in vitro and in vivo. *J. Microbiol. Epidemiol. Immunobiol.* **2019**, *6*, 56–64. [CrossRef]
17. Rubilar Panasiuk, C.T.; Barbieri, E.S.; Gázquez, A.; Avaro, M.; Vera Piombo, M.; Gittardi Calderón, A.A.; Seiler, E.N.; Fernandez, J.P.; Sepúlveda, L.R.; Chaar, F. In Silico Analysis of Sea Urchin Pigments as Potential Therapeutic Agents Against SARS-CoV-2: Main Protease (Mpro) as a Target. *ChemRxiv* **2020**. [CrossRef]
18. Barbieri, E.S.; Rubilar Panasiuk, C.T.; Gázquez, A.; Avaro, M.; Seiler, E.N.; Vera Piombo, M.; Gittardi Calderón, A.A.; Chaar, F.; Fernandez, J.P.; Sepúlveda, L.R. Sea Urchin Pigments as Potential Therapeutic Agents Against the Spike Protein of SARS-CoV-2 Based on in Silico Analysis. *ChemRxiv* **2020**. [CrossRef]
19. Mischenko, N.P.; Fedoreyev, S.A.; Pokhilo, N.D.; Anufriev, V.P.; Denisenko, V.A.; Glazunov, V.P. Echinamines A and B, first aminated hydroxynaphthazarins from the sea urchin *Scaphechinus mirabilis*. *J. Nat. Prod.* **2005**, *68*, 1390–1393. [CrossRef] [PubMed]
20. Vasileva, E.A.; Mishchenko, N.P.; Zadorozhny, P.A.; Fedoreyev, S.A. New aminonaphthoquinone from the sea urchins *Strongylocentrotus pallidus* and *Mesocentrotus nudus*. *Nat. Prod. Commun.* **2016**, *11*, 821–824. [CrossRef]
21. Zhou, D.Y.; Qin, L.; Zhu, B.W.; Wang, X.D.; Tan, H.; Yang, J.F.; Li, D.M.; Dong, X.P.; Wu, H.T.; Sun, L.M. Extraction and antioxidant property of polyhydroxylated naphthoquinone pigments from spines of purple sea urchin. *Food Chem.* **2011**, *129*, 1591–1597. [CrossRef]
22. Vasileva, E.A.; Mishchenko, N.P.; Fedoreyev, S.A. Diversity of polyhydroxynaphthoquinone pigments in North Pacific sea urchins. *Chem. Biodivers.* **2017**, *14*, e1700182. [CrossRef]
23. Hou, Y.; Vasileva, E.A.; Mishchenko, N.P.; Carne, A.; McConnell, M.; Bekhit, A.E.A. Extraction, structural characterization and stability of polyhydroxylated naphthoquinones from shell and spine of New Zealand sea urchin (*Evechinus chloroticus*). *Food Chem.* **2019**, *272*, 379–387. [CrossRef]
24. Powell, C.; Hughes, A.D.; Kelly, M.S.; Conner, S.; McDougall, G.J. Extraction and identification of antioxidant polyhydroxynaphthoquinone pigments from the sea urchin, *Psammechinus miliaris*. *LWT-Food Sci. Technol.* **2014**, *59*, 455–460. [CrossRef]
25. Soleimani, S.; Yousefzadi, M.; Moe, S. Antibacterial and antioxidant characteristics of pigments and coelomic fluid of sea urchin, *Echinodermata Mathaei* species, from the Persian Gulf. *J. Kerman Univ. Med. Sci.* **2015**, *22*, 614–628.

26. Kuwahara, R.; Hatate, H.; Yuki, T.; Murata, H.; Tanaka, R.; Hama, Y. Antioxidant property of polyhydroxylated naphthoquinone pigments from shells of purple sea urchin *Anthocidaris crassispina*. *LWT-Food Sci. Technol.* **2009**, *42*, 1296–1300. [CrossRef]
27. Brasseur, L.; Hennebert, E.; Fievez, L.; Caulier, G.; Bureau, F.; Tafforeau, L.; Flammang, P.; Gerbaux, P.; Eeckhaut, I. The roles of spinochromes in four shallow water tropical sea urchins and their potential as bioactive pharmacological agents. *Mar. Drugs* **2017**, *15*, 179. [CrossRef]
28. Pokhilo, N.D.; Shuvalova, M.I.; Lebedko, M.V.; Sopelnyak, G.I.; Yakubovskaya, A.Y.; Mischenko, N.P.; Fedoreyev, S.A.; Anufriev, V.P. Synthesis of Echinamines A and B, the first aminated hydroxynaphthazarins produced by the sea urchin *Scaphechinus mirabilis* and Its Analogues. *J. Nat. Prod.* **2006**, *69*, 1125–1129. [CrossRef] [PubMed]
29. Mel'man, G.I.; Mishchenko, N.P.; Denisenko, V.A.; Berdyshev, D.V.; Glazunov, V.P.; Anufriev, V.F. Amination of 2-hydroxy-and 2, 3-dihydroxynaphthazarins. Synthesis of echinamines A and B, metabolites produced by the sand dollar *Scaphechinus mirabilis*. *Russ. J. Org. Chem.* **2009**, *45*, 37–43. [CrossRef]
30. Pokhilo, N.D.; Yakubovskaya, A.Y.; Denisenko, V.A.; Anufriev, V.P. Regiospecificity in the reaction of 2,3-dichloronaphthazarins with azide anions. Synthesis of echinamine A—A metabolite produced by the sea urchin *Scaphechinus mirabilis*. *Tetrahedron Lett.* **2006**, *47*, 1385–1387. [CrossRef]
31. Polonik, S.G.; Polonik, N.S.; Denisenko, V.A.; Moiseenko, O.P.; Anufriev, V.F. Synthesis and transformation of 2-amino-3-hydroxynaphthazarin. *Russ. J. Org. Chem.* **2009**, *45*, 1410–1411. [CrossRef]
32. Polonik, N.S.; Anufriev, V.P.; Polonik, S.G. Short and Regiospecific Synthesis of Echinamine A—The Pigment of Sea Urchin *Scaphechinus mirabilis*. *Nat. Prod. Commun.* **2011**, *6*, 217–222.
33. Greenwood, J.R.; Calkins, D.; Sullivan, A.P.; Shelley, J.C. Towards the comprehensive, rapid, and accurate prediction of the favorable tautomeric states of drug-like molecules in aqueous solution. *J. Comput. Aided Mol. Des.* **2010**, *24*, 591–604. [CrossRef]
34. Shelley, J.C.; Cholleti, A.; Frye, L.L.; Greenwood, J.R.; Timlin, M.R.; Uchimaya, M. Epik: A software program for pK_a prediction and protonation state generation for drug-like molecules. *J. Comput. Aided Mol. Des.* **2007**, *21*, 681–691. [CrossRef]
35. Petukh, M.; Stefl, S.; Alexov, E. The role of protonation states in ligand-receptor recognition and binding. *Curr. Pharm. Des.* **2013**, *19*, 4182–4190. [CrossRef]
36. Dai, W.; Wu, Y.; Bi, J.; Wang, S.; Li, F.; Kong, W.; Barbier, J.; Cintrat, J.C.; Gao, F.; Gillet, D.; et al. Antiviral Effects of ABMA against Herpes Simplex Virus Type 2 In Vitro and In Vivo. *Viruses* **2018**, *10*, 119. [CrossRef]
37. Klysik, K.; Pietraszek, A.; Karewicz, A.; Nowakowska, M. Acyclovir in the Treatment of Herpes Viruses—A Review. *Curr. Med. Chem.* **2020**, *27*, 4118–4137. [CrossRef]
38. Tai, C.J.; Li, C.L.; Tai, C.J.; Wang, C.K.; Lin, L.T. Early Viral Entry Assays for the Identification and Evaluation of Antiviral Compounds. *J. Vis. Exp.* **2015**, *104*, e53124. [CrossRef]
39. Wang, G.; Hernandez, R.; Weninger, K.; Brown, D.T. Infection of cells by Sindbis virus at low temperature. *Virology* **2007**, *362*, 461–467. [CrossRef]
40. Akhtar, J.; Shukla, D. Viral entry mechanisms: Cellular and viral mediators of herpes simplex virus entry. *FEBS J.* **2009**, *276*, 7228–7236. [CrossRef]
41. Luo, Z.; Kuang, X.P.; Zhou, Q.Q.; Yan, C.Y.; Li, W.; Gong, H.B.; Kurihara, H.; Li, W.X.; Li, Y.F.; He, R.R. Inhibitory effects of baicalein against herpes simplex virus type 1. *Acta Pharm. Sin. B* **2020**, in press. [CrossRef]
42. Arii, J.; Kawaguchi, Y. The Role of HSV Glycoproteins in Mediating Cell Entry. In *Human Herpesviruses. Advances in Experimental Medicine and Biology*; Kawaguchi, Y., Mori, Y., Kimura, H., Eds.; Springer: Singapore, 2018; Volume 1045, pp. 3–21.
43. O'Donnell, C.D.; Kovacs, M.; Akhtar, J.; Valyi-Nagy, T.; Shukla, D. Expanding the role of 3-O sulfated heparan sulfate in herpes simplex virus type-1 entry. *Virology* **2010**, *397*, 389–398. [CrossRef]
44. Li, W.; Xu, C.; Hao, C.; Zhang, Y.; Wang, Z.; Wang, S.; Wang, W. Inhibition of herpes simplex virus by myricetin through targeting viral gD protein and cellular EGFR/PI3K/Akt pathway. *Antivir. Res.* **2020**, *177*, 104714. [CrossRef]
45. Mosmann, T. Rapid colorimetric assay for cellular growth and survival: Application to proliferation and cytotoxicity assays. *J. Immunol. Methods* **1983**, *65*, 55–63. [CrossRef]

46. Weislow, O.S.; Kiser, R.; Fine, D.L.; Bader, J.; Shoemaker, R.H.; Boyd, M.R. New soluble-formazan assay for HIV-1 cytopathic effects: Application to high-flux screening of synthetic and natural products for AIDS-antiviral activity. *J. Natl. Cancer Inst.* **1989**, *81*, 577–586. [CrossRef]
47. Killington, R.A.; Powell, K.L. Growth, assay, and purification of herpesviruses. In *Virology: A Practical Approach*; Mahy, B.W., Ed.; IRL Press: Oxford, UK, 1991; pp. 207–236.
48. Marcocci, M.E.; Amatore, D.; Villa, S.; Casciaro, B.; Aimola, P.; Franci, G.; Grieco, P.; Galdiero, M.; Palamara, A.T.; Mangoni, M.L.; et al. The Amphibian Antimicrobial Peptide Temporin B Inhibits In Vitro Herpes Simplex Virus 1 Infection. *Antimicrob. Agents Chemother.* **2018**, *62*, e02367. [CrossRef]
49. Cardozo, F.T.; Camelini, C.M.; Mascarello, A.; Rossi, M.J.; Nunes, R.J.; Barardi, C.R.; de Mendonca, M.M.; Simoes, C.M. Antiherpetic activity of a sulfated polysaccharide from *Agaricus brasiliensis* mycelia. *Antivir. Res.* **2011**, *92*, 108–114. [CrossRef]
50. Groom, C.R.; Bruno, I.J.; Lightfoot, M.P.; Ward, S.C. The Cambridge Structural Database. *Acta Cryst.* **2016**, *B72*, 171–179. [CrossRef]
51. Gerasimenko, A.V.; Fedoreev, S.A.; Mishchenko, N.P. Molecular and Crystal Structure of the Echinochrome Complex with Dioxane. *Krist. Russ. Crystallogr. Rep.* **2006**, *51*, 42–47. [CrossRef]
52. *Molecular Operating Environment (MOE)*; Chemical Computing Group ULC: Montreal, QC, Canada, 2019.

Publisher's Note: MDPI stays neutral with regard to jurisdictional claims in published maps and institutional affiliations.

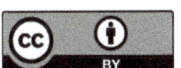

© 2020 by the authors. Licensee MDPI, Basel, Switzerland. This article is an open access article distributed under the terms and conditions of the Creative Commons Attribution (CC BY) license (http://creativecommons.org/licenses/by/4.0/).

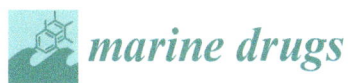

Article

Inspired by Sea Urchins: Warburg Effect Mediated Selectivity of Novel Synthetic Non-Glycoside 1,4-Naphthoquinone-6S-Glucose Conjugates in Prostate Cancer

Sergey A. Dyshlovoy [1,2,3,4,*,†], Dmitry N. Pelageev [2,3,†], Jessica Hauschild [1], Yurii E. Sabutskii [2], Ekaterina A. Khmelevskaya [2,3], Christoph Krisp [5], Moritz Kaune [1], Simone Venz [6,7], Ksenia L. Borisova [2], Tobias Busenbender [1], Vladimir A. Denisenko [2], Hartmut Schlüter [5], Carsten Bokemeyer [1], Markus Graefen [4], Sergey G. Polonik [2], Victor Ph. Anufriev [2] and Gunhild von Amsberg [1,4]

[1] Department of Oncology, Hematology and Bone Marrow Transplantation with Section Pneumology, Hubertus Wald-Tumorzentrum, University Medical Center Hamburg-Eppendorf, 20251 Hamburg, Germany; j.hauschild@uke.de (J.H.); moritz.kaune@stud.uke.uni-hamburg.de (M.K.); tobias.busenbender@gmx.de (T.B.); c.bokemeyer@uke.de (C.B.); g.von-amsberg@uke.de (G.v.A.)

[2] G.B. Elyakov Pacific Institute of Bioorganic Chemistry, Far-East Branch, Russian Academy of Sciences, 690022 Vladivostok, Russia; pelageev@mail.ru (D.N.P.); alixar2006@gmail.com (Y.E.S.); khea-96@mail.ru (E.A.K.); borisovaksenia@mail.ru (K.L.B.); vladenis@piboc.dvo.ru (V.A.D.); sergpol007@mail.ru (S.G.P.); anufriev@piboc.dvo.ru (V.P.A.)

[3] School of Natural Sciences, Far Eastern Federal University, 690091 Vladivostok, Russia

[4] Martini-Klinik, Prostate Cancer Center, University Hospital Hamburg-Eppendorf, 20251 Hamburg, Germany; graefen@martini-klinik.de

[5] Institute of Clinical Chemistry and Laboratory Medicine, Mass Spectrometric Proteomics, University Medical Center Hamburg-Eppendorf, 20251 Hamburg, Germany; c.krisp@uke.de (C.K.); hschluet@uke.de (H.S.)

[6] Department of Medical Biochemistry and Molecular Biology, University of Greifswald, 17489 Greifswald, Germany; simone.venz@uni-greifswald.de

[7] Interfacultary Institute of Genetics and Functional Genomics, Department of Functional Genomics, University of Greifswald, 17489 Greifswald, Germany

* Correspondence: s.dyshlovoy@uke.de or dyshlovoy@gmail.com; Tel.: +4940-7410-53591

† These authors equally contributed to this work.

Received: 16 April 2020; Accepted: 5 May 2020; Published: 11 May 2020

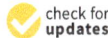

Abstract: The phenomenon of high sugar consumption by tumor cells is known as Warburg effect. It results from a high glycolysis rate, used by tumors as preferred metabolic pathway even in aerobic conditions. Targeting the Warburg effect to specifically deliver sugar conjugated cytotoxic compounds into tumor cells is a promising approach to create new selective drugs. We designed, synthesized, and analyzed a library of novel 6-S-(1,4-naphthoquinone-2-yl)-D-glucose chimera molecules (SABs)—novel sugar conjugates of 1,4-naphthoquinone analogs of the sea urchin pigments spinochromes, which have previously shown anticancer properties. A sulfur linker (thioether bond) was used to prevent potential hydrolysis by human glycoside-unspecific enzymes. The synthesized compounds exhibited a Warburg effect mediated selectivity to human prostate cancer cells (including highly drug-resistant cell lines). Mitochondria were identified as a primary cellular target of SABs. The mechanism of action included mitochondria membrane permeabilization, followed by ROS upregulation and release of cytotoxic mitochondrial proteins (AIF and cytochrome C) to the cytoplasm, which led to the consequent caspase-9 and -3 activation, PARP cleavage, and apoptosis-like cell death. These results enable us to further clinically develop these compounds for effective Warburg effect targeting.

Keywords: prostate cancer; thioglucoside conjugates; natural products; sea urchins; glucose uptake

1. Introduction

Chemotherapy remains an important treatment component for the vast majority of cancer patients. However, a lack of selectivity for tumor cells over normal cells frequently results in insufficient drug concentrations in the malignant tissue, systemic toxicity, and the development of drug resistance. Therefore, inexorable efforts have been made to develop targeted therapies allowing the release of cytotoxic activity in the region of interest while sparing healthy tissue. Potential therapeutic targets include cell surface antigens, growth receptors, key regulators of cellular signal transduction, and DNA repair defects [1]. Antibody drug conjugates (ADCs) consisting of an antibody linked to a biological active payload are under intensive investigation and first drugs are available in clinics, e.g., gemtuzumab ozogamicin in acute myeloid leukemia or brentuximab vedotin in relapsed Hodgkin´s lymphoma [2]. In urothelial carcinoma, nectin-4-targeted enfortumab vedotin has been recently accepted for priority review by the FDA [3]. On a similar note, radioisotope conjugated targeting antibodies are developed for imaging and radioimmunotherapy strategies. In fact, PSMA-ligand therapy with PSMA-linked α- or β-emitters are evaluated in clinical trials in prostate cancer and are applied to patients in every day's routine on individual bases [4]. Additional targeted therapies in prostate cancer include androgen-receptor (AR) targeting drugs such as abiraterone acetate, apalutamide, or enzalutamide as well as PARP-inhibitors in patients with DNA-repair defects [5].

Targeting the Warburg effect is an interesting novel treatment approach utilizing an increased sugar uptake of cancer cells to incorporate sugar conjugated cytotoxic compounds into tumor cells [6,7]. The high sugar demand of tumor cells results from the predominantly used metabolic pathway of glycolysis—even in aerobic conditions—which is energetically less efficient than oxidative phosphorylation found in healthy cells [8]. Thus, an overexpression of glycolytic enzymes in cytoplasm and glucose transporters (GLUTs) on the surface of cancer cells is frequently found in tumor cells in order to comply with the high sugar consumption [6,7].

Consequently, new compounds targeting the Warburg effect have been developed. In fact, sugar conjugates of docetaxel, busulfan, paclitaxel, and chlorambucil were found to be more selective to cancer cells in comparison with the non-conjugated "mother" molecules (reviewed in [6]). Furthermore, a glycosylated derivative of the alkylating agent ifosforamide—glufosfamide—has successfully passed clinical trials in human pancreatic, brain and CNS, lung cancer and soft tissue sarcoma [9].

More than 50% of the drugs currently available on the market are based on natural compounds and their synthetic derivatives [10]. Compared to compounds isolated from terrestrial sources, the marine-derived molecules are less studied [11,12]. At the same time, to date there are ten drugs approved for clinical use, seven of which are approved for the treatment of cancer and cancer-related conditions [13,14]. Spinochromes are an important family of polyhydroxynaphthoquinone secondary metabolites which were found in various sea urchin species. Due to their chemical diversity and promising pharmacological properties, these compounds attract the attention of scientific community as a base for development of new drugs [15,16]. Thus, spinochromes have revealed anti-allergic, anti-hypertensive, anti-diabetic, anti-oxidant, anti-inflammatory, and cardioprotective properties (reviewed in [15,16]). In general, biological effects of naphthoquinones are associated with generation of reactive oxygen species and modulation of redox signaling radical reactions [17] being either pro- or antioxidants or electrophiles [18]. Additionally, naphthazarins (5,8-dihydroxy-1,4-naphthoquinone derivatives), as well as other polymethoxylated natural and semisynthetic compounds possessing aromatic core, were reported to be potent anti-mitotic agents. Some of these compounds are capable of microtubule destabilizing and are therefore highly cytotoxic to cancer cells, representing an attractive starting point for further design as anticancer agents [19,20]. Thus, trimethyl ether of spinochrome D (tricrozarin B) inhibits a colony formation of human cancer HeLa S3 cells having IC$_{50}$ of 0.007 µg/mL [21].

Furthermore, our previous study also showed that methoxy derivatives of 1,4-naphthoquinones exhibit greater cytotoxicity compared to the corresponding unsubstituted hydroxy analogs [22].

In this study, in continuation of our research on sea urchin pigments [23–25], we synthesized and analyzed novel sugar conjugates of naturally derived and chemically modified hydroxyl-1,4-naphthoquinones related to the sea urchin spinochrome pigments. Recently, we identified several natural 1,4-naphthoquinones to be active in human drug-resistant prostate cancer cells [26] and were able to synthesize first conjugates with D-glucose possessing *in vitro* cytotoxic activity [22,26]. In the current study, we further modified the compounds bearing hydroxy-1,4-naphthoquinone scaffold and investigated their anticancer properties and the mechanism of action. Thus, to increase the selectivity of the identified natural 1,4-naphthoquinones via Warburg effect targeting, we conjugated these bioactive moieties with 6-mercaptoglucose. A glycoside bond is chemically reactive and may be easy degraded in the living system via enzyme-catalyzed hydrolysis. At the same time, thioglycosides have been reported to be more resistant to the enzyme-mediated degradation [27]. Therefore, we designed and synthesized a library of non-glycoside conjugates in order to increase stability of the target compounds under human body conditions; additionally, we introduced a novel sulfur linker (thioether bond) to prevent potential hydrolysis by the human glycoside-unspecific enzymes. It is important to note that an unsubstituted glycoside hydroxy group (at C1 position) is relevant for the stabilizing of the hydrogen bond interaction between glucose and GLUT-1 and therefore for successful uptake of the glucose conjugate via this system. In contrast, the conjugation of glucose at C6 position should have a minimal impact on the GLUT-1 mediated glucose uptake and therefore on the uptake of the synthesized compounds by the cancer cells. We were able to synthesize the new acetylated (protected) and non-acetylated (unprotected, containing free-glucose scaffold) thio-conjugates of 1,4-naphthoquinone and glucose. Human drug-resistant prostate cancer cells were chosen as the main model because of the known overexpression of GLUT-1. Here, we describe the synthesis of these new conjugates, as well as their Warburg effect-guided selective anticancer activity and mode of action.

2. Results

2.1. Design and Synthesis of the 6-S-(1,4-Naphthoquinon-2-yl)-D-Glucose Chimera Molecules

In continuation of the research on synthesis of bioactive 1,4-naphthoquinones, capable of selective activity towards human drug-resistance prostate cancer cells, we designed the chimera molecules consisting of cytotoxic 1,4-naphthoquinone pharmacophore and 6-thioglucose moiety. These derivatives are expected to exhibit selective cytotoxicity to cancer cells due to Warburg effect targeting and to be more stable in human body in comparison with conventional 1,4-naphthoquinone-glucosides due to the non-glycoside bond and thioether nature of the linker.

Thus, two different synthetic approaches were used for conjugation of naphthoquinones with 6-mercaptoglucose. We applied either: (a) a substitution reaction of halogenoquinones with readily available tetra-O-acetyl-6-mercaptoglucose in a basic condition (Figure 1A); or (b) an addition reaction of tetra-O-acetyl-6-mercaptoglucose to juglone, its acetate, or naphthazarin (Figure 1B). This was followed by saponification of the synthesized acetylated conjugates with MeONa/MeOH (Figure 1C).

Thus, halogenoquinones (Figure 1A) could be readily condensed with tetra-O-acetyl-6-mercaptoglucose in acetone solution with K_2CO_3, which resulted in acetylated conjugates **SAB-1, -3, -5, -7, -9, -11, -13, -15, -17, and -19** with the yields of about 60–70%. Note that chloroquinones, having an acidic β-hydroxyl group in the quinone core, did not react with tetra-O-acetyl-6-mercaptoglucose under the same conditions; therefore these reactions were performed in DMSO solution (yields ~80%).

As shown previously, reaction of thiols with juglone in EtOH gives exclusively 3-substituted products [28]. However, we observed that 5-acetyljuglone reacts with thiols giving the 2-substituted isomer as the main product of the reaction (Figure 1B). Boiling of naphthazarin excess with mercaptoglucose (molar ration 2:1) mainly gave 2-monosubstituted product **SAB-21** (Figure 1B).

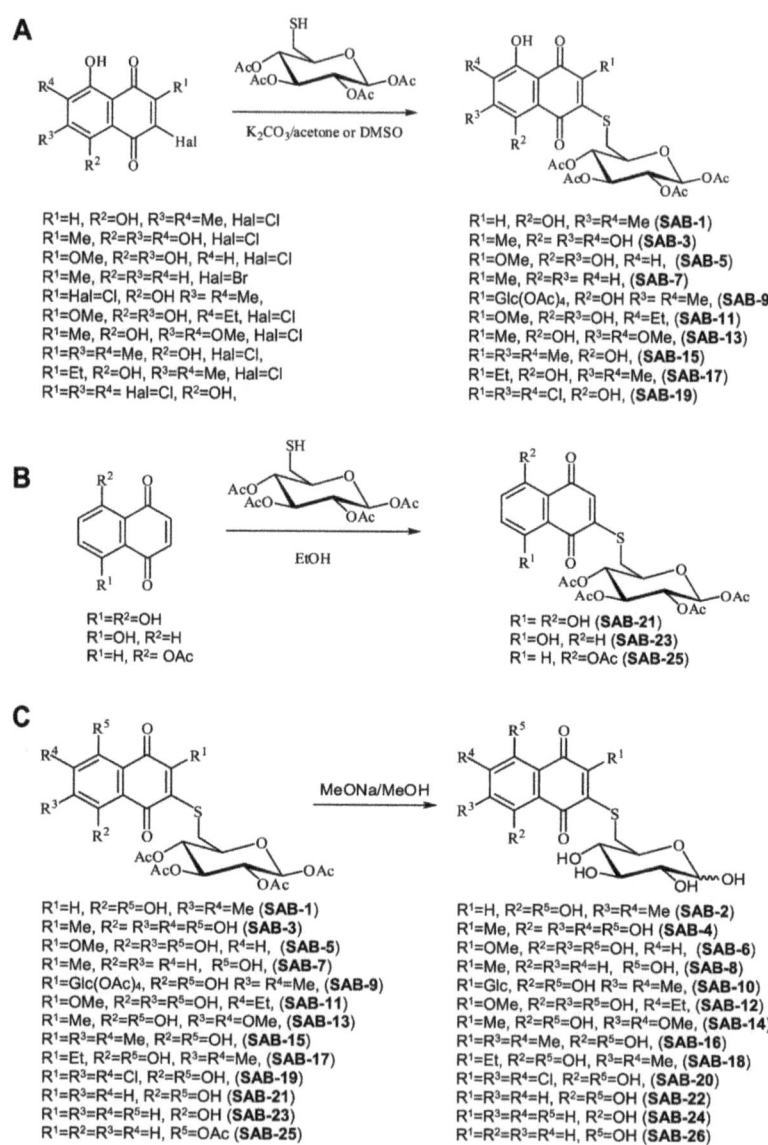

Figure 1. Scheme of synthesis: (**A**) synthesis of acetylated conjugates **SAB-1**, **-3**, **-5**, **-7**, **-9**, **-11**, **-13**, **-15**, **-17**, and **-19** from halogenoquinones with tetra-*O*-acetyl-6-mercaptoglucose; (**B**) synthesis of the acetylated conjugates **SAB-21**, **-23**, and **-25** from juglone derivatives and naphthazarin; and (**C**), synthesis of the deacetylated (unprotected) conjugates **SAB-2**, **-4**, **-6**, **-8**, **-10**, **-12**, **-14**, **-16**, **-18**, **-20**, **-22**, **-24**, and **-26** from the corresponding acetylated conjugates.

Further saponification of the synthesized acetylated conjugates by MeONa/MeOH led to the deprotected conjugates **SAB-2**, **-4**, **-6**, **-8**, **-10**, **-12**, **-14**, **-16**, **-18**, **-20**, **-22**, **-24**, and **-26** with the yields of 75–82% (Figure 1C). Thus, we were able to synthesize 26 compounds (14 pairs) containing either free or acetylated 6-thioglucose moiety (Figure 1A–C).

2.2. Evaluation of Cytotoxicity and Selectivity

First, we evaluated cytotoxic activity of the synthesized compounds in human drug-resistant prostate cancer PC-3 cells and human prostate non-cancer PNT2 cells. It has been reported that GLUT-1 is a main and the most abundant expressed receptor responsible for the glucose uptake in mammalian cells [7]. The expression of GLUT-1 in PC-3 was found to be higher in comparison with PNT2 cells (Figure 2A), thus these lines were considered a suitable model for the screening of Warburg-effect targeting substances (Figure 2B). Indeed, the selectivity of the conjugates bearing unprotected glucose residue (and therefore exhibiting increased affinity to GLUT-1) was significantly higher in comparison with acetylated derivatives (Figure 2C). Thus, we were able to identify one conjugate, **SAB-14**, to have a selectivity index (SI) > 2 (Figure 2B). For the further investigations, we selected **SAB-14** and **-13**—the acetylated derivative revealing a ~10-fold higher cytotoxicity and belonging to the same structural group as **SAB-14**. Both compounds were evaluated in five human prostate cancer cell lines known for different resistance profiles: LNCaP (AR-FL$^+$ and AR-V7$^-$, androgen-dependent, docetaxel-sensitive), 22Rv1 and VCaP (AR-FL$^+$ and AR-V7$^+$, androgen-independent, docetaxel-sensitive), and PC-3 and DU145 (AR-FL$^-$ and AR-V7$^-$, androgen-independent, docetaxel-resistant) [29,30]. In addition, five human non-cancer lines (PNT2, RWPE-1, HEK 293T, MRC-9, and HUVEC) were exposed to the derivates. In line with our previous results, both compounds were active and selective to human prostate cancer cells in comparison with non-cancer lines (Figure 2E). Note that **SAB-14**, bearing unprotected glucose moiety (Figure 2D), exhibited higher selectivity to the cancer cells (Figure 2E).

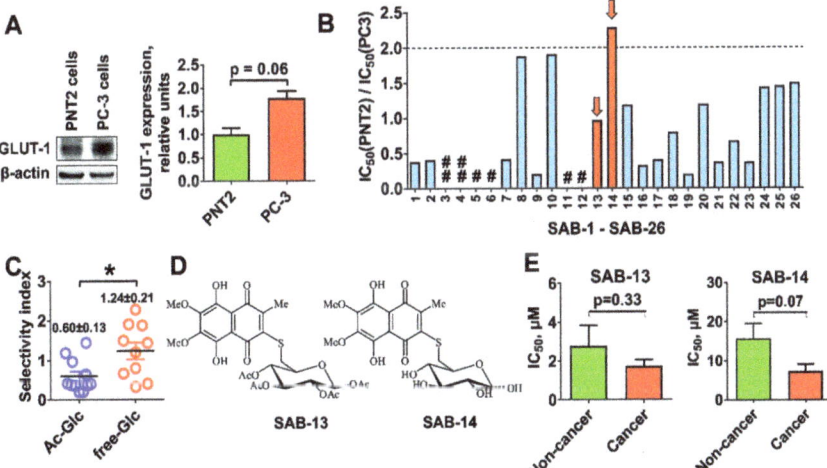

Figure 2. Cytotoxicity and selectivity of the synthesized compounds. (**A**) The Western blot examination of GLUT-1 expression in human prostate cancer PC-3 versus human prostate non-cancer PNT2 cells and its quantification. β-actin was used as a loading control (mean ± SEM; $n = 3$; Student's t-test). (**B**) Ratio of IC$_{50}$ (PNT2)/IC$_{50}$ (PC-3) indicated selective cytotoxicity towards human prostate cancer cells versus human prostate non-cancer cells. "#", IC$_{50}$ towards one of the tested cell line was >100 μM; "##", IC$_{50}$s (inhibition concentrations 50%) towards both tested cell line were >100 μM. (**C**) Pooled selectivity index (SI) value of acetylated derivatives (Ac-Glc) vs. non-acetylated derivatives (free-Glc) (mean ± SEM; $n \geq 10$; * $p < 0.05$, Student's t-test). For each compound, the SI was calculated as IC$_{50}$ (PNT2)/IC$_{50}$ (PC-3). (**D**) Structures of compounds **SAB-13** and **-14**. (**E**) The mean cytotoxicity of the most promising compounds **SAB-13** and **-14** in five prostate cancer (LNCaP, 22Rv1, VCaP, PC-3, and DU145) vs. five non-cancer (PNT2, RWPE-1, HEK 293T, MRC-9, and HUVEC) cell lines (mean ± SEM; $n = 5$; Student's t-test). Cells were treated for 48 h. The viability was measured by MTT assay.

2.3. Cytotoxicity Correlates with Glucose Uptake Rate in Prostate Cancer Cells

To examine whether synthesized compounds are able to target the Warburg effect, we accessed the glucose transporter-1 (GLUT-1) expression in the cells. Note that a mean GLUT-1 mRNA expression determined by qPCR was 1.6-fold higher in prostate cancer cells (LNCaP, 22Rv1, VCaP, PC-3, and DU145 cell lines) in comparison with human non-cancer cells (PNT2, RWPE-1, HEK 293T, MRC-9, and HUVEC cell lines), which correlated with the selectivity of the compounds (Figure 3A). Additionally, glucose depletion from culture medium resulted in increase of cytotoxic activity of both compounds (Figure 3B). Moreover, both compounds were able to inhibit glucose uptake in PC-3 cells, which was observed using two different detection methods (Figure 3C,D). Taken together, our results suggest that the novel compounds are concurrently ingested by the cells via the same GLUT-1 system as glucose and thus target the Warburg effect.

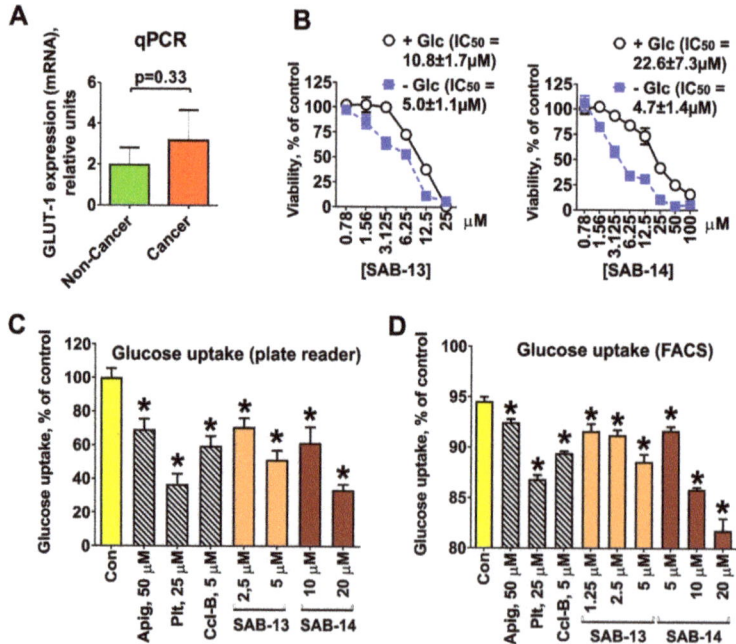

Figure 3. Cytotoxicity of the compounds is related to the Warburg effect. (**A**) The expression of the glucose transporter 1 mRNA (GLUT-1) in five human prostate cancer cell lines (LNCaP, 22Rv1, VCaP, PC-3, and DU145) versus four human non-cancer cell lines (PNT2, RWPE-1, HEK 293T, MRC-9, and HUVEC) (mean ± SEM; $n = 5$; Student's t-test). The expression was measured by qPCR. (**B**) The viability of PC-3 cells incubated with **SAB-13** and **-14** in glucose-free (−Glc) or in glucose-containing media (+Glc, 2 g/L). Cytotoxic activity was measured using MTT test following 24 h of treatment. (**C,D**) Concurrent inhibition of glucose uptake by the **SAB-13** and **-14**. PC-3 cells were treated with the compounds for 24 h and then the glucose uptake was measured using 2-NBDG-based assay either in cell culture by plate reader (**C**) or in single cells using flow cytometry technique (**D**) and then normalized to cell viability (mean ± SEM; $n = 3$; * $p < 0.05$, one-way ANOVA test). Apigenin (Apig), phloretin (Plt), and cytochalasin B (Ccl-B) were used as positive controls. The viability was measured by MTS assay (**B,C**) or by flow cytometry using PI staining (**D**).

2.4. SAB-13 and -14 Induce Caspase-Dependent Apoptosis

Pro-apoptotic signs such as phosphatidylserine externalization (Figure 4A–C) and PARP cleavage (Figure 4D) were found in the cells following 48 h treatment with **SAB-13** and **-14** at the concentrations which were close to IC$_{50}$s in the correspondent cell lines. In addition, cleavage of caspase-3 was observed (Figure 4D). Co-treatment with pan-caspase inhibitor zVAD antagonized the cytotoxic effects of **SAB-13** and **-14**, suggesting a caspase-dependent character of the induced apoptosis (Figure 4B). Furthermore, the cell cycle analysis revealed DNA fragmentation, another pro-apoptotic marker, detected as sub-G1 peak (Figure 4E). More detailed analysis of the generated data revealed a G2/M-cell cycle arrest under drug treatment (Figure 4F). This could be at least in part explained with the observed upregulation of p21 (Figure 4D), which may contribute both to the cycle arrest as well as to the induced apoptotic cell death [31].

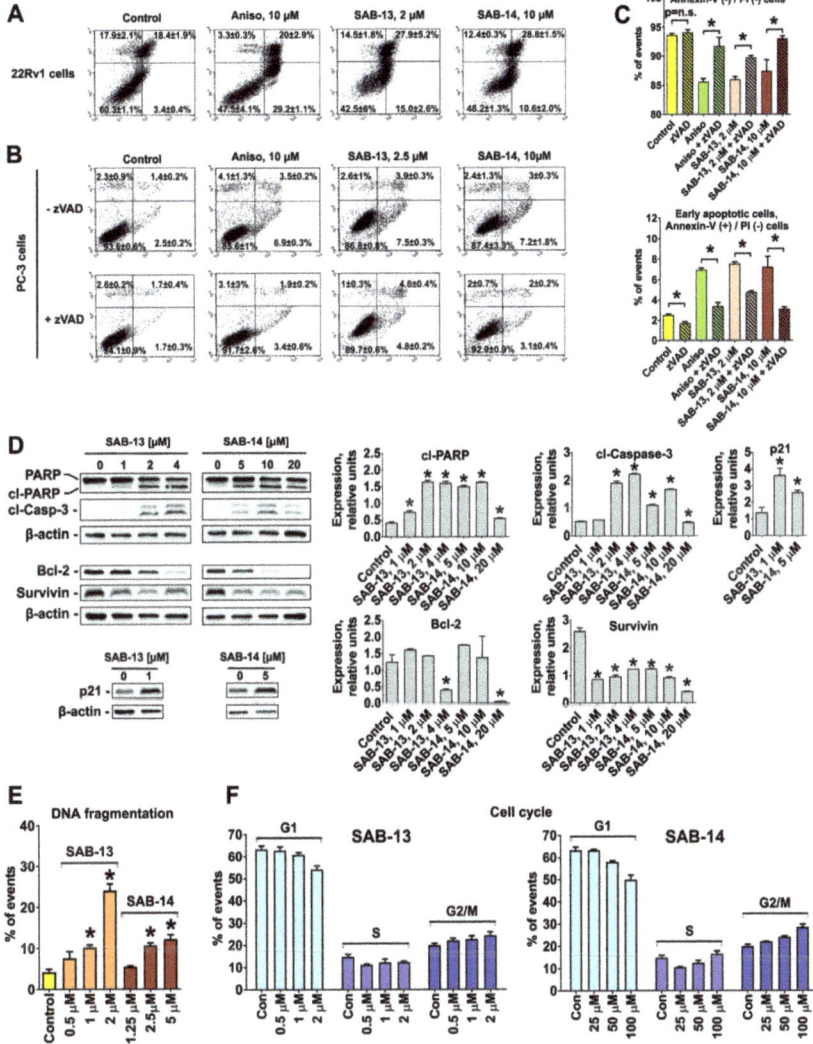

Figure 4. Pro-apoptotic activity of SAB-13 and SAB-14. (**A–C,E,F**), FACS analysis of the cells after 48 h treatment. Analysis of apoptosis induction in 22Rv1 (**A**) and PC-3 cells (**B**) using Annexin-V-FITC/propidium iodide (PI) double staining. PC-3 cells were pre-treated with 100 µM of pan-caspase inhibitor z-VAD(OMe)-fmk (zVAD) for 1 h and then treated with indicated concentrations

of the drugs for 48 h (**B**). Viable cells (Annexin-V-FITC(−)/PI(−), LL quadrant) or early apoptotic cells (Annexin-V-FITC(+)/PI(−), LR quadrant) were quantified using the Cell Quest Pro software (**C**) (mean ± SEM; $n = 3$; * $p < 0.05$, Student's t-test). (**D**) Western blotting analysis of the protein expression in 22Rv1 cells after 48 h of treatment. β-actin was used as a loading control (mean ± SEM; $n = 3$; one-way ANOVA test). Anisomycin (Aniso; treatment with 10 µM for 48 h) was used as a positive control. (**E**,**F**) Cell cycle analysis of 22Rv1 cells using PI staining, apoptotic cells were detected as sub-G1 population (**E**) (mean ± SEM; $n = 3$; * $p < 0.05$, one-way ANOVA test).

For this and further examinations, 22Rv1 cells were used as the main model. 22Rv1 cells express both AR-full length and AR-V7 [32]. The latter mediates resistance of prostate cancer to androgen receptor targeted therapies such as abiraterone or enzalutamide [33,34]. At the same time, PC-3 cells are AR-full length- and AR-V7-negative [32] and thus might be less relevant as clinical model for prostate cancer.

2.5. Effect of SAB-13 on the Proteome of Prostate Cancer Cells

To identify possible processes and molecular targets affected under the treatment, we investigated changes in proteome of 22Rv1 cells treated with **SAB-13**, as the most active compounds of the synthesized panel, at the concentration close to IC_{50}s in the correspondent cell line. The changes in the protein expression were examined using the LC-MS/MS method in DIA (data independent acquisition) mode. In total, 2163 proteins were identified and quantified. In total, 253 proteins had $1.5 \leq$ fold change $\leq 1/1.5$ and were significantly regulated ($p \leq 0.05$) (see Supplementary Materials Table S1). In fact, upregulation of 104 proteins and downregulation of 149 was detected following the treatment.

The proteomics data was analyzed using the Ingenuity Pathways Analysis software (IPA, QIAGEN Bioinformatics). Five top protein networks were constructed by IPA and the alteration of five kinases involved in several pro- and anti-apoptotic processes was predicted (Figure 5A, marked with red circle) and further validated in functional assays (Figure 5B). Thus, we showed a pronounced activation of ERK1/2, p38, and Akt kinases upon the treatment, while only slight phosphorylation of MEK1/2 and JNK1/2 kinases was observed (Figure 5B). Thus, alteration of ERK1/2, p38, and Akt may play an important role in the cellular effect mediated by the synthesized compounds. Note that the regulation (cleavage) of PARP and caspase (caspase-3), predicted in IPA analysis (Figure 5A), was confirmed experimentally as well (Figure 4D).

Next, gene ontology analysis and z-score algorithm were used to further predict the effect on biological processes/target (Figure 5C). Most of the proteins regulated under the treatment were located in cellular cytoplasm and nucleus, and were identified as enzymes (Figure 5C). Remarkably, the activity of several upstream regulators playing an important role in prostate cancer development and progression have been predicted to be affected by **SAB-13** (Figure 5D). Among them, the following are suppressed: E2F3 (transcription factor, its activity was reported to be associated with poor prostate cancer patients treatment prognosis [35]), ADRB (β-adrenergic receptor, its signaling is involved in the development of aggressive prostate cancer [36]), BRD4 (kinase, associated with tumor growth and metastatic potential of prostate cancer [37,38]), 25s proteasome (a promising and relevant target in a number of human cancers including prostate cancer [39]), and MYC (proto-oncogene, is involved in initiation and progression of a number of human cancers [40] and drives the development of the highly aggressive neuroendocrine prostate cancer [36]) (Figure 5D). Additionally, sirtuin and IL-8 signaling, as well as LXR/RXR and NO and ROS production in macrophages were proposed to be suppressed, while NER and EIF2 pathway, ILK signaling, and oxidative phosphorylation were predicted to be activated under the treatment (Figure 5E). At the same time, it is important to note that predicted activation of KDM5A and XBP1 and suppression of FOXO1 and RB1 were observed. These alterations may play a possible negative role in prostate cancer as undesirable effects of the drug, which is described elsewhere. Therefore, these effects should be carefully investigated before further development of these drugs for in-human trials.

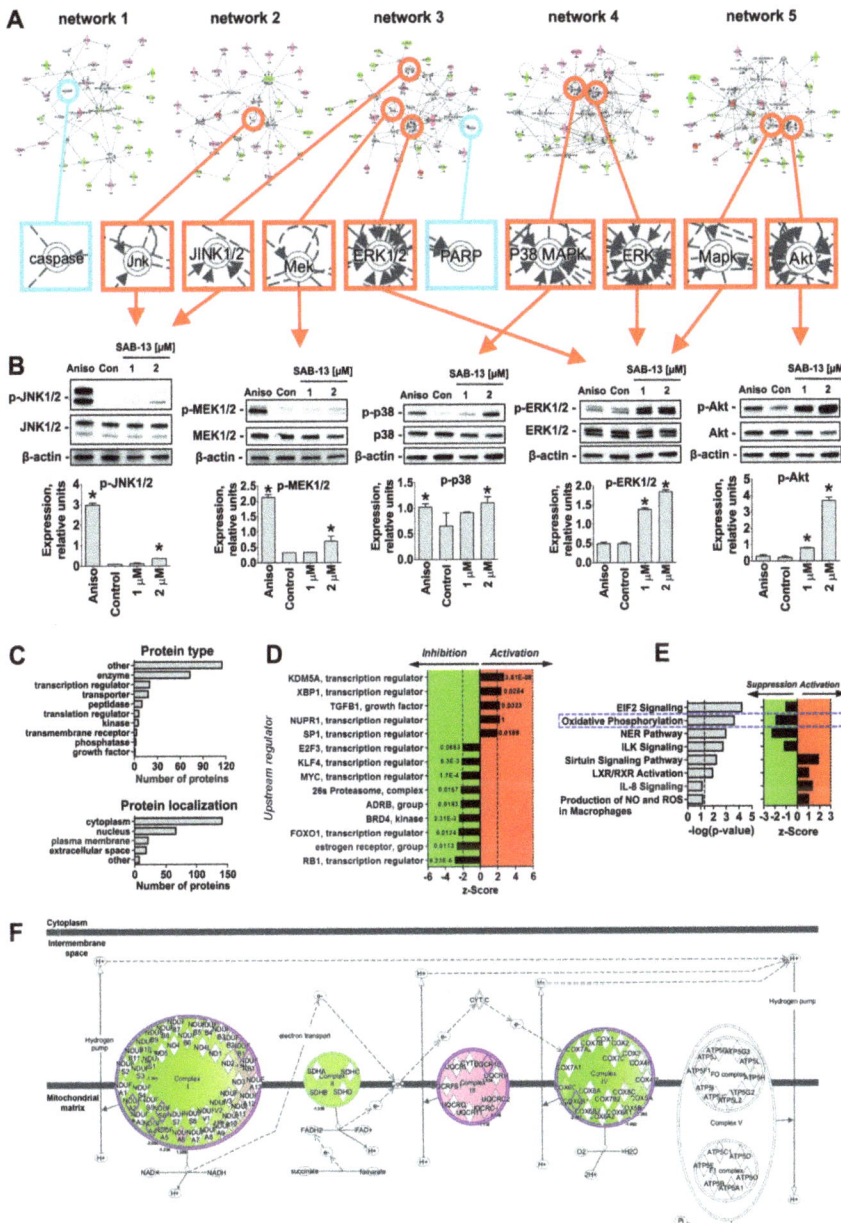

Figure 5. The effect of SAB-13 on proteome of prostate cancer cells. 22Rv1 cells were treated with **SAB-13** (2 µM, 48 h). The changes in proteome identified by LC-MS/MS and later analyzed using Ingenuity Pathway Analysis (IPA) software and z-score algorithm. (**A**) Hypothetical protein interaction networks between regulated proteins and the proteins predicted to be involved in interactions (constructed using IPA software). (**B**) Some kinases predicted to be affected under the treatment were further validated by

Western blotting (marked by red circle). The activation was observed 2 h after the treatment. β-actin was used as a loading control. The expression phospho-kinases was normalized to the non-phospho-kinases expression levels (mean ± SEM; $n = 3$; * $p < 0.05$; one-way ANOVA test). (**C**) Gene ontology analysis. (**D**) Top upstream targets and the calculated z-score of the effect (activation/inhibition), predicted by IPA. *p*-values of overlap is indicated on the graph (significance: $p < 0.05$, Fischer's exact test). (**E**) Top canonical pathways, predicted by IPA. The target/process is expected to be activated if z-score > 0 (red area) or suppressed if z-score < 0 (green area) (significance: $p < 0.05$, Fischer's exact test). (**F**) Representative scheme of oxidative phosphorylation. Affected proteins discovered by proteome analysis are marked with color.

Note that we discovered the alterations of protein components of four (out of five) main protein complexes located in the inner mitochondrial membrane and involved in the oxidative phosphorylation (see Table S1). These molecules were identified as parts of Complex I (genes *NDUFA4*, *NDUFS6*, *NDUFB1*, and *NDUFA2*), Complex II (gene *SDHB*), Complex III (gene *UQCR10*), and Complex IV (genes *COX6B1* and *COX17*). Therefore, oxidative phosphorylation was predicted to be inhibited/disrupted in **SAB-13**-treated cells (z-score = −1.89, *p*-value = 2.37×10^{-4}; Figure 5F).

2.6. SAB-13 and SAB-14 Induce Apoptosis via Mitochondria Targeting

Oxidative phosphorylation (or electron transport-linked phosphorylation) is a metabolic pathway of nutrients oxidation which takes place in mitochondria and ultimately results in ATP production in eukaryotic cells [41]. Thus, its disruption predicted by bioinformatical analysis of proteomics data may indicate mitochondria targeting by **SAB-13** and similar compounds. **SAB-13** was found to affect complexes I-IV, essential elements of oxidative phosphorylation machinery, which are located in the mitochondrial inner membrane. Consequently, we examined the effect of **SAB-13** on the mitochondrial membrane potential ($\Delta\Psi_m$) at the concentration close to IC_{50}. Significant and rapid loss of $\Delta\Psi_m$ was detected in the prostate cancer cells following both short- (2 h) and long-term (48 h) treatment (Figure 6A,B). Next, ROS production level was examined, which is known to be closely associated with mitochondrial integrity [42]. Indeed, a significant increase of the ROS level was observed 2 h after the treatment, simultaneously with $\Delta\Psi_m$ loss (Figure 6C,D). Moreover, pretreatment with an established antioxidant N-acetyl-L-cysteine could rescue the cells from the drug-induced apoptosis (Figure 6E). This confirms the cytotoxic effect of ROS generation under treatment. Additionally, we were able to show that caspase-9 (but not caspase-3) is activated shortly after treatment at the concentration close to IC_{50} (2 h, Figure 6F), whereas caspase-3 cleavage was observed after 48 h treatment (Figure 6G). Finally, the examination of different subcellular fractions revealed a redistribution of such pro-apoptotic proteins as cytochrome C and AIF (apoptosis inducing factor) from mitochondria to cytoplasm (Figure 7). This effect was accompanied by apoptosis induction, as indicated by cleaved PARP and cleaved caspase-3 as apoptotic markers (Figure 7). In conclusion, induced cancer cell apoptosis was strongly associated with targeting of mitochondria.

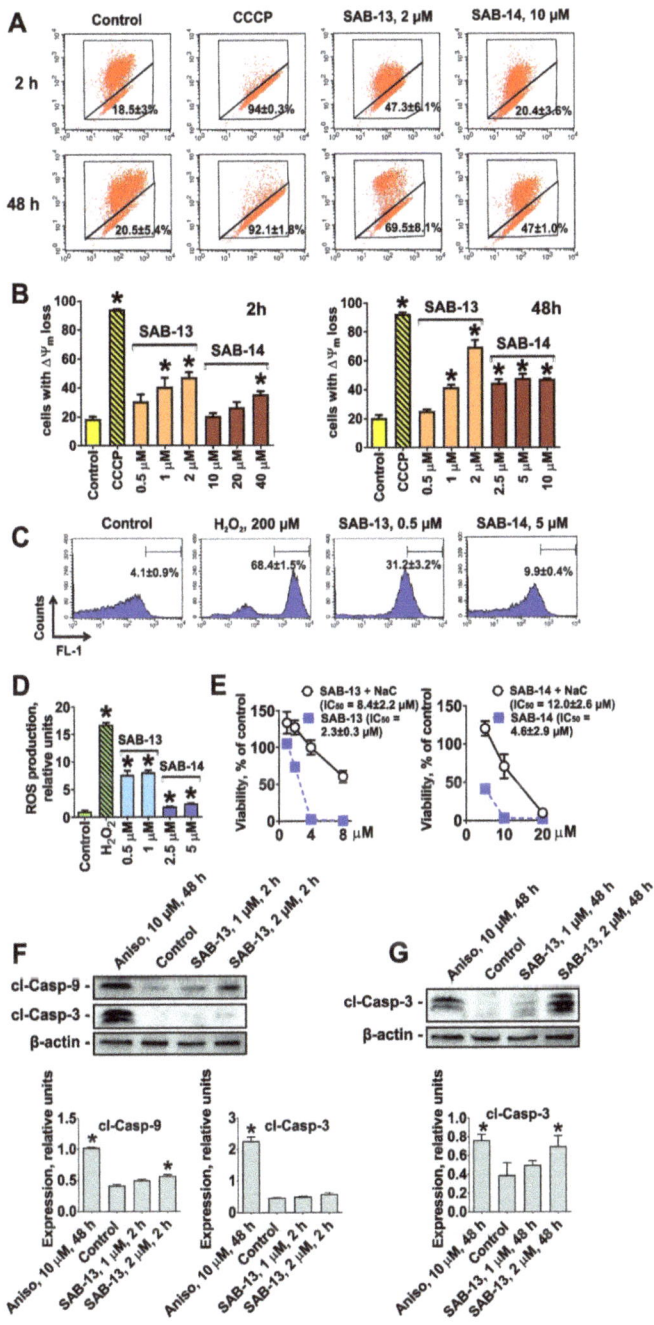

Figure 6. Effect of SAB-13 and SAB-14 on mitochondrial membrane potential and ROS production. (**A**,**B**) Effect of the drugs on mitochondrial membrane potential (MMP, $\Delta\Psi_m$). 22Rv1 cells were treated with the **SAB-13** or **SAB-14** for indicated time, harvested with trypsin, stained with JC-1, and measured

by FACS (**A**), and the cells containing depolarized mitochondria were quantified using the Cell Quest Pro software (**B**) (mean ± SEM; $n = 3$; * $p < 0.05$, one-way ANOVA test). CCCP (50 µM) was used as a positive control. (**C,D**) Effect on ROS production in 22Rv1 cells after 2 h of treatment. Cells were stained with CM-H$_2$DCFDA, treated with the drugs, harvested, and analyzed by FACS (**C**), and the ROS level was quantified using the Cell Quest Pro software (**D**) (mean ± SEM; $n = 3$; * $p < 0.05$, one-way ANOVA test). H$_2$O$_2$ (200 µM) was used as a positive control. (**E**) 22Rv1 cells were pre-treated with 1 mM NaC (N-acetyl-L-cysteine) for 1 h and then co-treated with the investigated drugs for 48 h FBS- and glucose-free media. Cell viability was measured by MTT assay, treatment time was 48 h. (**F,G**), Western blotting analysis of cleaved caspase-3 and -9 levels in 22Rv1 cells treated with **SAB-13** for 2 h (**F**) or 48 h (**G**). Anisomycin (Aniso) was used as a positive control. β-actin was used as a loading control (mean ± SEM; $n = 3$; one-way ANOVA test).

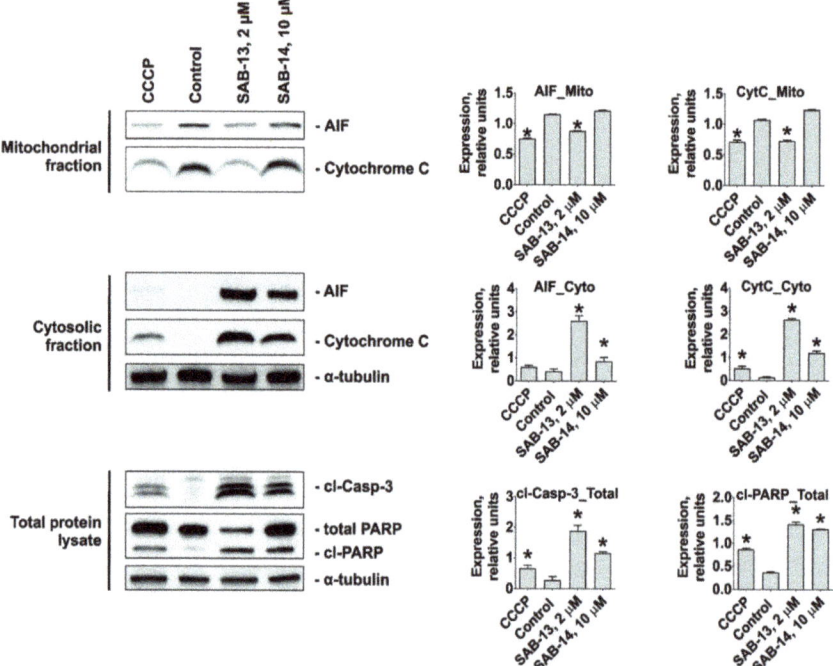

Figure 7. Quantification of the proteins in mitochondrial, cytoplasmic, and total fractions. 22Rv1 cells were treated with the drugs for 48 h, the proteins were extracted and fractionated using Cell Fractionation Kit (abcam). The mitochondrial (Mito), cytoplasmatic (Cyto) or total (Total) fractions were concentrated and analyzed by Western blotting. Cells treated with carbonyl cyanide 3-chlorophenylhydrazone (CCCP; 50 µM) were used as a positive control. α-tubulin was used as a loading control, the protein expression was normalized to α-tubulin expression levels either in cytosolic fraction or in the total protein lysate (mean ± SEM; $n = 3$; * $p < 0.05$; one-way ANOVA test).

3. Discussion

A significant percentage of prostate cancer patients initially respond to targeted (e.g., abiraterone acetate, enzalutamide, PARP-inhibitors, and PSMA-ligand therapy) or untargeted therapies (e.g., cabazitaxel, docetaxel, and radium-223) [43]. However, the majority of patients will experience an increasing loss of sensitivity to standard medications with each additional treatment line [44]. Primary as well as secondary drug-resistance are responsible for the limited treatment success and poor prognosis of patients suffering from advanced castration resistant prostate cancer (CRPC) [45]. Thus, expression of androgen receptor transcriptional variants of AR (AR-Vs), in particular AR-V7 [33], has been identified as an important mechanism of resistance to AR-targeted therapies. In addition, side effects caused by the damage of non-malignant cells limit the application of standard therapies in a mostly older and comorbid patient population. Thus, novel therapeutics capable of overcoming drug resistance while sparing side effects are urgently needed.

Conjugation of the cytotoxic molecule and the moiety, which is responsible for selective delivery of the active substance to cancer cells may increase specificity of the drug and to reduce its side effects. In the current study we conjugated bioactive 1,4-naphthoquinone scaffold, which has been previously shown to exhibit cytotoxic activity in human cancer cell lines, with a glucose moiety via a sulfur linker at C6 position using simple and effective methods. Note that the generated non-glycoside bond simplified the chemical synthesis of the compounds. Thus, we recently reported a number of O-glycosides of 1,4-naphthoquinones to undergo decomposition during the deacetylation step [46]. Moreover, we showed that some S-glycosides can convert into linear or angular tetracycles under the same conditions [46], whereas no undesired effects or side reactions were observed during the synthesis described in the current research. Thus, we used either: (i) a substitution reaction of the halogen atoms in 1,4-naphthoquinone derivatives by a sulfur atom of 6-mercaptoglucose derivative; or (ii) an addition reaction of 6-mercaptoglucose derivative to juglone, its acetate, or naphthazarin, followed by saponification of the acetylated conjugates.

This modification resulted in a higher specificity to cancer cells due to Warburg effect targeting as well as increased water solubility and therefore bioavailability of the synthesized molecules. An exchange of the ether linker to the thioether linker most likely will provide higher stability of the compounds in the human body [27] and a greater resistance to the enzymes mediated hydrolysis. The conjugation at C6 position of glucose molecule ensures the affinity of the synthesized conjugates to GLUT-1 and therefore its successful cellular uptake via this system. Furthermore, it should provide additional resistance to glycoside-specific enzymes due to the non-glycoside nature of the bond as well as novel sulfur linker.

Thus, we could synthesize 14 acetylated derivatives and 14 corresponding water-soluble unprotected (deacetylated) conjugates. Following a screening of the synthesized compounds, we chose two most promising candidates. Hence, **SAB-14** (6-((6-deoxy-6-S-D-glucopyranosyl)thio)-5,8-dihydroxy-7-methyl-2,3-dimethoxy-1,4-naphthoquinone) and its acetylated analog **SAB-13** (6-((1,2,3,4-tetra-O-acetyl-6-deoxy-β-D-glucopyranosyl)thio)-5,8-dihydroxy-7-methyl-2,3-dimethoxy-1,4-naphthoquinone) exhibited selectivity to human prostate cancer cells and were chosen for further investigations. The selectivity of these drugs was mediated by Warburg effect. This was confirmed by several experiments, namely correlation of selectivity to cancer cell lines with increased GLUT-1 expression in these cells, the increased cytotoxicity of the compounds in the glucose-depleted media, and the ability of the compounds to inhibit glucose uptake by the cells, which was confirmed with two different methods. Additionally, the compounds bearing unsubstituted glucose residue (e.g., **SAB-14**) were generally more selective in comparison with its acetylated analogs (e.g., **SAB-13**). This can be explained by the higher affinity of unprotected glucose residue to GLUT-1. These results strongly suggest the synthesized drugs were taken up by the same system, as glucose, i.e., glucose transporters (GLUTs).

The mechanism of anticancer activity of the natural 1,4-naphthoquinones and other related compounds includes generation of free superoxide radicals, which results in DNA damage and may lead to p53-independent cell death [22,47,48], as well as inhibition of topoisomerase-II [47,49,50]. Consequently, the examination of the mechanisms of anticancer activity of **SAB-13** and **-14** revealed an induction of caspase-dependent apoptosis. Additionally, we detected a G2/M arrest of the cancer cells under drug treatment, which could be related to the observed p21 upregulation in the treated cells. Pro-apoptotic effects of the synthesized conjugates were accompanied by downregulation of several anti-apoptotic proteins. Further investigation of the drug-mediated changes in cellular proteome as well as bioinformatical analysis of the data suggested mitochondria targeting as one of the central effects of **SAB-13**. Indeed, we were able to validate this effect in functional assays.

Thus, **SAB-13** is able to promote a generation of cytotoxic ROS and to induce a drop-down of mitochondrial membrane potential, which resulted in a release of cytotoxic mitochondrial proteins to cellular cytoplasm, caspases activation and ultimately cancer cell death (Figure 8). In addition, **SAB-13** activated caspase-9 shortly after treatment and prior to caspase-3 (Figure 8). It has been previously shown that the modification of existing drugs in order to assign them mitochondria-targeting properties (i.e., conjugation with the mitochondria-specific carrier molecule) significantly increases their activity towards cancer cells [51,52]. Moreover, these drugs were reported to be able to overcome the drug resistance to standard medications [51,52]. Despite the upregulated glycolysis (anaerobic respiration) in cancer cells in comparison to normal tissues, the oxidative phosphorylation (part of aerobic respiration machinery) was reported to be still active and even upregulated in different cancer entities [53]. Thus, oxidative phosphorylation has recently been identified as a new promising target in anticancer therapy promoting the therapeutic potential of the inhibitors of this biochemical process [41]. In fact, inhibitors of different steps of the oxidative phosphorylation cascade such as metformin, atovaquone, arsenic trioxide, carboxyamidotriazole, fenofibrate, and lonidamine have exhibited therapeutic efficacy in a number of clinical and preclinical studies for the treatment of different cancer types (reviewed in [53]). Thus, the combination of Warburg effect mediated selectivity and the simultaneous targeting of oxidative phosphorylation/mitochondria in cancer cells makes the synthesized conjugates promising agents in the therapy of the human CRPC and other cancers. Ongoing experiments will clarify if oxidative phosphorylation is a primary target of the drugs, or if the targeting of other mitochondrial components and functions cause a disruption of the oxidative phosphorylation along with other mitochondrial processes. In vivo experiments are currently in preparation to validate the above-described *in vitro* results.

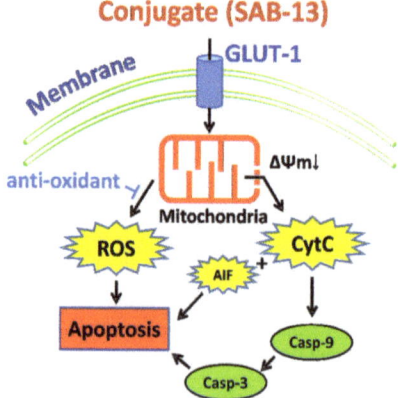

Figure 8. Suggested mechanism of anticancer activity *in vitro*.

4. Materials and Methods

4.1. Chemistry

4.1.1. General Chemistry (Reagents, Solvents and Equipment)

Reagents and solvents were purchased from Sigma (Taufkirchen, Germany) and Vekton (St. Petersburg, Russia). The initial quinones were purchased from Sigma or synthesized as described elsewhere. All reagents, initial quinones, and solvents were of analytical grade and used as received. The melting points were determined on a Boetius melting-point apparatus (Dresden, Germany) and are uncorrected. The ^{1}H and ^{13}C NMR spectra were recorded using Bruker Avance-300 (300 MHz), Bruker Avance III-500 HD (500 MHz), and Bruker Avance III-700 (700 MHz) spectrometers (Bruker

Corporation, Bremen, Germany) using CDCl$_3$ and DMSO-d$_6$ as the solvents with the signal of the residual non-deuterated solvent as the internal reference. The progress of reaction was monitored by thin-layer chromatography (TLC) on Sorbfil plates (IMID, Krasnodar, Russia) using the following solvent systems as eluents: hexane/benzene/acetone, 3:1:1 (v/v) (System A) and benzene/ethyl acetate/methanol, 7:4:2 (System B). Individual substances were isolated and purified using crystallization, column chromatography as well as preparative TLC on silica gel (Silicagel 60, 0.040–0.063 mm, Alfa Aesar, Karlsruhe, Germany) which was preliminarily treated with hydrochloric acid (pH = 2) in order to reduce a residual adsorption of quinones, followed by drying and activation by heating at 120 °C.

The initial quinone 6-chloro-5,8-dihydroxy-2,3-dimethoxy-7-methyl-1,4-naphthoquinone was synthesized from the commercially available reagents as described below. A solution of diazomethane in Et$_2$O (0.2 M) was added dropwise to a stirring solution of 6-chloro-2,3,5,8-tetrahydroxy-7-methyl-1,4-naphthoquinone (299 mg, 1.0 mmol) in 1,4-dioxane (50 mL), until TLC indicated completion of dimethoxylated product with R_f = 0.70 (system A) formation. The reaction mixture was evaporated in vacuo and the solid was recrystallized from methanol. Red-brown solid; yield 75% (224 mg); mp 179-181 °C; R_f = 0.70 (A). ^{1}H NMR (CDCl$_3$, 500 MHz) δ: 2.42 (s, 3H, -CH$_3$), 4.12 (s, 3H, -OCH$_3$), 4.13 (s, 3H, -OCH$_3$), 12.94 (s, 1H, C(8)-OH), 13.04 (s, 1H, C(5)-OH). ^{13}C NMR (125 MHz, CDCl$_3$) δ: 13.5 (-CH$_3$), 61.7 (2 × -OCH$_3$), 108.0 (C-8a), 108.4 (C-4a), 134.2 (C-6), 139.0 (C-7), 147.6, 148.0, 156.3 (C-5), 159.2 (C-8), 181.8 (C-4), 181.9 (C-1); IR (CHCl$_3$) $ν_{max}$: 3003, 2954, 2855, 1605, 1457, 1432, 1418, 1401, 1379, 1286, 1188, 1158, 1138, 1113, 1053 cm^{-1}. HRMS (EI): m/z [M − H]$^−$ calcd for C$_{13}$H$_{10}$ClO$_6$: 297.0171; found: 297.0168.

1,2,3,4-Tetra-O-acetyl-6-deoxy-6-thio-β-D-glucopyranose, used for the synthesis of the conjugates, was synthesized from the commercially available reagents as described below. Potassium metabisulfite (4.37 g, 19.65 mmol, 1.5 eq) was added to a refluxing solution of 1,2,3,4-tetra-O-acetyl-6-deoxy-β-D-glucopyranosyl-6-isothiouronium iodide (7.0 g, 13.1 mmol) in mixture of water (75 mL) and chloroform (75 mL). The reaction mixture was refluxed for 2 h, cooled to room temperature. The organic layer was separated. The aqueous layer was extracted with chloroform (2 × 50 mL). The organic layers were combined, dried over NaSO$_4$, filtered, and the solvent evaporated under vacuum. The residue was recrystallized from MeOH to give pure crystalline product. White solid; yield 57.4% (2.74 g); mp 109-111 °C; R_f = 0.51 (A). ^{1}H NMR (500 MHz, CDCl$_3$) δ: 1.75 (dd, J = 9.6, 7.5 Hz, 1H, -SH), 2.01 (s, 3H, -COCH$_3$), 2.03 (s, 3H, -COCH$_3$), 2.05 (s, 3H, -COCH$_3$), 2.12 (s, 3H, -COCH$_3$), 2.62 (m, H-6a), 2.71 (m, H-6b), 3.96 (ddd, J = 9.7, 6.5, 3.0 Hz, 1H, H-5), 5.11 (t, J = 9.7 Hz, 1H, H-4), 5.12 (t, J = 9.4 Hz, 1H, H-2), 5.25 (t, J = 9.4 Hz, 1H, H-3), 5.71 (t, J = 8.4 Hz, 1H, H-1). ^{13}C NMR (125 MHz, CDCl$_3$) δ: 20.5 (2 × -COCH$_3$), 20.6 (-COCH$_3$), 20.8 (-COCH$_3$), 25.8 (C-6), 70.3 (C-2), 70.4 (C-4), 72.8 (C-3), 75.0 (C-5), 91.7 (C-1), 169.0 (-COCH$_3$), 169.2 (-COCH$_3$), 169.5 (-COCH$_3$), 170.1 (-COCH$_3$). IR (CHCl$_3$) $ν_{max}$: 3056, 3006, 1759, 1602, 1429, 1370, 1250, 1192, 1079, 1038 cm^{-1}. HRMS (ESI): m/z [M + Na]$^+$ calcd for C$_{14}$H$_{20}$NaO$_9$S: 387.0720; found: 387.0717.

4.1.2. General Procedure for Synthesis of the Acetylated Conjugates **SAB-1**, **-7**, **-9**, **-13**, **-15**, **-17**, and **-19** in Acetone Solution (Figure 1A)

Finely powdered potassium carbonate (0.415 g, 3.0 mmol) was added to a solution of the correspondent quinone, (1.0 mmol) and tetra-O-acetyl-6-mercaptoglucose (0.368 g, 1.01 mmol) in acetone (120 mL). The mixture was stirred at room temperature until reaction completed (3 h, controlled by TLC), acidified with HCl, and concentrated in vacuo. The residue was purified by column chromatography (silica gel, hexane/acetone, 10:1) to give products **1**, **7**, **9**, **13**, **15**, **17**, and **19**.

2-(1,2,3,4-Tetra-O-acetyl-6-deoxy-β-D-glucopyranos-6-ylthio)-5,8-dihydroxy-6,7-dimethyl-1,4-naphthoquinone (**SAB-1**). Red solid; yield 406 mg (70%); mp 203–205 °C; R_f = 0.33 (A). ^{1}H NMR (CDCl$_3$, 500 MHz) δ: 2.02 (s, 3H, -COCH$_3$), 2.03 (s, 3H, -COCH$_3$), 2.08 (s, 3H, -COCH$_3$), 2.13 (s, 3H, -COCH$_3$), 2.22 (s, 3H, C(7)-CH$_3$), 2.23 (s, 3H, C(6)-CH$_3$), 3.05 (dd, J = 14.0, 7.0 Hz, 1H, H-6′a), 3.13 (dd, J = 14.0, 3.2 Hz, 1H, H-6′b), 3.97 (ddd, J = 9.5, 7.0, 3.2 Hz, 1H, H-5′), 5.11 (t, J = 9.5 Hz, 1H, H-4′), 5.14 (dd, J = 9.5, 8.2 Hz, 1H, H-2′), 5.28 (t, J = 9.5 Hz, 1H, H-3′), 5.73 (d, J = 8.2 Hz, 1H, H-1′), 6.75 (s, 1H, H-3), 13.01 (s, 1H,

C(8)-O$\underline{\text{H}}$), 13.02 (s, 1H, C(5)-O$\underline{\text{H}}$). ^{13}C NMR (125 MHz, CDCl$_3$) δ: 12.3 (C(7)-$\underline{\text{C}}$H$_3$), 12.5 (C(6)-$\underline{\text{C}}$H$_3$), 20.5 (2 × -CO$\underline{\text{C}}$H$_3$), 20.6 (-CO$\underline{\text{C}}$H$_3$), 20.7 (-CO$\underline{\text{C}}$H$_3$), 32.0 (C-6′), 70.1 (C-2′), 71.0 (C-4′), 72.6 (C-3′), 73.4 (C-5′), 91.5 (C-1′), 108.5 (C-4a), 109.4 (C-8a), 125.6 (C-3), 139.9 (C-7), 142.0 (C-6), 148.6 (C-2), 168.8 (-$\underline{\text{C}}$OCH$_3$), 169.2 (-$\underline{\text{C}}$OCH$_3$), 169.4 (C-5), 169.6 (-$\underline{\text{C}}$OCH$_3$), 170.0 (-$\underline{\text{C}}$OCH$_3$), 170.6 (C-8), 171.8 (C-1), 173.0 (C-4). IR (CHCl$_3$) v_{max}: 2942, 1760, 1599, 1555, 1431, 1371 cm^{-1}. HRMS (EI): m/z [M + Na]$^+$ calcd for C$_{26}$H$_{28}$O$_{13}$SNa: 603.1143; found: 603.1142.

2-(1,2,3,4-Tetra-O-acetyl-6-deoxy-β-D-glucopyranos-6-ylthio)-5-hydroxy-3-methyl-1,4-naphthoquinone (**SAB-7**). Yellow solid; yield 385 mg (70%); mp 160–161 °C; R_f = 0.38 (A). ^{1}H NMR (CDCl$_3$, 500 MHz) δ: 1.62 (s, 3H, -CO$\underline{\text{C}}$H$_3$), 1.97 (s, 3H, -CO$\underline{\text{C}}$H$_3$), 1.98 (s, 3H, -CO$\underline{\text{C}}$H$_3$), 2.05 (s, 3H, -CO$\underline{\text{C}}$H$_3$), 2.36 (s, 3H, C(3)-CH$_3$), 3.22 (dd, J = 14.8, 2.3 Hz, 1H, H-6′a), 3.54 (dd, J = 14.8, 8.3 Hz, 1H, H-6′b), 3.82 (ddd, J = 9.4, 8.3, 2.3 Hz, 1H, H-5′), 4.98 (t, J = 9.4 Hz, 1H, H-4′), 5.00 (dd, J = 9.4, 8.3 Hz, 1H, H-2′), 5.17 (t, J = 9.4 Hz, 1H, H-3′), 5.49 (d, J = 8.3 Hz, 1H, H-1′), 7.21 (dd, J = 7.2, 2.2, 1H, H-6), 7.56 (t, J = 7.2, 1H, H-7), 7.58 (dd, J = 7.2, 2.2, 1H, H-8), 12.15 (s, 1H, C(5)-O$\underline{\text{H}}$). ^{13}C NMR (CDCl$_3$, 500 MHz) δ: 14.5 (C(3)-$\underline{\text{C}}$H$_3$), 19.9 (-CO$\underline{\text{C}}$H$_3$), 20.5 (-CO$\underline{\text{C}}$H$_3$), 20.5 (-CO$\underline{\text{C}}$H$_3$), 20.6 (-CO$\underline{\text{C}}$H$_3$), 33.8 (C-6′), 70.0 (C-2′), 70.6 (C-4′), 72.6 (C-3′), 76.4 (C-5′), 91.5 (C-1′), 114.9 (C-4a), 119.6 (C-8), 123.8 (C-6), 133.0 (C-8a), 135.7 (C-7), 146.4 (C-3), 147.2 (C-2), 161.3 (C-5), 168.6 (-$\underline{\text{C}}$OCH$_3$), 169.1 (-$\underline{\text{C}}$OCH$_3$), 169.4 (-$\underline{\text{C}}$OCH$_3$), 170.0 (-$\underline{\text{C}}$OCH$_3$), 180.2 (C-1), 187.2 (C-4).IR (CHCl$_3$) v_{max}:3096, 2944, 1760, 1667, 1632; 1599, 1572, 1457, 1430, 1367cm^{-1}. HRMS (ESI): m/z [M + Na]$^+$ calcd for C$_{25}$H$_{26}$O$_{12}$SNa: 573.1037; found: 573.1040.

2,3-Di(1,2,3,4-tetra-O-acetyl-6-deoxy-β-D-glucopyranos-6-ylthio)-5,8-dihydroxy-6,7-dimethyl-1,4-naphthoquinone (**SAB-9**). Red solid; yield 258 mg (65%, recovery of starting quinone was 166 mg (58%)); mp 202–205 °C; R_f = 0.76 (A). ^{1}H NMR (CDCl$_3$, 700 MHz) δ: 1.81 (s, 6H, 2×-CO$\underline{\text{C}}$H$_3$), 1.99 (s, 6H, 2 × -CO$\underline{\text{C}}$H$_3$), 2.00 (s, 6H, 2 × -CO$\underline{\text{C}}$H$_3$), 2.08 (s, 6H, 2 × -CO$\underline{\text{C}}$H$_3$), 2.26 (s, 6H, C(6)-CH$_3$, C(7)-CH$_3$), 3.47 (dd, J = 14.5, 8.7 Hz, 2H, H-6′a, H-6″a), 3.52 (dd, J = 14.5, 2.4 Hz, 2H, H-6′b, H-6″b), 4.05 (ddd, J = 9.5, 8.7, 2.4 Hz, 2H, H-5′, H-5″), 4.96 (t, J = 9.5 Hz, 2H, H-4′, H-4″), 5.05 (dd, J = 9.5, 8.4 Hz, 2H, H-2′, H-2″), 5.32 (t, J = 9.5 Hz, 2H, H-3′, H-3″), 5.72 (d, J = 8.4 Hz, 2H, H-1′, H-1″), 13.23 (s, 2H, C(5)-O$\underline{\text{H}}$, C(8)-O$\underline{\text{H}}$). ^{13}C NMR (176 MHz, CDCl$_3$) δ: 12.4 (C(6)-$\underline{\text{C}}$H$_3$, C(7)-$\underline{\text{C}}$H$_3$), 20.3 (2×-CO$\underline{\text{C}}$H$_3$), 20.6 (2 × -CO$\underline{\text{C}}$H$_3$), 20.6 (2 × -CO$\underline{\text{C}}$H$_3$), 20.7 (2 × -CO$\underline{\text{C}}$H$_3$), 35.4 (C-6′, C-6″), 70.4 (C-2′, C-2″), 71.3 (C-4′, C-4″), 72.5 (C-3′, C-3″), 75.6 (C-5′, C-5″), 91.3 (C-1′, C-1″), 109.3 (C-4a, C-8a), 138.6 (C-6, C-7), 145.5 (C-2, C-3), 161.7 (C-5, C-8), 168.8 (2 × -$\underline{\text{C}}$OCH$_3$), 169.2 (2 × -$\underline{\text{C}}$OCH$_3$), 169.7 (2 × -$\underline{\text{C}}$OCH$_3$), 170.1 (2 × -$\underline{\text{C}}$OCH$_3$), 178.7 (C-1, C-4). IR (CHCl$_3$) v_{max}: 3053, 2946, 1759, 1600, 1487, 1427, 1370 cm^{-1}. HRMS (EI): m/z [M + Na]$^+$ calcd for C$_{40}$H$_{46}$O$_{22}$S$_2$Na: 965.1814;found: 965.1807.

6-(1,2,3,4-Tetra-O-acetyl-6-deoxy-β-D-glucopyranos-6-ylthio)-5,8-dihydroxy-7-methyl-2,3-dimethoxy-1,4-naphthoquinone (**SAB-13**). Dark red solid; yield 457 mg (73%); mp 96–98 °C; R_f = 0.35 (A). ^{1}H NMR (CDCl$_3$, 500 MHz) δ: 1.99 (s, 6H, 2 × -CO$\underline{\text{C}}$H$_3$), 2.00 (s, 3H, -CO$\underline{\text{C}}$H$_3$), 2.02 (s, 3H, -CO$\underline{\text{C}}$H$_3$), 2.51 (s, 3H, -CH$_3$), 3.16 (dd, J = 14.5, 8.1 Hz, 1H, H-6′a), 3.36 (dd, J = 14.5, 2.5 Hz, 1H, H-6′b), 3.71 (ddd, J = 9.5, 8.1, 2.5 Hz, 1H, H-5′), 4.12 (s, 3H, -OCH$_3$), 4.13 (s, 3H, -OCH$_3$), 4.98 (t, J = 9.5 Hz, 1H, H-4′), 5.05 (dd, J = 8.3, 9.5 Hz, 1H, H-2′), 5.17 (t, J = 9.5 Hz, 1H, H-3′), 5.60 (t, J = 8.3 Hz, 1H, H-1′), 13.02 (s, 1H, C(8)-O$\underline{\text{H}}$), 13.43 (s, 1H, C(5)-O$\underline{\text{H}}$). ^{13}C NMR (125 MHz, CDCl$_3$) δ: 15.0 (-$\underline{\text{C}}$H$_3$), 20.5 (3×-CO$\underline{\text{C}}$H$_3$), 20.6 (-CO$\underline{\text{C}}$H$_3$), 34.5 (C-6′), 61.6 (-O$\underline{\text{C}}$H$_3$), 61.7 (-O$\underline{\text{C}}$H$_3$), 70.2 (C-2′), 70.9 (C-4′), 72.6 (C-3′), 74.9 (C-5′), 91.4 (C-1′), 107.8 (C-4a), 108.5 (C-8a), 136.7 (C-6), 144.7 (C-7), 147.8 (C-3), 147.9 (C-2), 160.0 (C-8), 161.3 (C-5), 168.6 (-$\underline{\text{C}}$OCH$_3$), 169.2 (-$\underline{\text{C}}$OCH$_3$), 169.5 (-$\underline{\text{C}}$OCH$_3$), 170.0 (-$\underline{\text{C}}$OCH$_3$), 180.7 (C-1), 181.0 (C-4). IR (CHCl$_3$) v_{max}: 3698, 3610, 3026, 2947, 1760, 1602, 1558, 1455, 1433, 1392, 1374, 1286, 1250, 1192, 1136, 1114, 1077, 1038 cm^{-1}. HRMS (ESI): m/z [M + Na]$^+$ calcd for C$_{27}$H$_{30}$NaO$_{15}$S: 649.1198; found: 649.1195.

6-(1,2,3,4-Tetra-O-acetyl-6-deoxy-β-D-glucopyranos-6-ylthio)-5,8-dihydroxy-2,3,7-trimethyl-1,4-naphthoquinone (**SAB-15**). Dark red solid; yield 421 mg (71%); mp 148–151 °C; R_f = 0.52 (A). ^{1}H NMR (CDCl$_3$, 500 MHz) δ: 1.88 (s, 3H, -CO$\underline{\text{C}}$H$_3$), 1.99 (s, 6H, 2 × -CO$\underline{\text{C}}$H$_3$), 2.03 (s, 3H, -CO$\underline{\text{C}}$H$_3$), 2.24 (s, 3H, -CH$_3$), 2.25 (s, 3H, -CH$_3$), 2.46 (s, 3H, -CH$_3$), 3.30 (dd, J = 14.6, 7.5 Hz, 1H, H-6′a), 3.34 (dd, J = 14.6, 3.2 Hz, 1H, H-6′b), 3.77 (ddd, J = 9.6, 7.5, 3.2 Hz, 1H, H-5′), 4.98 (t, J = 9.6 Hz, 1H, H-4′), 5.03 (dd, J = 9.6,

8.3 Hz, 1H, H-2′), 5.18 (t, J = 9.6 Hz, 1H, H-3′), 5.59 (t, J = 8.3 Hz, 1H, H-1′), 13.34 (s, 1H, C(8)-OH), 13.46 (s, 1H, C(5)-OH). ^{13}C NMR (125 MHz, CDCl$_3$) δ: 12.4 (2×-CH$_3$), 15.1 (-CH$_3$), 20.3 (-COCH$_3$), 20.5 (2×-COCH$_3$), 20.6 (-COCH$_3$), 34.5 (C-6′), 70.2 (C-2′), 70.8 (C-4′), 72.6 (C-3′), 75.4 (C-5′), 91.5 (C-1′), 109.1 (C-4a), 109.4 (C-8a), 140.4 (C-6), 140.8 (C-3), 141.1 (C-2), 146.7 (C-7), 168.6 (-COCH$_3$), 169.2 (-COCH$_3$), 169.5 (-COCH$_3$), 170.1 (-COCH$_3$), 171.3 (C-8), 171.6 (C-1, C-5), 171.9 (C-4). IR (CHCl$_3$) ν_{max}: 3705, 3609, 3026, 2944, 1760, 1600, 1559, 1429, 1396, 1373, 1340, 1302, 1250, 1219, 1192, 1121, 1077, 1039 cm^{-1}. HRMS (ESI): m/z [M + Na]$^+$ calcd for C$_{27}$H$_{30}$NaO$_{13}$S: 617.1299; found: 617.1297.

6-(1,2,3,4-Tetra-O-acetyl-6-deoxy-β-D-glucopyranos-6-ylthio)-7-ethyl-5,8-dihydroxy-2,3-dimethyl-1,4-naphthoquinone (**SAB-17**). Dark red solid; yield 481 mg (79%); mp 179–182 °C; R_f = 0.59 (A). ^{1}H NMR (CDCl$_3$, 500 MHz) δ: 1.15 (t, J = 7.6 Hz, 1H, -CH$_2$CH$_3$), 1.89 (s, 3H, -COCH$_3$), 1.99 (s, 6H, 2 × -COCH$_3$), 2.03 (s, 3H, -COCH$_3$), 2.24 (s, 6H, 2 × -CH$_3$), 3.02 (q, J = 7.6 Hz, 2H, -CH$_2$CH$_3$), 3.30 (dd, J = 14.5, 7.7 Hz, 1H, H-6′a), 3.34 (dd, J = 14.5, 3.0 Hz, 1H, H-6′b), 3.77 (ddd, J = 9.6, 7.7, 3.0 Hz, 1H, H-5′), 4.98 (t, J = 9.6 Hz, 1H, H-4′), 5.04 (dd, J = 9.6, 8.3 Hz, 1H, H-2′), 5.18 (t, J = 9.6 Hz, 1H, H-3′), 5.60 (t, J = 8.3 Hz, 1H, H-1′), 13.36 (s, 1H, C(8)-OH), 13.49 (s, 1H, C(5)-OH). ^{13}C NMR (125 MHz, CDCl$_3$) δ: 12.4 (2 × -CH$_3$), 13.6 (-CH$_2$CH$_3$), 20.3 (-COCH$_3$), 20.5 (2 × -COCH$_3$), 20.6 (-COCH$_3$), 22.4 (-CH$_2$CH$_3$), 34.5 (C-6′), 70.2 (C-2′), 70.9 (C-4′), 72.6 (C-3′), 75.3 (C-5′), 91.4 (C-1′), 109.2 (C-4a), 109.7 (C-8a), 139.7 (C-6), 140.9 (C-3), 141.3 (C-2), 152.1 (C-7), 168.5 (-COCH$_3$), 169.2 (-COCH$_3$), 169.5 (-COCH$_3$), 170.0 (-COCH$_3$), 170.8 (C-8), 171.7 (C-5), 171.9 (C-1), 172.1 (C-4). IR (CHCl$_3$) ν_{max}: 3668, 3601, 3028, 2937, 2875, 1760, 1600, 1556, 1456, 1372, 1338, 1303, 1282, 1249, 1194, 1124, 1076, 1039 cm^{-1}. HRMS (ESI): m/z [M + Na]$^+$ calcd for C$_{28}$H$_{32}$NaO$_{13}$S: 631.1456; found: 631.1453.

2-(1,2,3,4-Tetra-O-acetyl-6-deoxy-β-D-glucopyranos-6-ylthio)-3,6,7-trichloro-5,8-dihydroxy-1,4-naphthoquinone (**SAB-19**). Purple solid; yield 420 mg (64%); mp 156–159 °C; R_f = 0.48 (A). ^{1}H NMR (CDCl$_3$, 700 MHz) δ: 1.79 (s, 3H, -COCH$_3$), 1.99 (s, 3H, -COCH$_3$), 2.00 (s, 3H, -COCH$_3$), 2.06 (s, 3H, -COCH$_3$), 3.39 (dd, J = 14.7, 2.6 Hz, 1H, H-6′a), 3.66 (dd, J = 14.7, 8.0 Hz, 1H, H-6′b), 3.89 (ddd, J = 9.8, 8.0, 2.6 Hz, 1H, H-5′), 5.02 (t, J = 9.8 Hz, 1H, H-4′), 5.03 (dd, J = 9.4, 8.4 Hz, 1H, H-2′), 5.20 (t, J = 9.4 Hz, 1H, H-3′), 5.54 (t, J = 8.4 Hz, 1H, H-1′), 12.96 (s, 2H, C(5)-OH, C(8)-OH). ^{13}C NMR (176 MHz, CDCl$_3$) δ: 20.2 (-COCH$_3$), 20.5 (2×-COCH$_3$), 20.6 (-COCH$_3$), 34.6 (C-6′), 70.0 (C-2′), 70.7 (C-4′), 72.5 (C-3′), 75.6 (C-5′), 91.7 (C-1′), 109.5 (C-4a), 109.7 (C-8a), 135.4 (C-6, C-7), 141.3 (C-3), 146.3 (C-2), 159.4 (C-8), 160.0 (C-5), 168.5 (-COCH$_3$), 169.1 (-COCH$_3$), 169.5 (-COCH$_3$), 170.0 (-COCH$_3$), 173.3 (C-4), 177.8 (C-1). IR (CHCl$_3$) ν_{max}: 3697, 3605, 3026, 2944, 1761, 1616, 1559, 1523, 1404, 1371, 1271, 1248, 1192, 1076, 1041 cm^{-1}. HRMS (ESI): m/z [M + Na]$^+$ calcd for C$_{24}$H$_{21}$Cl$_3$NaO$_{13}$S: 676.9660; found: 676.9655.

4.1.3. General Procedure for Synthesis of the Acetylated Conjugates **SAB-3**, **-5**, and **-11** in DMSO Solution (Figure 1A)

The tetra-O-acetyl-6-mercaptoglucose (0.368 g, 1.01 mmol) and finely powdered potassium carbonate (0.415 g, 3.0 mmol) was added to a solution of correspondent quinone (1.0 mmol) in DMSO (20 mL). The mixture was stirred at room temperature until reaction completed (3 h, controlled by TLC), diluted with H$_2$O (200 mL), acidified with HCl, and extracted with AcOEt (3 × 100 mL). The extract was washed with water (2 × 50 mL), dried with anhydrous Na$_2$SO$_4$, and concentrated in vacuo. The residue was purified by column chromatography (silica gel, hexane/acetone, 10:1) to give products **3**, **5**, and **11**.

6-(1,2,3,4-Tetra-O-acetyl-6-deoxy-β-D-glucopyranos-6-ylthio)-2,3,5,8-tetrahydroxy-7-methyl-1,4-naphthoquinone (**SAB-3**). Red solid; yield 467 mg (78%); mp 207–211 °C; R_f = 0.12 (A). ^{1}H NMR (CDCl$_3$, 500 MHz) δ: 1.99 (s, 3H, -COCH$_3$), 2.00 (s, 6H, 2 × COCH$_3$), 2.02 (s, 3H, -COCH$_3$), 2.49 (s, 3H, C(7)-CH$_3$), 3.16 (dd, J = 14.5, 8.0 Hz, 1H, H-6′a), 3.33 (dd, J = 14.5, 2.6 Hz, 1H, H-6′b), 3.76 (ddd, J = 9.4, 8.0, 2.6 Hz, 1H, H-5′), 5.00 (t, J = 9.4 Hz, 1H, H-4′), 5.06 (dd, J = 9.4, 8.3 Hz, 1H, H-2′), 5.19 (t, J = 9.4 Hz, 1H, H-3′), 5.62 (d, J = 8.3 Hz, 1H, H-1′), 6.82 (br.s, 2H, C(2)-OH, C(3)-OH), 12.24 (s, 1H, C(5)-OH), 12.70 (s, 1H, C(8)-OH). ^{13}C NMR (CDCl$_3$, 125 MHz) δ: 15.0 (C(7)-CH$_3$), 20.5 (3×-COCH$_3$), 20.6 (-COCH$_3$), 34.7 (C-6′), 70.2 (C-2′), 70.9 (C-4′), 72.6 (C-3′), 74.9 (C-5′), 91.5 (C-1′), 106.2 (C-8a), 107.0 (C-4a), 136.3 (C-6), 137.8 (C-2 *), 138.0 (C-3 *), 144.3 (C-7), 156.5 (C-8), 157.9 (C-5), 168.7 (-COCH$_3$), 169.2 (-COCH$_3$), 169.5 (-COCH$_3$),

170.1 (-COCH$_3$), 182.4 (C-4), 182.7 (C-1). IR (CHCl$_3$) ν_{max}: 3432, 2944, 1760, 1693, 1626, 1594, 1556, 1419, 1373, 1310 cm^{-1}. HRMS (ESI): m/z [M + Na]$^+$ calcd for C$_{25}$H$_{26}$O$_{15}$SNa 621.0885; found: 621.0882. *—The assignment of signal is ambiguous.

7-(1,2,3,4-Tetra-O-acetyl-6-deoxy-β-D-glucopyranos-6-ylthio)-2,5,8-trihydroxy-6-methoxy-1,4-naphthoquinone (**SAB-5**). Red solid; yield 461 mg (77%); mp 109–112 °C; R_f = 0.20 (A). ^{1}H NMR (CDCl$_3$, 500 MHz) δ: 1.90 (s, 3H, -COCH$_3$), 1.89 (s, 3H, -COCH$_3$), 1.99 (s, 3H, -COCH$_3$), 2.03 (s, 3H, -COCH$_3$), 3.13 (dd, J = 14.5, 2.8 Hz, 1H, H-6′a), 3.29 (dd, J = 14.5, 7.7 Hz, 1H, H-6′b), 3.83 (ddd, J = 9.5, 7.7, 2.8 Hz, 1H, H-5′), 4.22 (s, 3H, C(6)-OCH$_3$), 5.02 (t, J = 9.5 Hz, 1H, H-4′), 5.04 (dd, J = 9.5, 8.3 Hz, 1H, H-2′), 5.19 (t, J = 9.5 Hz, 1H, H-3′), 5.59 (d, J = 8.3 Hz, 1H, H-1′), 6.42 (s, 1H, H-3), 7.39 (br s, 1H, C(2)-OH), 12.65 (s, 1H, C(8)-OH), 13.17 (s, 1H, C(5)-OH). ^{13}C NMR (CDCl$_3$, 125 MHz) δ: 20.4 (-COCH$_3$), 20.5 (2×-COCH$_3$), 20.6 (-COCH$_3$), 33.8 (C-6′), 61.9 (C(6)-OCH$_3$), 70.2 (C-2′), 70.9 (C-4′), 72.6 (C-3′), 75.6 (C-5′), 91.4 (C-1′), 107.6 (C-8a), 109.0 (C-4a), 110.2 (C-3), 126.2 (C-7), 157.0 (C-2), 160.3 (C-6), 160.5 (C-5), 168.3 (C-8), 168.5 (-COCH$_3$), 169.2 (-COCH$_3$), 169.5 (-COCH$_3$), 170.1 (-COCH$_3$), 170.4 (C-1), 180.4 (C-4). IR (CHCl$_3$) ν_{max}: 3514, 3404, 2945, 1760, 1659, 1604, 1553, 1445, 1397, 1370, 1349 cm^{-1}. HRMS (ESI): m/z [M + Na]$^+$ calcd for C$_{25}$H$_{26}$O$_{15}$SNa 621.0885; found: 621.0881.

7-(1,2,3,4-Tetra-O-acetyl-6-deoxy-β-D-glucopyranos-6-ylthio)-3-ethyl-2,5,8-trihydroxy-6-methoxy-1,4-naphthoquinone (**SAB-11**). Red solid; yield 501 mg (80%); mp 167–171 °C; R_f = 0.33 (A). ^{1}H NMR (CDCl$_3$, 700 MHz) δ: 1.13 (t, J = 7.5, 3H, -CH$_2$CH$_3$), 1.93 (s, 3H, -COCH$_3$), 1.98 (s, 3H, -COCH$_3$), 1.99 (s, 3H, -COCH$_3$), 2.02 (s, 3H, -COCH$_3$), 2.62 (q, J = 7.5, 2H, -CH$_2$CH$_3$), 4.17 (s, 3H, C(6)-OCH$_3$), 3.16 (dd, J = 14.2, 2.8 Hz, 1H, H-6′a), 3.24 (dd, J = 14.2, 7.7 Hz, 1H, H-6′b), 3.81 (ddd, J = 9.5, 7.7, 2.8 Hz, 1H, H-5′), 5.02 (t, J = 9.5 Hz, 1H, H-4′), 5.04 (dd, J = 9.5, 8.2 Hz, 1H, H-2′), 5.18 (t, J = 9.5 Hz, 1H, H-3′), 5.61 (d, J = 8.2 Hz, 1H, H-1′), 7.41 (br s, 1H, C(2)-OH), 12.56 (s, 1H, C(8)-OH), 13.47 (s, 1H, C(5)-OH). ^{13}C NMR (176 MHz, CDCl$_3$) δ: 12.6 (-CH$_2$CH$_3$), 16.2 (-CH$_2$CH$_3$), 20.4 (-COCH$_3$), 20.5 (2×-COCH$_3$), 20.6 (-COCH$_3$), 34.1 (C-6′), 61.7 (C(6)-OCH$_3$), 70.3 (C-2′), 70.9 (C-4′), 72.6 (C-3′), 75.4 (C-5′), 91.4 (C-1′), 106.2 (C-8a), 110.0 (C-4a), 125.3 (C-7), 126.4 (C-3), 153.7 (C-2), 155.3 (C-5), 159.7 (C-6), 162.6 (C-8), 168.5 (-COCH$_3$), 169.2 (-COCH$_3$), 169.5 (-COCH$_3$), 170.0 (-COCH$_3$), 176.8 (C-1), 185.2 (C-4). IR (CHCl$_3$) ν_{max}: 3408, 2976, 2941, 2878, 1760, 1598, 1555, 1460 cm^{-1}. HRMS (EI): m/z [M + Na]$^+$ calcd for C$_{27}$H$_{30}$O$_{15}$SNa: 649.1198; found: 649.1192.

4.1.4. Procedure for Synthesis of Naphthazarin Derivative SAB-21 (Figure 1B)

Tetra-O-acetyl-6-mercaptoglucose (190 mg, 0.52 mmol) was added to the refluxing solution of naphthazarin (190 mg, 1.0 mmol) in 30 mL of EtOH during 30 min. The reaction mixture was refluxed for 1.5 h, concentrated in vacuo. The residue was purified by column chromatography (silica gel, hexane/acetone, 10:1) to give the product **21**. Naphthazarin recovery was 44% (83 mg).

2-(1,2,3,4-Tetra-O-acetyl-6-deoxy-β-D-glucopyranos-6-ylthio)-5,8-dihydroxy-1,4-naphthoquinone (**SAB-21**). Purple solid; yield 167 mg (54%); mp 207–210 °C; R_f = 0.38 (A). ^{1}H NMR (CDCl$_3$, 500 MHz) δ: 2.02 (s, 6H, -COCH$_3$), 2.03 (s, 3H, -COCH$_3$), 2.08 (s, 3H, -COCH$_3$), 2.13 (s, 3H, -COCH$_3$), 3.02 (dd, J = 14.1, 6.9 Hz, 1H, H-6′a), 3.10 (dd, J = 14.1, 3.2 Hz, 1H, H-6′b), 3.96 (ddd, J = 9.5, 6.9, 3.2 Hz, 1H, H-5′), 5.11 (t, J = 9.5 Hz, 1H, H-4′), 5.14 (dd, J = 9.5, 8.4 Hz, 1H, H-2′), 5.26 (t, J = 9.4 Hz, 1H, H-3′), 5.71 (t, J = 8.4 Hz, 1H, H-1′), 6.68 (s, 1H, H-3), 7.21 (dd, J = 9.4 Hz, 1H, H-7), 7.27 (dd, J = 9.4 Hz, 1H, H-6), 12.11 (s, 1H, C(8)-OH), 12.57 (s, 1H, C(5)-OH). ^{13}C NMR (125 MHz, CDCl$_3$) δ: 20.5 (2×-COCH$_3$), 20.6 (-COCH$_3$), 20.7 (-COCH$_3$), 31.9 (C-6′), 70.1 (C-2′), 71.0 (C-4′), 72.5 (C-3′), 73.3 (C-5′), 91.6 (C-1′), 111.1 (C-4a), 111.5 (C-8a), 128.1 (C-3), 128.8 (C-7), 130.8 (C-6), 154.2 (C-2), 158.5 (C-5), 159.4 (C-8), 168.8 (-COCH$_3$), 169.1 (-COCH$_3$), 169.6 (-COCH$_3$), 170.0 (-COCH$_3$), 183.6 (C-1), 183.9 (C-4). IR (CHCl$_3$) ν_{max}: 3695, 3600, 3054, 2928, 1761, 1607, 1577, 1556, 1455, 1409, 1371, 1338, 1240, 1221, 1193, 1109, 1077, 1039 cm^{-1}. HRMS (ESI): m/z [M + Na]$^+$ calcd for C$_{24}$H$_{24}$NaO$_{13}$S: 575.0830; found: 575.0829.

4.1.5. General Procedure for Synthesis of Juglone Derivatives 23 and 25 (Figure 1B)

Tetra-O-acetyl-6-mercaptoglucose (0.367 g, 1.01 mmol) was added to a suspension of juglone or juglone acetate (1.0 mmol) in EtOH (65 mL). The reaction mixture was stirred at room temperature for 12 h and concentrated in vacuo. The residue was purified by column chromatography (silica gel, hexane/acetone, 10:1) to give the products **23** and **25**.

2-(1,2,3,4-Tetra-O-acetyl-6-deoxy-β-D-glucopyranos-6-ylthio)-8-hydroxy-1,4-naphthoquinone (**SAB-23**). Yellow solid; yield 349 mg (65%); mp 188–191 °C; R_f = 0.39 (A). ^{1}H NMR (CDCl$_3$, 500 MHz) δ: 2.02 (s, 3H, -COCH$_3$), 2.03 (s, 3H, -COCH$_3$), 2.07 (s, 3H, -COCH$_3$), 2.12 (s, 3H, -COCH$_3$), 3.00 (dd, J = 14.0, 7.0 Hz, 1H, H-6′a), 3.07 (dd, J = 14.0, 3.2 Hz, 1H, H-6′b), 3.95 (ddd, J = 9.6, 7.0, 3.2 Hz, 1H, H-5′), 5.10 (d, J = 9.6 Hz, 1H, H-4′), 5.14 (dd, J = 9.5, 8.3 Hz, 1H, H-2′), 5.26 (d, J = 9.5 Hz, 1H, H-3′), 5.71 (d, J = 8.3 Hz, 1H, H-1′), 6.64 (s, 1H, H-3), 7.23 (dd, J = 8.0, 1.5 Hz, 1H, H-7), 7.60 (dd, J = 7.4, 1.5 Hz, 1H, H-5), 7.62 (dd, J = 8.0, 7.4 Hz, 1H, H-6), 11.65 (s, 3H, C(8)-OH). ^{13}C NMR (125 MHz, CDCl$_3$) δ: 20.5 (2 × -COCH$_3$), 20.6 (-COCH$_3$), 20.7 (-COCH$_3$), 31.8 (C-6′), 70.1 (C-2′), 71.0 (C-4′), 72.6 (C-3′), 73.3 (C-5′), 91.6 (C-1′), 114.7 (8a), 119.3 (C-5), 123.9 (C-7), 128.7 (C-3), 132.0 (C-4a), 137.1 (C-6), 153.3 (C-2), 161.9 (C-8), 168.8 (-COCH$_3$), 169.1 (-COCH$_3$), 169.6 (-COCH$_3$), 170.0 (-COCH$_3$), 180.8 (C-4), 186.8 (C-1). IR (CHCl$_3$) ν_{max}: 3700, 3600, 2942, 1761, 1634, 1601, 1562, 1457, 1427, 1369, 1273, 1246, 1194, 1169, 1140, 1078, 1039 cm^{-1}. HRMS (ESI): m/z [M + Na]$^+$ calcd for C$_{24}$H$_{24}$NaO$_{12}$S: 536.0881; found: 536.0880.

2-(1,2,3,4-Tetra-O-acetyl-6-deoxy-β-D-glucopyranos-6-ylthio)-5-acetoxy-1,4-naphthoquinone (**SAB-25**). Yellow solid; yield 353 mg (61%); mp 172–175 °C; R_f = 0.30 (A). ^{1}H NMR (CDCl$_3$, 500 MHz) δ: 2.02 (s, 6H, 2 × -COCH$_3$), 2.06 (s, 3H, -COCH$_3$), 2.11 (s, 3H, -COCH$_3$), 2.43 (s, 3H, -COCH$_3$′), 2.97 (dd, J = 14.1, 7.1 Hz, 1H, H-6′a), 3.03 (dd, J = 14.1, 3.2 Hz, 1H, H-6′b), 3.93 (ddd, J = 9.6, 7.1, 3.2 Hz, 1H, H-5′), 5.09 (d, J = 9.6 Hz, 1H, H-4′), 5.12 (dd, J = 9.5, 8.3 Hz, 1H, H-2′), 5.24 (d, J = 9.3 Hz, 1H, H-3′), 5.70 (d, J = 8.3 Hz, 1H, H-1′), 6.54 (s, 1H, H-3), 7.37 (dd, J = 8.0, 1.2 Hz, 1H, H-6), 7.71 (dd, J = 8.0, 7.8 Hz, 1H, H-7), 8.06 (dd, J = 7.8, 1.3 Hz, 1H, H-8). ^{13}C NMR (125 MHz, CDCl$_3$) δ: 20.5 (2 × -COCH$_3$), 20.6 (-COCH$_3$), 20.7 (-COCH$_3$), 21.1 (-COCH$_3$′), 31.7 (C-6′), 70.1 (C-2′), 71.0 (C-4′), 72.6 (C-3′), 73.4 (C-5′), 91.5 (C-1′), 123.2 (4a), 125.5 (C-8), 129.3 (C-3), 130.2 (C-6), 133.6 (C-8a), 134.2 (C-7), 149.6 (C-5), 152.2 (C-2), 168.8 (-COCH$_3$), 169.1 (-COCH$_3$), 169.3 (-COCH$_3$), 169.6 (-COCH$_3$), 170.0 (-COCH$_3$), 180.2 (C-4), 181.2 (C-1). IR (CHCl$_3$) ν_{max}: 3700, 3600, 3016, 2942, 1761, 1671, 1650, 1600, 1566, 1541, 1522, 1457, 1370, 1337, 1247, 1193, 1106, 1078, 1039 cm^{-1}. HRMS (ESI): m/z [M + Na]$^+$ calcd for C$_{26}$H$_{26}$NaO$_{13}$S: 601.0986; found: 601.0982.

4.1.6. General Procedure for Synthesis of Deacetylated Conjugates SAB-2, -4, -6, -8, -10, -12, -14, -16, -18, -20, -22, -24, and -26 (Figure 1C, Saponification of the Acetylated Conjugates)

A solution of MeONa (0.9 mL of a 1.06 N) in MeOH was added to a stirring suspension of appropriate acetylated conjugate (0.3 mmol) in anhydrous MeOH (20 mL). The reaction mixture was stirred for 30 min, neutralized with HCl, concentrated in vacuo. The residue was purified by preparative TLC (silica gel, benzene/ethyl acetate/methanol 7:4:2 (v/v)) to give the products.

2-(6-Deoxy-D-glucopyranos-6-ylthio)-5,8-dihydroxy-6,7-dimethyl-1,4-naphthoquinone (**SAB-2**). Red solid; yield 93 mg (75%); R_f = 0.70 (B). α-anomer: ^{1}H NMR (500 MHz, DMSO-d$_6$) δ: 2.14 (s, 3H, C(7)-CH$_3$), 2.15 (s, 3H, C(6)-CH$_3$), 3.02 (dd, J = 13.3, 8.4 Hz, 1H, H-6′a), 3.09 (dd, J = 9.9, 8.7Hz, 1H, H-4′), 3.19 (dd, J = 9.6, 3.6 Hz, 1H, H-2′), 3.36 (dd, J = 13.3, 2.4 Hz, 1H, H-6′b), 3.45 (dd, J = 9.6, 8.7 Hz, 1H, H-3′), 3.84 (ddd, J = 9.9, 8.4, 2.4 Hz, 1H, H-5′), 4.93 (d, J = 3.6 Hz, 1H, H-1′), 6.90 (s, 1H, H-3), 12.83 (s, 1H, C(8)-OH), 13.10 (s, 1H, C(5)-OH). ^{13}C NMR (125 MHz, DMSO-d$_6$) δ: 12.1 (C(7)-CH$_3$), 12.3 (C(6)-CH$_3$), 32.8 (C-6′), 69.3 (C-5′), 72.3 (C-2′), 72.7 (C-3′), 73.7 (C-4′), 92.6 (C-1′), 107.9 (C-4a), 109.0 (C-8a), 124.7 (C-3), 138.7 (C-7), 141.1 (C-6), 151.3 (C-2), 166.3 (C-5), 167.5 (C-8), 173.4 (C-1), 174.7 (C-4). β-anomer: ^{1}H NMR (500 MHz, DMSO-d$_6$) δ: 2.14 (s, 3H, C(7)-CH$_3$), 2.15 (s, 3H, C(6)-CH$_3$), 2.95 (dd, J = 8.8, 7.7 Hz, 1H, H-2′), 3.03 (dd, J = 14.0, 8.0 Hz, 1H, H-6′a), 3.11 (t, J = 8.8 Hz, 1H, H-4′), 3.17 (t, J = 8.8 Hz, 1H, H-3′), 3.38 (dd, J = 14.0, 2.5 Hz, 1H, H-6′b), 3.40 (ddd, J = 8.8, 8.0, 2.5 Hz, 1H, H-5′),

4.34 (d, J = 7.7 Hz, 1H, H-1′), 6.89 (s, 1H, H-3), 12.82 (s, 1H, C(8)-O$\underline{H}$), 13.10 (s, 1H, C(5)-O$\underline{H}$). ^{13}C NMR (125 MHz, DMSO-d$_6$) δ: 12.1 (C(7)-$\underline{C}$H$_3$), 12.3 (C(6)-$\underline{C}$H$_3$), 32.6 (C-6′), 73.1 (C-4′), 73.6 (C-5′), 74.8 (C-2′), 76.2 (C-3′), 97.1 (C-1′), 107.9 (C-4a), 109.0 (C-8a), 124.8 (C-3), 138.7 (C-7), 141.1 (C-6), 151.1 (C-2), 166.1 (C-5), 167.3 (C-8), 173.6 (C-1), 174.9 (C-4). HRMS (ESI): m/z [M + Na]$^+$ calcd for C$_{18}$H$_{20}$O$_9$SNa: 435.0720; found: 435.0720.

6-(6-Deoxy-D-glucopyranos-6-ylthio)-2,3,5,8-tetrahydroxy-7-methyl-1,4-naphthoquinone (**SAB-4**). Red solid; yield 101 mg (78%); R_f = 0.57 (B). α-anomer: ^{1}H NMR (DMSO-d$_6$, 300 MHz) δ: 2.43 (s, 3H, C(7)-CH$_3$), 3.00 (dd, J = 13.7, 8.0 Hz, 1H, H-6′a), 3.08 (t, J = 9.2Hz, 1H, H-4′), 3.14 (dd, J = 9.3, 3.4Hz, 1H, H-2′), 3.38 (t, J = 9.3 Hz, 1H, H-3′), 3.39 (dd, J = 13.7, 2.6 Hz, 1H, H-6′b), 3.71 (ddd, J = 9.3, 8.0, 2.6 Hz, 1H, H-5′), 4.83 (d, J = 3.4 Hz, 1H, H-1′), 10.53 (br s, 2H, C(2)-O$\underline{H}$, C(3)-O$\underline{H}$), 12.88 (s, 1H, C(5)-O$\underline{H}$), 13.20 (s, 1H, C(8)-O$\underline{H}$). ^{13}C NMR (DMSO-d$_6$, 75 MHz) δ: 14.9 (C(7)-$\underline{C}$H$_3$), 36.6 (C-6′), 70.8 (C-5′), 72.4 (C-2′), 72.8 (C-3′), 73.2 (C-4′), 92.4 (C-1′), 106.8 (C-8a), 107.7 (C-4a), 136.3 (C-6), 141.3 (C-2*), 141.4 (C-3*), 141.9 (C-7), 154.9 (C-8), 157.1 (C-5), 183.2 (C-4), 183.5 (C-1). β-anomer: ^{1}H NMR (DMSO-d$_6$, 300 MHz) δ: 2.43 (s, 3H, C(7)-CH$_3$), 2.89 (dd, J = 8.8, 7.7Hz, 1H, H-2′), 2.95 (dd, J = 13.3, 8.2 Hz, 1H, H-6′a), 3.02 (t, J = 8.8 Hz, 1H, H-4′), 3.07 (t, J = 8.8 Hz, 1H, H-3′), 3.18 (ddd, J = 8.8, 8.2, 2.2 Hz, 1H, H-5′), 3.35 (dd, J = 13.3, 2.2 Hz, 1H, H-6′b), 4.24 (d, J = 7.7 Hz, 1H, H-1′), 10.53 (br s, 2H, C(2)-O$\underline{H}$, C(3)-O$\underline{H}$), 12.88 (s, 1H, C(5)-O$\underline{H}$), 13.20 (s, 1H, C(8)-O$\underline{H}$).^{13}C NMR (DMSO-d$_6$, 75 MHz) δ: 14.9 (C(7)-$\underline{C}$H$_3$), 36.8 (C-6′), 72.8 (C-4′), 74.9 (C-2′), 75.3 (C-5′), 76.4 (C-3′), 97.1 (C-1′), 106.9 (C-8a), 107.8 (C-4a), 135.9 (C-6), 141.3 (C-2*), 141.4 (C-3*), 142.1 (C-7), 154.9 (C-8), 157.1 (C-5), 183.1 (C-4), 183.3 (C-1). HRMS (ESI): m/z [M + Na]$^+$ calcd for C$_{17}$H$_{18}$O$_{11}$SNa: 453.0462; found: 453.0459. *–The assignment of signal is ambiguous.

7-(6-Deoxy-D-glucopyranos-6-ylthio)-2,5,8-trihydroxy-6-methoxy-1,4-naphthoquinone (**SAB-6**). Red solid; yield 97 mg (75%), R_f = 0.81(B). α-anomer: ^{1}H NMR (500 MHz, DMSO-d$_6$) δ: 3.06 (t, J = 9.2 Hz, 1H, H-4′), 3.12 (dd, J = 13.0, 8.2 Hz, 1H, H-6′a), 3.13 (dd, J = 9.2, 3.6 Hz, 1H, H-2′), 3.39 (t, J = 9.2 Hz, 1H, H-3′), 3.45 (dd, J = 13.0, 2.6 Hz, 1H, H-6′b), 3.77 (ddd, J = 9.2, 8.2, 2.6 Hz, 1H, H-5′), 4.06 (s, 3H, C(6)-OCH$_3$), 4.84 (d, J = 3.6 Hz, 1H, H-1′), 6.39 (s, 1H, H-3), 11.90 (br s, 1H, C(2)-O$\underline{H}$), 12.95 (s, 1H, C(8)-O$\underline{H}$), 13.08 (s, 1H, C(5)-O$\underline{H}$).^{13}C NMR (125 MHz, DMSO-d$_6$) δ: 35.7 (C-6′), 61.2 (C(6)-O$\underline{C}$H$_3$), 70.8 (C-5′), 72.3 (C-2′), 72.8 (C-3′), 73.1 (C-4′), 92.4 (C-1′), 107.1 (C-8a), 109.4 (C-4a), 109.8 (C-3), 130.2 (C-7), 158.9 (C-6), 159.2 (C-2), 165.0 (C-8), 165.7 (C-5), 173.4 (C-1), 174.8 (C-4). β-anomer: ^{1}H NMR (500 MHz, DMSO-d$_6$) δ: 2.89 (dd, J = 9.0, 7.7 Hz, 1H, H-2′), 3.06 (t, J = 9.0 Hz, 1H, H-4′), 3.09 (t, J = 9.0 Hz, 1H, H-3′), 3.11 (dd, J = 13.3, 8.0 Hz, 1H, H-6′a), 3.28 (ddd, J = 9.0, 8.0, 2.4 Hz, 1H, H-5′), 3.46 (dd, J = 13.3, 2.4 Hz, 1H, H-6′b), 4.07 (s, 3H, C(6)-OCH$_3$), 4.26 (d, J = 7.7 Hz, 1H, H-1′), 6.38 (s, 1H, H-3), 11.90 (br s, 1H, C(2)-O$\underline{H}$), 12.96 (s, 1H, C(8)-O$\underline{H}$), 13.08 (s, 1H, C(5)-O$\underline{H}$). ^{13}C NMR (125 MHz, DMSO-d$_6$) δ: 35.5 (C-6′), 61.3 (C(6)-O$\underline{C}$H$_3$), 72.7 (C-4′), 74.9 (C-2′), 75.4 (C-5′), 76.4 (C-3′), 97.0 (C-1′), 107.3 (C-8a), 109.5 (C-4a), 109.8 (C-3), 129.7 (C-7), 159.0 (C-6), 159.2 (C-2), 165.3 (C-8), 165.5 (C-5), 173.2 (C-1), 174.0 (C-4). HRMS (ESI): m/z [M + Na]$^+$ calcd for C$_{17}$H$_{18}$O$_{11}$SNa: 453.0462; found: 453.0458.

2-(6-Deoxy-D-glucopyranos-6-ylthio)-5-hydroxy-3-methyl-1,4-naphthoquinone (**SAB-8**). Red solid; yield 86 mg (75%); R_f = 0.77 (B). α-anomer: ^{1}H NMR (700 MHz, DMSO-d$_6$) δ: 2.24 (s, 3H, C(3)-CH$_3$), 3.03 (dd, J = 9.2, 3.6 Hz, 1H, H-2′), 3.04 (t, J = 9.2 Hz, 1H, H-4′), 3.26 (dd, J = 13.6, 8.0 Hz, 1H, H-6′a), 3.36 (t, J = 9.2 Hz, 1H, H-3′), 3.48 (dd, J = 13.6, 2.5 Hz, 1H, H-6′b), 3.74 (ddd, J = 9.2, 8.0, 2.5 Hz, 1H, H-5′), 4.81 (d, J = 3.6 Hz, 1H, H-1′), 7.29 (d, J = 8.0, 1H, H-6), 7.50 (d, J = 8.0, 1H, H-8), 7.69 (t, J = 8.0, 1H, H-7), 11.98 (s, 1H, C(5)-O$\underline{H}$). ^{13}C NMR (175 MHz, DMSO-d$_6$) δ: 14.4 (C(3)-$\underline{C}$H$_3$), 35.7 (C-6′), 71.3 (C-5′), 72.5 (C-2′), 72.6 (C-3′), 72.8 (C-4′), 92.3 (C-1′), 114.8 (C-4a), 119.1 (C-8), 123.4 (C-6), 133.1 (C-8a), 136.1 (C-7), 144.5 (C-3), 148.7 (C-2), 160.2 (C-5), 180.1 (C-1), 186.8 (C-4). β-anomer: ^{1}H NMR (700 MHz, DMSO-d$_6$) δ: 2.26 (s, 3H, C(3)-CH$_3$), 2.84 (dd, J = 8.2, 7.7 Hz, 1H, H-2′), 3.04 (t, J = 8.2 Hz, 1H, H-4′), 3.07 (t, J = 8.2 Hz, 1H, H-3′), 3.25 (dd, J = 13.3, 7.5 Hz, 1H, H-6′a), 3.28 (ddd, J = 8.2, 7.5, 2.1 Hz, 1H, H-5′), 3.52 (dd, J = 13.3, 2.1 Hz, 1H, H-6′b), 4.26 (d, J = 7.7 Hz, 1H, H-1′), 7.28 (d, J = 8.0, 1H, H-6), 7.51 (d, J = 8.0, 1H, H-8), 7.71 (t, J = 8.0, 1H, H-7), 11.99 (s, 1H, C(5)-O$\underline{H}$).^{13}C NMR (175 MHz, DMSO-d$_6$) δ: 14.5 (C(3)-$\underline{C}$H$_3$), 35.8 (C-6′), 72.4 (C-4′), 74.8 (C-2′), 75.4 (C-5′), 76.2 (C-3′), 97.0 (C-1′),

114.9 (C-4a), 119.2 (C-8), 123.5 (C-6), 133.0 (C-8a), 136.1 (C-7), 145.2 (C-3), 149.3 (C-2), 160.2 (C-5), 180.1 (C-1), 186.9 (C-4). HRMS (ESI): m/z [M + Na]$^+$ calcd for $C_{17}H_{18}O_8SNa$: 405.0615; found: 405.0618.

2,3-Di(6-deoxy-D-glucopyranos-6-ylthio)-5,8-dihydroxy-6,7-dimethyl-1,4-naphthoquinone (**SAB-10**). Dark red solid; yield 142 mg (78%); R_f = 0.04 (B). ^{1}H NMR (500 MHz, DMSO-d$_6$) δ: α-anomer: 2.13 (s, 6H, (C(6,7)-CH$_3$), 3.06 (t, J = 9.1 Hz, 2H, H-4′), 3.11 (dd, J = 13.2, 8.4 Hz, 2H, H-6a′), 3.12 (dd, J = 9.1, 3.4 Hz, 2H, H-2′), 3.39 (dd, J = 9.1 Hz, 2H, H-3′), 3.44 (dd, J = 13.2, 2.3 Hz, 2H, H-6b′), 3.77 (ddd, J = 9.1, 8.4, 2.3 Hz, 2H, H-5′), 4.77 (d, J = 3.4 Hz, 2H, H-1′), 13.08 (br s, 2H, C(5,8)-OH); β-anomer: 2.13 (s, 6H, (C(6,7)-CH$_3$), 2.89 (dd, J = 8.2, 7.7Hz, 2H, H-2′), 3.05 (t, J = 8.2 Hz, 2H, H-4′), 3.08 (dd, J = 13.3, 7.7 Hz, 2H, H-6a′), 3.09 (dd, J = 8.2 Hz, 2H, H-3′), 3.27 (ddd, J = 8.2, 7.7, 2.0 Hz, 2H, H-5′), 3.45 (dd, J = 13.3, 2.0 Hz, 2H, H-6b′), 4.26 (d, J = 7.7 Hz, 2H, H-1′), 13.08 (br s, 2H, C(5,8)-OH); ^{13}C NMR (125 MHz, DMSO-d$_6$) δ: carbohydrate moiety: α-anomer: 35.9 (C-6′), 70.8 (C-5′), 72.3 (C-2′), 72.8 (C-3′), 73.2 (C-4′), 92.4 (C-1′), β-anomer: 35.7 (C-6′), 72.7 (C-4′), 74.9 (C-2′), 75.4 (C-5′), 76.4 (C-3′), 97.0 (C-1′); naphthoquinone moiety: 12.5 ((C-6,7)-CH$_3$), 109.1 (C-4a,8a), 138.6 (C-2,3), 147.3 (C-6,7), 161.0 (C-5,8), 177.5 (C-4,8); HRMS (ESI): m/z [M + Na]$^+$ calcd for $C_{24}H_{30}O_{14}S_2Na$: 629.0969; found: 629.0976.

7-(6-Deoxy-D-glucopyranos-6-ylthio)-3-ethyl-2,5,8-trihydroxy-6-methoxy-1,4-naphthoquinone (**SAB-12**). Red solid; yield 113 mg (82%); R_f = 0.26 (B). α-anomer: ^{1}H NMR (500 MHz, DMSO-d$_6$) δ: 1.03 (t, J = 7.5, 3H, -CH$_2$CH$_3$), 2.49 (q, 2H, -CH$_2$CH$_3$), 3.06 (t, J = 9.1 Hz, 1H, H-4′), 3.11 (dd, J = 13.2, 8.4 Hz, 1H, H-6′a), 3.12 (dd, J = 9.1, 3.4Hz, 1H, H-2′), 3.39 (dd, J = 9.1 Hz, 1H, H-3′), 3.44 (dd, J = 13.2, 2.3 Hz, 1H, H-6′b), 3.77 (ddd, J = 9.1, 8.4, 2.3 Hz, 1H, H-5′), 4.02 (s, 3H,C(6)-OCH$_3$), 4.84 (d, J = 3.4 Hz, 1H, H-1′), 11.35 (br s, 1H, C(2)-OH), 12.92 (s, 1H, C(8)-OH), 13.51 (s, 1H, C(5)-OH). ^{13}C NMR (125 MHz, DMSO-d$_6$) δ: 12.6 (-CH$_2$CH$_3$), 15.7 (-CH$_2$CH$_3$), 35.9 (C-6′), 61.0 (C(6)-OCH$_3$), 70.8 (C-5′), 72.3 (C-2′), 72.8 (C-3′), 73.2 (C-4′), 92.4 (C-1′), 107.1 (C-8a), 108.9 (C-4a), 125.6 (C-3), 128.4 (C-7), 156.1 (C-2), 157.3 (C-5), 158.1 (C-6), 164.8 (C-8), 174.3 (C-1), 181.5 (C-4). β-anomer: ^{1}H NMR (500 MHz, DMSO-d$_6$) δ: 1.03 (t, J = 7.5, 3H, -CH$_2$CH$_3$), 2.49 (q, 2H, -CH$_2$CH$_3$), 2.89 (dd, J = 8.2, 7.7Hz, 1H, H-2′), 3.05 (t, J = 8.2 Hz, 1H, H-4′), 3.08 (dd, J = 13.3, 7.7 Hz, 1H, H-6′a), 3.09 (dd, J = 8.2 Hz, 1H, H-3′), 3.27 (ddd, J = 8.2, 7.7, 2.0 Hz, 1H, H-5′), 3.45 (dd, J = 13.3, 2.0 Hz, 1H, H-6′b), 4.02 (s, 3H,C(6)-OCH$_3$), 4.26 (d, J = 7.7 Hz, 1H, H-1′), 11.35 (br s, 1H, C(2)-OH), 12.92 (s, 1H, C(8)-OH), 13.51 (s, 1H, C(5)-OH).^{13}C NMR (125 MHz, DMSO-d$_6$) δ: 12.6 (-CH$_2$CH$_3$), 15.7 (-CH$_2$CH$_3$), 35.7 (C-6′), 61.1 (C(6)-OCH$_3$), 72.7 (C-4′), 74.9 (C-2′), 75.4 (C-5′), 76.4 (C-3′), 97.1 (C-1′), 107.2 (C-8a), 108.7 (C-4a), 125.6 (C-3), 127.9 (C-7), 156.1 (C-2), 157.4 (C-5), 158.2 (C-6), 164.6 (C-8), 174.5 (C-1), 181.7 (C-4). HRMS (ESI): m/z [M + Na]$^+$ calcd for $C_{19}H_{22}O_{11}SNa$: 481.0775; found: 481.0778.

6-(6-Deoxy-D-glucopyranos-6-ylthio)-5,8-dihydroxy-7-methyl-2,3-dimethoxy-1,4-naphthoquinone (**SAB-14**). Purple solid; yield 85 mg (62%), R_f = 0.46 (B). α-anomer: ^{1}H NMR (500 MHz, DMSO-d$_6$) δ: 2.43 (s, 3H, C(7)-CH$_3$), 3.04 (m, 1H, H-4′), 3.06 (dd, J = 13.6, 7.6 Hz, 1H, H-6′a), 3.11 (m, 1H, H-2′), 3.36 (m, 1H, H-3′),3.42 (dd, J = 13.6, 2.3Hz, 1H, H-6′b), 3.70 (m, 1H, H-5′), 4.01 (s, 3H,-OCH$_3$), 4.02 (s, 3H,-OCH$_3$), 4.48 (d, J = 6.6Hz, 1H, C(2′)-OH), 4.68 (d, J = 4.8Hz, 1H, C(3′)-OH), 4.81 (t, J = 4.8 Hz, 1H, H-1′), 4.94 (d, J = 5.7 Hz, 1H, C(4′)-OH), 6.27 (d, J = 4.8Hz, 1H, C(1′)-OH), 12.92 (s, 1H, C(8)-OH), 13.21 (s, 1H, C(5)-OH). ^{13}C NMR (125 MHz, DMSO-d$_6$) δ:15.0 (C(7)-CH$_3$), 36.8 (C-6′), 61.4 (2× -OCH$_3$), 70.8 (C-5′), 72.3 (C-2′), 72.8 (C-3′), 73.1 (C-4′), 92.4 (C-1′), 107.8 (C-4a), 108.5 (C-8a), 138.2 (C-6), 142.9 (C-7), 147.8 (C-3), 147.9 (C-2), 158.8 (C-8), 160.6 (C-5), 180.5 (C-1), 180.7 (C-4). β-anomer:^{1}H NMR (500 MHz, DMSO-d$_6$) δ: 2.43 (s, 3H,C(7)-CH$_3$), 2.88 (m, 1H, H-2′), 3.04 (m, 3H,H-4′,H-3′, H-6′a), 3.20 (m, 1H, H-5′), 3.41 (dd, J = 13.5, 2.1 Hz, 1H, H-6′b), 4.01 (s, 3H,-OCH$_3$), 4.02 (s, 3H,-OCH$_3$), 4.23 (dd, J = 7.6, 6.4 Hz, 1H, H-1′), 4.84 (d, J = 4.8 Hz, 1H, C(2′)-OH), 4.86 (d, J = 4.4 Hz, 1H, C(3′)-OH), 4.99 (d, J = 5.0 Hz, 1H, C(4′-OH), 6.56 (d, J = 6.8 Hz, 1H, C(1′)-OH), 12.92 (s, 1H, C(8)-OH), 13.21 (s, 1H, C(5)-OH). ^{13}C NMR (125 MHz, DMSO-d$_6$) δ:15.0 (C(7)-CH$_3$), 36.8 (C-6′), 61.4 (2×-OCH$_3$), 72.7 (C-4′), 74.9 (C-2′), 75.3 (C-5′), 76.4 (C-3′), 97.1 (C-1′), 107.8 (C-4a), 108.5 (C-8a), 138.2 (C-6), 142.9 (C-7), 147.8 (C-3), 147.9 (C-2), 158.8 (C-8), 160.6 (C-5), 180.5 (C-1), 180.7 (C-4). HRMS (ESI): m/z [M + Na]$^+$ calcd for $C_{19}H_{22}NaO_{11}S$: 481.0775; found: 481.0775.

2-(6-Deoxy-D-glucopyranos-6-ylthio)-5,8-dihydroxy-3,6,7-trimethyl-1,4-naphthoquinone (**SAB-16**). Dark red solid; yield 78 mg (61%); R_f = 0.53 (B). α-anomer: ^{1}H NMR (500 MHz, DMSO-d_6) δ: 2.17 (s, 6H, C(6)-C$\underline{H}_3$, C(7)-C$\underline{H}_3$), 2.36 (s, 3H, C(3)-C$\underline{H}_3$), 3.04 (dd, J = 9.9, 8.7Hz, 1H, H-4′), 3.08 (dd, J = 9.6, 3.6Hz, 1H, H-2′), 3.14 (dd, J = 14.0, 7.7 Hz, 1H, H-6′a), 3.36 (dd, J = 9.6, 8.7 Hz, 1H, H-3′), 3.49 (dd, J = 14.0, 2.6 Hz, 1H, H-6′b), 3.73 (ddd, J = 9.9, 7.7, 2.6 Hz, 1H, H-5′), 4.78 (d, J = 3.6 Hz, 1H, H-1′), 13.23 (s, 1H, C(5)-O$\underline{H}$), 13.28 (s, 1H, C(8)-O$\underline{H}$). ^{13}C NMR (125 MHz, DMSO-d_6) δ: 12.2 (C(6)-$\underline{C}H_3$, C(7)-$\underline{C}H_3$), 14.9 (C(3)-$\underline{C}H_3$), 36.5 (C-6′), 70.9 (C-5′), 72.2 (C-2′), 72.6 (C-3′), 72.9 (C-4′), 92.3 (C-1′), 108.8 (C-8a), 109.0 (C-4a), 139.9 (C-6*), 140.2 (C-7*), 142.8 (C-2), 145.1 (C-3), 169.0 (C-5), 169.2 (C-8), 172.3 (C-4), 172.7 (C-1). β-anomer: ^{1}H NMR (500 MHz, DMSO-d_6) δ: 2.17 (s, 6H, C(6)-C$\underline{H}_3$, C(7)-C$\underline{H}_3$), 2.37 (s, 3H, C(3)-C$\underline{H}_3$), 2.87 (dd, J = 8.8, 7.7Hz, 1H, H-2′), 3.04 (t, J = 8.8Hz, 1H, H-4′), 3.07 (t, J = 8.8 Hz, 1H, H-3′), 3.15 (dd, J = 14.0, 7.6 Hz, 1H, H-6′a), 3.25 (ddd, J = 8.8, 7.6, 2.5 Hz, 1H, H-5′), 3.48 (dd, J = 14.0, 2.5 Hz, 1H, H-6′b), 4.23 (d, J = 7.7 Hz, 1H, H-1′), 13.23 (s, 1H, C(5)-O$\underline{H}$), 13.29 (s, 1H, C(8)-O$\underline{H}$). ^{13}C NMR (125 MHz, DMSO-d_6) δ: 12.2 (C(6)-$\underline{C}H_3$, C(7)-$\underline{C}H_3$), 14.9 (C(3)-$\underline{C}H_3$), 36.3 (C-6′), 72.5 (C-4′), 74.8 (C-2′), 75.3 (C-5′), 76.2 (C-3′), 96.9 (C-1′), 108.9 (C-8a), 109.1 (C-4a), 140.0 (C-6*), 140.2 (C-7*), 142.4 (C-2), 145.4 (C-3), 169.2 (C-5), 169.5 (C-8), 172.1 (C-4), 172.5 (C-1). HRMS (ESI): m/z [M + Na]$^+$ calcd for $C_{19}H_{22}NaO_9S$: 449.0877; found: 449.0873. *—The assignment of signal is ambiguous.

2-(6-Deoxy-D-glucopyranos-6-ylthio)-5,8-dihydroxy-3-ethyl-6,7-dimethyl-1,4-naphthoquinone (**SAB-18**). Dark red solid; yield 82 mg (62%); R_f = 0.56 (B). α-anomer: ^{1}H NMR (500 MHz, DMSO-d_6) δ: 1.09 (t, J = 7.5 Hz, 3H, -CH$_2$C$\underline{H}_3$), 2.16 (s, 6H, C(6)-C$\underline{H}_3$, C(7)-C$\underline{H}_3$), 2.92 (q, J = 7.5 Hz, 2H, -C$\underline{H}_2$CH$_3$), 3.03 (dd, J = 9.9, 8.7Hz, 1H, H-4′), 3.10 (dd, J = 9.6, 3.6Hz, 1H, H-2′), 3.17 (dd, J = 14.0, 7.7 Hz, 1H, H-6′a), 3.36 (dd, J = 9.6, 8.7 Hz, 1H, H-3′), 3.50 (dd, J = 14.0, 2.6 Hz, 1H, H-6′b), 3.75 (ddd, J = 9.9, 7.7, 2.6 Hz, 1H, H-5′), 4.79 (d, J = 3.6 Hz, 1H, H-1′), 13.24 (s, 1H, C(5)-O$\underline{H}$), 13.31 (s, 1H, C(8)-O$\underline{H}$). ^{13}C NMR (125 MHz, DMSO-d_6) δ: 12.2 (C(6)-$\underline{C}H_3$, C(7)-$\underline{C}H_3$), 13.3 (-CH$_2\underline{C}H_3$), 21.9 (-$\underline{C}H_2$CH$_3$), 36.5 (C-6′), 70.9 (C-5′), 72.2 (C-2′), 72.6 (C-3′), 73.0 (C-4′), 92.3 (C-1′), 108.9 (C-8a), 109.3 (C-4a), 140.2 (C-6*), 140.6 (C-7*), 142.0 (C-2), 149.9 (C-3), 170.5 (C-4*), 170.5 (C-5*), 170.7 (C-8*), 171.6 (C-1). β-anomer: ^{1}H NMR (500 MHz, DMSO-d_6) δ: 1.09 (t, J = 7.5 Hz, 3H, -CH$_2$C$\underline{H}_3$), 2.16 (s, 6H, C(6)-C$\underline{H}_3$, C(7)-C$\underline{H}_3$), 2.87 (dd, J = 8.8, 7.7 Hz, 1H, H-2′), 2.92 (q, J = 7.5 Hz, 2H, -C$\underline{H}_2$CH$_3$), 3.03 (t, J = 8.8 Hz, 1H, H-4′), 3.07 (t, J = 8.8 Hz, 1H, H-3′), 3.15 (dd, J = 14.0, 7.6 Hz, 1H, H-6′a), 3.26 (ddd, J = 8.8, 7.6, 2.5 Hz, 1H, H-5′), 3.52 (dd, J = 14.0, 2.5 Hz, 1H, H-6′b), 4.23 (d, J = 7.7 Hz, 1H, H-1′), 13.24 (s, 1H, C(5)-O$\underline{H}$), 13.33 (s, 1H, C(8)-O$\underline{H}$). ^{13}C NMR (125 MHz, DMSO-d_6) δ: 12.2 (2C, C(6)-$\underline{C}H_3$, C(7)-$\underline{C}H_3$), 13.3 (-CH$_2\underline{C}H_3$), 21.8 (-$\underline{C}H_2$CH$_3$), 36.3 (C-6′), 72.7 (C-4′), 74.8 (C-2′), 75.4 (C-5′), 76.2 (C-3′), 96.9 (C-1′), 109.0 (C-8a), 109.3 (C-4a), 140.3 (C-6*), 140.6 (C-7*), 141.5 (C-2), 150.2 (C-3), 170.3 (C-5*), 170.7 (C-4*), 170.9 (C-8*), 171.4 (C-1). HRMS (ESI): m/z [M + Na]$^+$ calcd for $C_{20}H_{24}NaO_9S$: 463.1033; found: 463.1028. *–The assignment of signal is ambiguous.

2-(6-Deoxy-D-glucopyranos-6-ylthio)-3,6,7-trichloro-5,8-dihydroxy-1,4-naphthoquinone (**SAB-20**). Purple solid; yield 69 mg (47%); R_f = 0.66 (B). α-anomer: ^{1}H NMR (500 MHz, DMSO-d_6) δ: 3.10 (m,2H,H-2′,H-4′), 3.39 (t, J = 9.4 Hz, 1H, H-3′), 3.48 (dd, J = 13.4, 7.5 Hz, 1H, H-6′a), 3.69 (dd, J = 13.5, 2.1 Hz, 1H, H-6′b), 3.81 (m, 1H, H-5′), 4.75 (d, J = 3.7 Hz, 1H, H-1′), 4.78 (s, 1H, C(4′)-O$\underline{H}$), 5.05 (br s, 2H, C(2′)-O$\underline{H}$, C(3′)-O$\underline{H}$), 6.33 (br s, 1H,C(1′)-O$\underline{H}$), 12.49 (br s, 2H, C(5)-O$\underline{H}$, C(8)-O$\underline{H}$). ^{13}C NMR (125 MHz, DMSO-d_6) δ: 36.5 (C-6′), 71.0 (C-5′), 72.2 (C-2′), 72.7 (C-3′), 73.0 (C-4′), 96.9 (C-1′), 111.1 (C-4a), 111.6 (C-8a), 132.3 (C-7), 132.7 (C-6), 138.4 (C-3), 148.6 (C-2), 156.7 (C-8), 157.1 (C-5), 174.0 (C-1), 178.2 (C-4). β-anomer: ^{1}H NMR (500 MHz, DMSO-d_6) δ: 2.83 (m, 1H, H-2′), 3.10 (m, 2H,H-3′,H-4′), 3.34 (m, 1H, H-5′), 3.48 (dd, J = 13.4, 7.5 Hz, 1H, H-6′a), 3.71 (dd, J = 13.5, 2.1 Hz, 1H, H-6′b), 4.21 (d, J = 7.7 1H, H-1′), 4.18 (d, J = 5.2 Hz, 1H, C(4′)-O$\underline{H}$), 5.05 (br s, 2H, C(2′)-O$\underline{H}$, C(3′)-O$\underline{H}$), 6.48 (br s, 1H,C(1′)-O$\underline{H}$), 12.49 (br s, 2H, C(5)-O$\underline{H}$, C(8)-O$\underline{H}$). ^{13}C NMR (125 MHz, DMSO-d_6) δ: 36.1 (C-6′), 72.3 (C-4′), 74.7 (C-2′), 75.3 (C-5′), 76.1 (C-3′), 92.4 (C-1′), 110.9 (C-4a), 111.5 (C-8a), 132.2 (C-7), 132.6 (C-6), 138.0 (C-3), 148.6 (C-2), 156.2 (C-8), 156.9 (C-5), 173.3 (C-1), 177.5 (C-4). HRMS (ESI): m/z [M + Na]$^+$ calcd for $C_{16}H_{13}Cl_3NaO_9S$: 508.9238; found: 508.9234.

2-(6-Deoxy-D-glucopyranos-6-ylthio)-5,8-dihydroxy-1,4-naphthoquinone (**SAB-22**). Purple solid; yield 75 mg (65%); R_f = 0.48 (B). α-anomer: ^{1}H NMR (500 MHz, DMSO-d$_6$) δ: 3.06 (dd, *J* = 13.6, 7.6 Hz, 1H, H-6′a), 3.08 (m, 1H, H-4′), 3.18 (m, 1H, H-2′), 3.34 (dd, *J* = 13.6, 2.1Hz, 1H, H-6′b), 3.44 (m, 1H, H-3′), 3.86 (m, 1H, H-5′), 4.56 (d, *J* = 6.6Hz, 1H, C(2′)-OH), 4.77 (d, *J* = 4.9Hz, 1H, C(3′)-OH), 4.92 (t, *J* = 4.2 Hz, 1H, H-1′), 5.29 (d, *J* = 5.4Hz, 1H, C(4′)-OH), 6.42 (d, *J* = 4.7Hz, 1H, C(1′)-OH), 6.87 (s, 1H, H-3), 7.34 (d, *J* = 9.4 Hz, 1H, H-7), 7.40 (d, *J* = 9.4Hz, 1H, H-6), 11.86 (s, 1H, C(8)-OH), 12.59 (s, 1H, C(5)-OH). ^{13}C NMR (125 MHz, DMSO-d$_6$) δ: 32.9 (C-6′), 69.1 (C-5′), 72.2 (C-2′), 72.7 (C-3′), 73.6 (C-4′), 92.6 (C-1′), 111.2 (C-4a), 111.7 (C-8a), 127.3 (C-3), 128.6 (C-7), 130.4 (C-6), 157.0 (C-2), 157.6 (C-5), 157.5 (C-8), 183.8 (C-1), 184.2 (C-4). β-anomer: ^{1}H NMR (500 MHz, DMSO-d$_6$) δ: 2.94 (m, 1H, H-2′), 3.04 (dd, *J* = 13.5, 7.9 Hz, 1H, H-6′a), 3.11 (m, 1H, H-4′), 3.16 (m, 1H, H-3′), 3.35 (dd, *J* = 13.5, 2.1 Hz, 1H, H-6′b), 3.41 (m, 1H, H-5′), 4.34 (dd, *J* = 7.5, 6.9 Hz, 1H, H-1′), 4.91 (d, *J* = 4.8 Hz, 1H, C(2′)-OH), 4.96 (d, *J* = 4.7 Hz, 1H, C(3′)-OH), 5.33 (d, *J* = 5.0 Hz, 1H, C(4′)-OH), 6.71 (d, *J* = 6.6 Hz, 1H, C(1′)-OH), 6.87 (s, 1H, H-3), 7.34 (d, *J* = 9.4 Hz, 1H, H-7), 7.40 (d, *J* = 9.4Hz, 1H, H-6), 11.86 (s, 1H, C(8)-OH), 12.59 (s, 1H, C(5)-OH). ^{13}C NMR (125 MHz, DMSO-d$_6$) δ: 32.6 (C-6′), 73.1 (C-4′), 73.5 (C-5′), 74.8 (C-2′), 76.2 (C-3′), 97.1 (C-1′), 111.2 (C-4a), 111.7 (C-8a), 127.4 (C-3), 128.6 (C-7), 130.4 (C-6), 155.5 (C-2), 156.9 (C-5), 157.5 (C-8), 183.8 (C-1), 184.3 (C-4). HRMS (ESI): *m/z* [M + Na]$^+$ calcd for C$_{16}$H$_{16}$NaO$_9$S: 407.0407; found: 407.0402.

2-(6-Deoxy-D-glucopyranos-6-ylthio)-8-hydroxy-1,4-naphthoquinone (**SAB-24**). Yellow solid; yield 74 mg (64%); R_f = 0.46 (B). α-anomer: ^{1}H NMR (500 MHz, DMSO-d$_6$) δ: 2.99 (dd, *J* = 13.4, 8.2 Hz, 1H, H-6′a), 3.09 (m, 1H, H-4′), 3.18 (m, 1H, H-2′), 3.31 (dd, *J* = 13.4, 2.6 Hz, 1H, H-6′b), 3.44 (m, 1H, H-3′), 3.86 (m, 1H, H-5′), 4.56 (d, *J* = 6.6 Hz, 1H, C(2′)-OH), 4.78 (d, *J* = 5.0 Hz, 1H, C(3′)-OH), 4.92 (t, *J* = 4.4 Hz, 1H, H-1′), 5.28 (d, *J* = 5.3 Hz, 1H, C(4′)-OH), 6.42 (d, *J* = 4.6 Hz, 1H, C(1′)-OH), 6.81 (s, 1H, H-3), 7.30 (d, *J* = 8.4, 0.8 Hz, 1H, H-7), 7.50 (d, *J* = 7.4, 0.8Hz, 1H, H-5), 7.75 (dd, *J* = 8.4, 7.4 Hz, 1H, H-6), 11.46 (s, 1H, C(8)-OH). ^{13}C NMR (125 MHz, DMSO-d$_6$) δ: 32.7 (C-6′), 69.2 (C-5′), 72.2 (C-2′), 72.7 (C-3′), 73.6 (C-4′), 92.5 (C-1′), 114.9 (C-8a), 118.7 (C-5), 123.5 (C-7), 127.7 (C-3), 132.1 (C-4a), 137.3 (C-6), 154.6 (C-2), 160.5 (C-8), 180.4 (C-4), 186.2 (C-1). β-anomer: ^{1}H NMR (500 MHz, DMSO-d$_6$) δ: 2.94 (m, 1H, H-2′), 2.98 (m, 1H, H-4′), 3.03 (dd, *J* = 13.4, 7.7 Hz, 1H, H-6′a), 3.14 (m, 1H, H-3′), 3.33 (dd, *J* = 13.4, 2.3 Hz, 1H, H-6′b), 3.40 (m, 1H, H-5′), 4.33 (dd, *J* = 7.5, 6.6 Hz, 1H, H-1′), 4.91 (d, *J* = 4.8 Hz, 1H, C(2′)-OH), 4.96 (d, *J* = 4.7 Hz, 1H, C(3′)-OH), 5.33 (d, *J* = 5.1 Hz, 1H, C(4′)-OH), 6.71 (d, *J* = 6.6 Hz, 1H, C(1′)-OH), 6.81 (s, 1H, H-3), 7.30 (d, *J* = 8.4, 0.8 Hz, 1H, H-7), 7.50 (d, *J* = 7.4, 0.8Hz, 1H, H-5), 7.75 (dd, *J* = 8.4, 7.4 Hz, 1H, H-6), 11.46 (s, 1H, C(8)-OH). ^{13}C NMR (125 MHz, DMSO-d$_6$) δ: 32.5 (C-6′), 73.1 (C-4′), 73.5 (C-5′), 74.8 (C-2′), 76.2 (C-3′), 97.1 (C-1′), 114.9 (C-8a), 118.7 (C-5), 123.5 (C-7), 127.8 (C-3), 132.1 (C-4a), 137.3 (C-6), 154.3 (C-2), 160.5 (C-8), 180.4 (C-4), 186.2 (C-1). HRMS (ESI): *m/z* [M + Na]$^+$ calcd for C$_{16}$H$_{16}$NaO$_8$S: 391.0458; found: 391.0455.

2-(6-Deoxy-D-glucopyranos-6-ylthio)-5-hydroxy-1,4-naphthoquinone (**SAB-26**). Yellow solid; yield 65 mg (59%); R_f = 0.46 (B). α-anomer:^{1}H NMR (500 MHz, DMSO-d$_6$) δ: 3.01 (dd, *J* = 13.4, 8.1 Hz, 1H, H-6′a), 3.08 (m, 1H, H-4′), 3.18 (m, 1H, H-2′), 3.32 (dd, *J* = 13.4, 2.4Hz, 1H, H-6′b), 3.44 (m, 1H, H-3′), 3.87 (m, 1H, H-5′), 4.56 (d, *J* = 6.7Hz, 1H, C(2′)-OH), 4.77 (d, *J* = 4.9Hz, 1H, C(3′)-OH), 4.92 (t, *J* = 4.2 Hz, 1H, H-1′), 5.28 (d, *J* = 5.4Hz, 1H, C(4′)-OH), 6.42 (d, *J* = 4.8Hz, 1H, C(1′)-OH), 6.81 (s, 1H, H-3), 7.36 (d, *J* = 8.4, 1.0 Hz, 1H, H-6), 7.56 (d, *J* = 7.5, 1.0Hz, 1H, H-8), 7.71 (dd, *J* = 8.4, 7.5Hz, 1H, H-7), 12.12 (s, 1H, C(5)-OH). ^{13}C NMR (125 MHz, DMSO-d$_6$) δ: 32.9 (C-6′), 69.1 (C-5′), 72.2 (C-2′), 72.7 (C-3′), 73.6 (C-4′), 92.6 (C-1′), 114.4 (C-4a), 119.3 (C-8), 124.8 (C-6), 126.8 (C-3), 131.7 (C-8a), 136.1 (C-7), 156.1 (C-2), 160.5 (C-5), 181.2 (C-1), 186.6 (C-4). β-anomer:^{1}H NMR (500 MHz, DMSO-d$_6$) δ: 2.94 (m, 1H, H-2′), 3.02 (dd, *J* = 13.4, 7.9 Hz, 1H, H-6′a), 3.10 (m, 1H, H-4′), 3.16 (m, 1H, H-3′), 3.35 (dd, *J* = 13.4, 2.3 Hz, 1H, H-6′b), 3.41 (m, 1H, H-5′), 4.34 (dd, *J* = 7.6, 6.6 Hz, 1H, H-1′), 4.91 (d, *J* = 4.6 Hz, 1H, C(2′)-OH), 4.95 (d, *J* = 4.8 Hz, 1H, C(3′)-OH), 5.33 (d, *J* = 5.1 Hz, 1H, C(4′)-OH), 6.70 (d, *J* = 6.7 Hz, 1H, C(1′)-OH), 6.81 (s, 1H, H-3), 7.36 (d, *J* = 8.4, 1.0 Hz, 1H, H-6), 7.56 (d, *J* = 7.5, 1.0Hz, 1H, H-8), 7.71 (dd, *J* = 8.4, 7.5Hz, 1H, H-7), 12.12 (s, 1H, C(5)-OH). ^{13}C NMR (125 MHz, DMSO-d$_6$) δ: 32.6 (C-6′), 73.1 (C-4′), 73.5 (C-5′), 74.8 (C-2′), 76.2 (C-3′), 97.1 (C-1′), 114.4 (C-4a), 119.3 (C-8), 124.8 (C-6), 126.9 (C-3), 131.7

(C-8a), 136.1 (C-7), 155.9 (C-2), 160.5 (C-5), 181.2 (C-1), 186.6 (C-4). HRMS (ESI): m/z [M + Na]$^+$ calcd for $C_{16}H_{16}NaO_8S$: 391.0458; found: 391.0455. * The assignment of signal is ambiguous.

4.2. Biology

4.2.1. General Biology (Reagents and Antibodies)

Annexin-V-FITC was purchased from BD Bioscience (San Jose, CA, USA). MTT (3-(4,5-dimethylthiazol-2-yl)-2,5-diphenyltetrazolium bromide) and propidium iodide (PI) from Sigma (Taufkirchen, Germany). cOmplete™ *EASY*packs protease inhibitors cocktail and PhosSTOP™ *EASY*packs – from Roche (Mannheim, Germany). Anisomycin was from NeoCorp (Weilheim, Germany). z-VAD(OMe)-fmk was from Enzo Life Sciences (Farmingdale, NY, USA). H_2O_2 was from Carl Roth (Karlsruhe, Germany). CCCP (2-[2-(3-chlorophenyl)hydrazinylyidene]propanedinitrile) was from Sigma (Taufkirchen, Germany). JC-1 (5,5′,6,6′-tetrachloro-1,1′,3,3′-tetraethylbenzimidazolylcarbocyanine iodide) was from AdiloGen Life Science (Epalinges, Switzerland). N-acetylcystein was from MedChemExpress (Monmouth Junction, NJ, USA). Primary and secondary antibodies used are listed in Table 1.

Table 1. List of antibodies used.

Antibodies	Clonality	Source	Cat.-No.	Dilution	Manufacturer
anti-AIF	mAb	rabbit	#5318	1:1000	Cell Signaling
anti-Akt	pAb	rabbit	#9272	1:1000	Cell Signaling
anti-Bcl-2	pAb	rabbit	#2876	1:1000	Cell Signaling
anti-cleaved Caspase-3	mAb	rabbit	#9664	1:1000	Cell Signaling
anti-cleaved Caspase-9	mAb	rabbit	#20750	1:1000	Cell Signaling
anti-cytochrome C	mAb	rabbit	#11940	1:1000	Cell Signaling
anti-ERK1/2	mAb	mouse	#9107	1:2000	Cell Signaling
anti-GLUT1	mAb	rabbit	#12939	1:1000	Cell Signaling
anti-JNK1/2	mAb	rabbit	#9258	1:1000	Cell Signaling
anti-MEK1/2	pAb	rabbit	#9122	1:1000	Cell Signaling
anti-mouse IgG-HRP		sheep	NXA931	1:10,000	GE Healthcare
anti-p21$^{Waf1/Cip1}$	mAb	rabbit	#2947	1:1000	Cell Signaling
anti-p38	mAb	rabbit	#9212	1:1000	Cell Signaling
anti-PARP	pAb	rabbit	#9542	1:1000	Cell Signaling
anti-phospho-Akt	mAb	rabbit	#4058	1:1000	Cell Signaling
anti-phospho-ERK1/2	mAb	rabbit	#4377	1:1000	Cell Signaling
anti-phospho-JNK1/2	mAb	rabbit	#4668	1:1000	Cell Signaling
anti-phospho-MEK1/2	mAb	rabbit	#2338	1:1000	Cell Signaling
anti-phospho-p38	mAb	rabbit	#4511	1:1000	Cell Signaling
anti-rabbit IgG-HRP		goat	#7074	1:5000	Cell Signaling
anti-Survivin	pAb	rabbit	NB500-201	1:1000	Novus
anti-α-Tubulin	mAb	mouse	T5168	1:5000	Sigma-Aldrich
anti-β-Actin-HRP	pAb	goat	sc-1616	1:10,000	Santa Cruz

4.2.2. Cell Lines and Culture Conditions

The human prostate cancer cell lines PC-3, DU145, 22Rv1, and LNCaP, as well as human prostate non-cancer cell lines RWPE-1 and PNT2 were purchased from ATCC (Manassas, VA, USA). The human prostate cancer cell line VCaP was purchased from ECACC (Salisbury, UK). HEK 293T (human embryonic kidney cells), MRC-9 (human fibroblast cells) and HUVEC (human umbilical vascular endothelial cells, passage 11) were a gift from Prof. Sonja Loges (University Medical Center Hamburg-Eppendorf, Hamburg, Germany). All the cells had a passage number ≤ 30. Authentification of all cell lines used was recently performed by commercial service (Multiplexion GmbH, Heidelberg, Germany).

Cells were cultured as monolayers at 37 °C in a humidified atmosphere with 5% (v/v) CO_2 in the correspondent culture medium: 10% FBS/RPMI medium (RPMI medium supplemented with Glutamax™-I (gibco® Life technologies™, Paisley, UK) containing 10% fetal bovine serum (FBS, gibco® Life technologies™) and 1% penicillin/streptomycin (Invitrogen)) for PNT2, LNCaP,

22Rv1, PC-3, and DU145 and cells; 10% FBS/DMEM medium (DMEM medium supplemented with Glutamax™-I (gibco® Life technologies™) containing 10% FBS and 1% penicillin/streptomycin (gibco® Life technologies™)) for VCaP, MRC-9, and HEK 293 cells; Keratinocyte Serum Free Medium (K-SFM) kit (gibco® Life technologies™, Paisley, UK, Cat. #17005-042) supplied with BPE and hEGF for RWPE-1 cells; and Clonetics® EGM™-2 SingleQuots® medium (Lonza, Walkersville, MD, USA) containing 10% FBS for HUVEC cells. Cells were continuously kept in culture for a maximum of 3 months, and were regularly checked for stable phenotype and mycoplasma infection.

4.2.3. MTT Assay

Cell viability was determined by MTT assay. Cells were pre-incubated overnight in 96-well plates (6×10^3 cells/well in 100 µL/well). Then, the medium was replaced with fresh medium containing the determined compounds (100 µL/well), and cells were incubated for the indicated time. Next, 10 µL/well of (3-(4,5-dimethylthiazol-2-yl)-2,5-diphenyltetrazolium bromide) reagent were added. After 2–4 h of incubation, the media was aspirated and the plates were dried. Fifty microliters per well of DMSO were added to each well and the cell viability was measured using Infinite F200PRO reader (TECAN, Männedorf, Switzerland). Results were calculated by The GraphPad Prism software v. 7.05 (GraphPad Prism software Inc., La Jolla, CA, USA) and are represented as IC_{50} of the compounds against control cells treated with the solvent alone.

4.2.4. Quantitative Real-Time PCR (qPCR)

GLUT-1 gene expression in different cell lines was measured by qPCR. Cells were seeded in Petri dishes (1×10^6 cells per ø 10 cm dish in 5 mL of media for 22Rv1) in 10% FBS/RPMI media and incubated overnight. Cells were harvested by scratching, washed, and homogenized using QIAshredder (Cat. #79654, QIAGEN, Hilden, Germany). The total RNA was isolated using PureLink® RNA Mini Kit (Cat. # 12183018A, Invitrogen, Carlsbad, CA, USA) with the on-column DNA digestion using PureLink™ DNase (Cat. # 12185-010, Invitrogen). RNA was diluted up to 30 µL and 2 µg of RNA was transcribed into cDNA using Maxima First Strand cDNA Synthesis Kit for RT-qPCR (Cat. # K1642, Thermo Scientific, Vilnius, Lithuania). qPCR was performed using 2X KAPA SYBR FAST qPCR Master Mix Optimized for Roche LightCycler 480 (Cat. # KK4609, KAPA biosystems, Worburn, MA, USA) according to the manufacturer's recommendations. For each reaction, 20 ng of template cDNA and 2 pmol of primers were used. The expression of human GLUT-1 and GAPDH genes were analyzed using primers, purchased from by Eurofins MWG-Biotech AG (Ebersberg, Germany). Primers sequences and melting temperatures (Tm): GLUT-1: forward AAC TCT TCA GCC AGG GTC CAC, reverse CAC AGT GAA GAT GAT GAA GAC, Tm = 60 °C; GAPDH: forward TGC ACC ACC AAC TGC TTA, reverse GAG GCA GGG ATG ATG TTC, Tm = 56 °C. The PCR conditions were 30 s 95 °C, followed by 40 cycles of 15 s 95 °C, 5 s Tm, and 26 s 72 °C (measurement of fluorescence). Melting curve analysis (10 s 95 °C, 60 s 65 °C, and 1 s 97 °C) was performed directly after PCR run. Relative gene expression was calculated using the $2^{-\Delta\Delta CT}$ method.

4.2.5. Glucose Uptake Assay

The effects of the synthesized substance on glucose uptake were evaluated using the Glucose Uptake Cell-Based Assay Kit (Cayman chemicals, Ann Arbor, MI, USA) and two different methods. (a) Plate reader-based measurement: PC-3 cells (12×10^3 cells/well) were seeded in two 96-well plates, incubated overnight, and treated with the investigated drugs in 100 µL/well of glucose-free 0.1% FBS/RPMI media for 24 h. Then, the 10 µL/well of either 2-NBDG solution (2-deoxy-2-[(7-nitro-2,1,3-benzoxadiazol-4-yl)amino]-D-glucose, 5 mg/mL, for glucose uptake measurements) or vehicle solution (for cell viability measurements) in glucose-free 0.1% FBS/RPMI media were added to each well. After 6 h of incubation, the cells were carefully washed twice with PBS (200 µL/well). Then, for glucose uptake measurements, the 100 µL/well of PBS were added and the fluorescence was measured using Infinite F200PRO reader (TECAN, Männedorf, Switzerland); or, for the cell viability measurements, 100 µL/well of media containing MTS reagent were added to the cells and viability was measured as described before [54]. Glucose uptake rate was normalized to the cell viability measured by MTS assay in order to measure the uptake rate exclusively in the viable cells. (b) FACS-based readout: The experiment was performed as described before [26]. In brief, the PC-3 cells were seeded into 12-well plates and treated with the investigated compounds for 24 h in RPMI media (glucose-free, 0.1% FBS). The plates were then incubated with 2-NBDG solution, the cells were harvested by trypsination, washed, stained with PI, and analyzed using a flow cytometry.

4.2.6. Analysis of Cell Cycle Progression and DNA Fragmentation

The effects on cell cycle progression and DNA fragmentation were analyzed by flow cytometry using PI staining as described previously [55]. Cells (2×10^5 cells/well) were pre-incubated overnight in 6-well plates. Then, cells were treated with the substances in 2 mL of fresh culture media/well for 48 h. Cells were harvested by trypsination, fixed in 70% EtOH, stained with PI, and analyzed by FACS Calibur (BD Bioscience, San Jose, CA, USA). The results were quantified using BD Bioscience Cell Quest Pro v.5.2.1. software (BD Bioscience, San Jose, CA, USA). The sub-G1 population was considered to reflect apoptotic cells (containing fragmented DNA).

4.2.7. Analysis of Apoptosis (Annexin-V-FITC/PI Double Staining)

To examine induction of drug-induced apoptosis FACS-based analysis with Annexin-V-FITC and propidium iodide (PI) double staining was performed as previously described [56,57]. Cells were seeded in 6-well plates (2×10^5 cells/well) and incubated overnight. Treatment with the substances was performed in 2 mL fresh culture media/well for 48 h. Cells were harvested by trypsination, stained with Annexin-V-FITC and PI for 15 min, and analyzed using FACS Calibur (BD Bioscience, San Jose, CA, USA). The results were quantified using BD Bioscience Cell Quest Pro v.5.2.1. software (BD Bioscience, San Jose, CA, USA).

4.2.8. Western Blotting

Cells (10^6 cells/well) were seeded in Petri dishes (ø 6 cm) and incubated overnight. The cells were treated with the investigational drugs in fresh culture media (5 mL/dish) for 48 h. Then, cells were harvested by scratching and lysed in the lysis buffer (1% NP-40, 50 mM Tris-HCl (pH 7.6), 0.88% NaCl, 0.25% sodium cholate, 1 mM Na_3VO_4, 0.1 mM PMSF, protease inhibitors cocktail (cOmplete Mini EDTA-free EASYpacks, Roche, Mannheim, Germany)). Proteins were extracted and diluted with lysis buffer and loading dye, heated 5 min at 99 °C and subjected to electrophoresis in gradient Mini-PROTEAN® TGX Stain-Free™ gels (Bio-Rad, Hercules, CA, USA). Proteins were transferred from gel to 0.2 µm pore PVDF membrane using Trans-Blot® Turbo™ RTA Mini PVDF Trans kit (Bio-Rad) and Trans-Blot® Turbo™ Blotting System (Bio-Rad) according to the manufactures protocol. The membrane was blocked (5% BSA in 0.05% Tween-20/TBS), treated with primary and secondary antibodies, and the signals were detected using the ECL chemiluminescence system (Thermo Scientific, Rockford, IL, USA). All procedures were performed according to the manufacturer's protocols. The antibodies used are listed in Table 1.

4.2.9. Proteomics

The sample preparation and proceeding, data acquisition and analysis have been described previously [26]. In brief, 22Rv1 cells (4×10^6 cells/bottle in 20 mL/bottle) were seeded and incubated in T75 culture bottles overnight. Then, the cells were treated 2 µM of **SAB-13** or equal volume with vehicle (DMSO) for 48 h. Treatment was performed in triplicates. Cells were harvested by scratching, washed with ice-cold PBS (2×10 mL) and flash-frozen. The samples were further proceeded (for details, see [26]) and digested by trypsin. Peptides were separated on a 25 cm C18 reversed phase column (BEH C18 Column, 130Å, 1.7 µm, 75 µm × 250 mm, Waters Corporation, Milford, MS, USA) within a 60 min gradient from 2%–30% acetonitrile (equilibration buffer: 0.1% formic acid; elution buffer:

99.9% acetonitrile and 0.1% formic acid) buffer at a flow rate of 250 nL/min using a nano-UPLC system (Acquity, Waters Corporation, Milford, MS, USA) and full recovery autosampler vials, coupled via electrospray ionization (ESI) to a tandem mass spectrometer equipped with a quadrupole and an orbitrap (QExactive, Thermo Fisher Scientific, Bremen, Germany), using MS/MS mode in DDA (data dependent acquisition) and DIA (data independent acquisition). The peptide library necessary for DIA analysis was generated by DDA-LC-MS/MS of 1 randomly selected sample per biological triplicate. The peptides were identified with the search engine Sequest (integrated in the Proteome Discoverer software version 2.0, Thermo Fischer Scientific) using the human Uniprot protein database (EMBL; Hinxton Cambridge, UK, release December 2018). All samples were acquired in DIA mode and data extraction with the peptide library was performed using the Skyline software (version 4.2, MacCoss Lab Washington University, Seattle, WA, USA). Peptides with a dot-product (dotP) of 0.85 and above were considered for further analysis and the peptide areas were summed to protein areas. Statistical analysis (data normalization, Student's t-tests, principal component analysis, hierarchical clustering) was performed using the Perseus software (version 1.5.8, Max-Planck Institute of Biochemistry, Munich, Germany). Proteins were considered to be significantly different in abundance if a $1.5 \leq$ fold change $\leq 1/1.5$ and p-value ≤ 0.05 was detected (Student's t-test).

4.2.10. Bioinformatical Analysis

Bioinformatical analysis of the proteomics data was performed using the Ingenuity Pathways Analysis (IPA) (release 46901286, QIAGEN Bioinformatics, Venlo, The Netherlands). The list of significantly regulated proteins discovered by global proteome analysis were proceeded by IPA software to access protein interaction networks, gene ontology, relevant biological molecules, and processes affected by the drug, as previously described [58]. The shortest hypothetical pathway networks were constructed, showing the most relevant direct and indirect interactions of the regulated proteins and the proteins predicted to be involved in the interactions. z-Score algorithm was used to identify biological functions which are expected to be suppressed (z-score < 0) or activated (z-score > 0) upon treatment in cancer cells. The p-values were calculated by IPA software using the Fischer's exact test according to the software's protocols.

4.2.11. Analysis of Intracellular ROS Level

Intracellular ROS levels were accessed using the ROS-sensitive CM-H_2DCFDA reagent (Cat. No. C6827, Molecular probes, Invitrogen, Eugene, OR, USA). The experiment was performed as previously described with slight modifications [59]. In brief, 22Rv1 cells (10^5 cells/well) were seeded in 12-well plates and incubated overnight. The media was changed with freshly made pre-warmed staining solution (4 µM CM-H_2DCFDA/PBS, 0.5 mL/well) and incubated in the dark (37 °C, 5% CO_2) for 30 min. Then, the staining solution was exchanged with 1 mL/well of pre-warmed PBS containing the investigated compounds or H_2O_2 (positive control) at the indicated concentrations and the cells were incubated for 2 h. Next, the cells were trypsinized, resuspended in pre-warmed PBS (200 µL/sample) and immediately analyzed by FACS according to the manufacture's protocol.

4.2.12. Analysis of Mitochondrial Membrane Potential ($\Delta\Psi_m$)

The drop down of mitochondrial membrane potential ($\Delta\Psi_m$) was measured using staining with $\Delta\Psi_m$-sensitive JC-1 dye (5,5′,6,6′-Tetrachloro-1,1′,3,3′-tetraethyl-imidacarbocyanine iodide) and flow cytometry technique. Cells (10^5 cells/well) were seeded in 12-well plates and incubated overnight. Then, the media was changed to PBS (1 mL/well) containing the investigational drugs and the cells were incubated for 2 h (37 °C, 5% CO_2, in the dark). The cells were trypsinized, pelleted, resuspended in 100 µL of 2 µM JC-1/PBS, incubated for 1 h (37 °C, 5% CO_2, in the dark), and analyzed by flow cytometry technique.

4.2.13. Cell Fractionation

The separation of cellular nuclear, mitochondrial, and cytosolic fractions was performed using the Cell Fractionation Kit ab109719 (abcam, Cambridge, MA, USA). 22Rv1 cells (4×10^6 cells/bottle) were seeded in T75 culture bottles (in 20 mL/bottle) and incubated overnight. Cells were treated for 48 h and harvested by scratching. Further procedures were performed as previously described with slight modifications [59]. Nuclear fractions were homogenized using QIAshedder kit (QUIAGEN, Hilden, Germany). Cytosolic and mitochondrial fractions were concentrated using Amicon® Ultra-2 Centrifugal Filter device (Cat. No. UFC203024, Merck, Darmstadt, Germany).

4.2.14. Data and Statistical Analysis

For statistical analyses of all the datasets (apart from proteomics data), the GraphPad Prism software v. 7.05 was used (GraphPad Prism software Inc., La Jolla, CA, USA). Data are presented as mean ± SEM. The unpaired Student's t-test or one-way ANOVA followed by Dunnett's post-hoc tests were used for comparison of two or several groups, correspondently. Dunnett's post-hoc test was used to compare each of a number of a multiple treatment with a single control. All experiments were performed in in triplicates ($n = 3$, biological replicates) unless otherwise stated. Differences were considered to be statistically significant (*) if $p < 0.05$.

5. Conclusions

We were able to synthesize novel 6-S-(1,4-naphthoquinone-2-yl)-D-glucose chimera molecules, the derivatives of the sea urchin pigments spinochromes. The compounds exhibited a Warburg effect mediated selectivity to human prostate cancer cells (including highly drug resistant cell lines) and effectively inhibited the oxidative phosphorylation. Mitochondria were identified as a primary cellular target of these compounds. The mechanism of action included mitochondrial membrane permeabilization, followed by ROS upregulation and release of cytotoxic mitochondrial proteins (AIF and cytochrome C) to the cytoplasm, which lead to the consequent caspase-9 and -3 activation, PARP cleavage and apoptosis-like cell death.

Supplementary Materials: The following are available online at http://www.mdpi.com/1660-3397/18/5/251/s1, Table S1: List of proteins regulated in 22Rv1 cells under the SAB-13 treatment and discovered by proteomics.

Author Contributions: Conception and design, S.A.D., D.N.P., and G.v.A.; Development of methodology, S.A.D., and D.N.P.; Acquisition of data, S.A.D., D.N.P., J.H., Y.E.S., K.L.B., C.K., M.K., S.V., E.A.K., T.B., V.A.D., and S.G.P.; Artwork, S.A.D.; Analysis and interpretation of data, S.A.D., D.N.P., J.H., Y.E.S., C.K., M.K., K.L.B., S.V., E.A.K., T.B., V.A.D., M.G., H.S., C.B., S.G.P., V.P.A., and G.v.A.; Writing of the manuscript—original draft preparation, S.A.D., D.N.P., and G.v.A.; Writing of the manuscript—review and editing, All authors; Fundraising, G.v.A.; Review and/or revision of the final version of the manuscript, All authors; and Study supervision, S.A.D., S.G.P. and G.v.A. All authors have read and agreed to the published version of the manuscript.

Funding: This study was supported by a grant of the Hamburger Krebsgesellschaft and Russian Foundation for Basic Research (RFBR) grant No 18-33-00460_mol_a. The study was carried out using the equipment of the Collective Facilities Center "The Far Eastern Center for Structural Molecular Research (NMR/MS) PIBOC FEB RAS".

Acknowledgments: We would like to thank Tina Rohlfing and Bianca Sievers (University Medical Center Hamburg-Eppendorf) for technical support of the biological part of this research; Roman S. Popov (G.B. Elyakov Pacific Institute of Bioorganic Chemistry) for the measurements of MS of synthesized compounds; Valery P. Glazunov (G.B. Elyakov Pacific Institute of Bioorganic Chemistry) for recording IR spectra; and Maxim S. Kokoulin (G.B. Elyakov Pacific Institute of Bioorganic Chemistry) for assistance in spectral signal assignment.

Conflicts of Interest: The authors declare no conflict of interest.

References

1. Peng, X.; Pentassuglia, L.; Sawyer, D.B. Emerging anticancer therapeutic targets and the cardiovascular system: Is there cause for concern? *Circ. Res.* **2010**, *106*, 1022–1034. [CrossRef] [PubMed]

2. Coats, S.; Williams, M.; Kebble, B.; Dixit, R.; Tseng, L.; Yao, N.-S.; Tice, D.A.; Soria, J.-C. Antibody–Drug Conjugates: Future Directions in Clinical and Translational Strategies to Improve the Therapeutic Index. *Clin. Cancer Res.* **2019**, *25*, 5441. [CrossRef] [PubMed]
3. McGregor, B.A.; Sonpavde, G. Enfortumab Vedotin, a fully human monoclonal antibody against Nectin 4 conjugated to monomethyl auristatin E for metastatic urothelial Carcinoma. *Expert Opin. Investig. Drugs* **2019**, *28*, 821–826. [CrossRef] [PubMed]
4. Chakravarty, R.; Siamof, C.M.; Dash, A.; Cai, W. Targeted α-therapy of prostate cancer using radiolabeled PSMA inhibitors: A game changer in nuclear medicine. *Am. J. Nucl. Med. Mol. Imag.* **2018**, *8*, 247–267.
5. Adashek, J.J.; Jain, R.K.; Zhang, J. Clinical Development of PARP Inhibitors in Treating Metastatic Castration-Resistant Prostate Cancer. *Cells* **2019**, *8*, 860. [CrossRef]
6. Calvaresi, E.C.; Hergenrother, P.J. Glucose conjugation for the specific targeting and treatment of cancer. *Chem. Sci.* **2013**, *4*, 2319–2333. [CrossRef]
7. Hossain, F.; Andreana, P.R. Developments in carbohydrate-based cancer therapeutics. *Pharmaceuticals* **2019**, *12*, 84. [CrossRef]
8. Vander Heiden, M.G.; Cantley, L.C.; Thompson, C.B. Understanding the Warburg effect: The metabolic requirements of cell proliferation. *Science* **2009**, *324*, 1029–1033. [CrossRef]
9. NIH, Studies Found for: Glufosfamide. 2019. Available online: https://clinicaltrials.gov/ct2/results?cond=glufosfamide&term=&cntry=&state=&city=&dist= (accessed on 31 December 2019).
10. Newman, D.J.; Cragg, G.M. Natural products as sources of new drugs from 1981 to 2014. *J. Nat. Prod.* **2016**, *79*, 629–661. [CrossRef]
11. Molinski, T.F.; Dalisay, D.S.; Lievens, S.L.; Saludes, J.P. Drug development from marine natural products. *Nat. Rev. Drug Discov.* **2009**, *8*, 69–85. [CrossRef]
12. Stonik, V.A. Marine natural products: A way to new drugs. *Acta Nat.* **2009**, *2*, 15–25. [CrossRef]
13. Dyshlovoy, S.A.; Honecker, F. Marine Compounds and Cancer: The First Two Decades of XXI Century. *Mar. Drugs* **2019**, *18*, 20. [CrossRef] [PubMed]
14. Mayer, A. Marine Pharmaceutical: The Clinical Pipeline. 2019. Available online: https://www.midwestern.edu/departments/marinepharmacology/clinical-pipeline.xml (accessed on 16 April 2020).
15. Shikov, A.N.; Pozharitskaya, O.N.; Krishtopina, A.S.; Makarov, V.G. Naphthoquinone pigments from sea urchins: Chemistry and pharmacology. *Phytochem. Rev.* **2018**, *17*, 509–534. [CrossRef]
16. Aminin, D.; Polonik, S. 1,4-Naphthoquinones: Some Biological Properties and Application. *Chem. Pharm. Bull.* **2020**, *68*, 46–57. [CrossRef]
17. Klotz, L.-O.; Hou, X.; Jacob, C. 1,4-naphthoquinones: From oxidative damage to cellular and inter-cellular signaling. *Molecules* **2014**, *19*, 14902–14918. [CrossRef]
18. Kumagai, Y.; Shinkai, Y.; Miura, T.; Cho, A.K. The chemical biology of naphthoquinones and its environmental implications. *Annu. Rev. Pharmacol. Toxicol.* **2012**, *52*, 221–247. [CrossRef]
19. Acharya, B.R.; Bhattacharyya, S.; Choudhury, D.; Chakrabarti, G. The microtubule depolymerizing agent naphthazarin induces both apoptosis and autophagy in A549 lung cancer cells. *Apoptosis* **2011**, *16*, 924–939. [CrossRef]
20. Jordan, M.A.; Wilson, L. Microtubules as a target for anticancer drugs. *Nat. Rev. Cancer* **2004**, *4*, 253–265. [CrossRef]
21. Masuda, K.; Funayama, S.; Komiyama, K.; Umezawa, I. Constituents of Tritonia crocosmaeflora, II. Tricrozarin B, an antitumor naphthazarin derivative. *J. Nat. Prod.* **1987**, *50*, 958–960. [CrossRef]
22. Pelageev, D.N.; Dyshlovoy, S.A.; Pokhilo, N.D.; Denisenko, V.A.; Borisova, K.L.; Keller-von Amsberg, G.; Bokemeyer, C.; Fedorov, S.N.; Honecker, F.; Anufriev, V.P. Quinone-carbohydrate nonglucoside conjugates as a new type of cytotoxic agents: Synthesis and determination of *in vitro* activity. *Eur. J. Med. Chem.* **2014**, *77*, 139–144. [CrossRef]
23. Balaneva, N.N.; Shestak, O.P.; Anufriev, V.F.; Novikov, V.L. Synthesis of Spinochrome D, A Metabolite of Various Sea-Urchin Species. *Chem. Nat. Compd.* **2016**, *52*, 213–217. [CrossRef]
24. Pelageev, D.N.; Anufriev, V.P. Synthesis of Mirabiquinone A: A Biquinone from the Sea Urchin Scaphechinus mirabilis and Related Compounds. *Synthesis* **2016**, *48*, 761–764.
25. Sabutskii, Y.E.; Denisenko, V.A.; Polonik, S.G. The Acid-Catalyzed 2-O-Alkylation of Substituted 2-Hydroxy-1,4-naphthoquinones by Alcohols: Versatile Preparative Synthesis of Spinochrome D and Its 6-Alkoxy Derivatives. *Synthesis* **2018**, *50*, 3738–3748.

26. Dyshlovoy, S.A.; Pelageev, D.N.; Hauschild, J.; Borisova, K.L.; Kaune, M.; Krisp, C.; Venz, S.; Sabutskii, Y.E.; Khmelevskaya, E.A.; Busenbender, T.; et al. Successful Targeting of the Warburg Effect in Prostate Cancer by Glucose-Conjugated 1,4-Naphthoquinones. *Cancers* **2019**, *11*, 1690. [CrossRef]
27. Driguez, H. Thiooligosaccharides as Tools for Structural Biology. *ChemBioChem* **2001**, *2*, 311–318. [CrossRef]
28. Thomson, R.H. Studies in the Juglone Series. III. Addition Reactions. *J. Org. Chem.* **1951**, *16*, 1082–1090. [CrossRef]
29. Tamaki, H.; Harashima, N.; Hiraki, M.; Arichi, N.; Nishimura, N.; Shiina, H.; Naora, K.; Harada, M. Bcl-2 family inhibition sensitizes human prostate cancer cells to docetaxel and promotes unexpected apoptosis under caspase-9 inhibition. *Oncotarget* **2014**, *5*, 11399–11412. [CrossRef]
30. Liu, C.; Zhu, Y.; Lou, W.; Nadiminty, N.; Chen, X.; Zhou, Q.; Shi, X.B.; de Vere White, R.W.; Gao, A.C. Functional p53 determines docetaxel sensitivity in prostate cancer cells. *Prostate* **2013**, *73*, 418–427. [CrossRef]
31. Karimian, A.; Ahmadi, Y.; Yousefi, B. Multiple functions of p21 in cell cycle, apoptosis and transcriptional regulation after DNA damage. *DNA Repair* **2016**, *42*, 63–71. [CrossRef]
32. Dyshlovoy, S.A.; Otte, K.; Tabakmakher, K.M.; Hauschild, J.; Makarieva, T.N.; Shubina, L.K.; Fedorov, S.N.; Bokemeyer, C.; Stonik, V.A.; von Amsberg, G. Synthesis and anticancer activity of the derivatives of marine compound rhizochalin in castration resistant prostate cancer. *Oncotarget* **2018**, *9*, 16962–16973. [CrossRef]
33. Antonarakis, E.S.; Lu, C.; Wang, H.; Luber, B.; Nakazawa, M.; Roeser, J.C.; Chen, Y.; Mohammad, T.A.; Fedor, H.L.; Lotan, T.L.; et al. AR-V7 and resistance to enzalutamide and abiraterone in prostate cancer. *N. Engl. J. Med.* **2014**, *371*, 1028–1038. [CrossRef] [PubMed]
34. Nelson, P.S. Targeting the androgen receptor in prostate cancer—A resilient foe. *N. Engl. J. Med.* **2014**, *371*, 1067–1069. [CrossRef] [PubMed]
35. Foster, C.S.; Falconer, A.; Dodson, A.R.; Norman, A.R.; Dennis, N.; Fletcher, A.; Southgate, C.; Dowe, A.; Dearnaley, D.; Jhavar, S.; et al. factor E2F3 overexpressed in prostate cancer independently predicts clinical outcome. *Oncogene* **2004**, *23*, 5871–5879. [CrossRef] [PubMed]
36. Braadland, P.R.; Ramberg, H.; Grytli, H.H.; Taskén, K.A. β-Adrenergic Receptor Signaling in Prostate Cancer. *Front. Oncol.* **2015**, *4*, 375. [CrossRef] [PubMed]
37. Shafran, J.S.; Andrieu, G.P.; Gyorffy, B.; Denis, G.V. BRD4 regulates metastatic potential of castration-resistant prostate cancer through AHNAK. *Mol. Cancer Res.* **2019**, *17*, 1627–1638. [CrossRef]
38. Tan, Y.; Wang, L.; Du, Y.; Liu, X.; Chen, Z.; Weng, X.; Guo, J.; Chen, H.; Wang, M.; Wang, X. Inhibition of BRD4 suppresses tumor growth in prostate cancer via the enhancement of FOXO1 expression. *Int. J. Oncol.* **2018**, *53*, 2503–2517. [CrossRef]
39. Frankland-Searby, S.; Bhaumik, S.R. The 26S proteasome complex: An attractive target for cancer therapy. *Biochim. Biophys. Acta* **2012**, *1825*, 64–76. [CrossRef]
40. Koh, C.M.; Bieberich, C.J.; Dang, C.V.; Nelson, W.G.; Yegnasubramanian, S.; De Marzo, A.M. MYC and Prostate Cancer. *Genes Cancer* **2010**, *1*, 617–628. [CrossRef]
41. Sica, V.; Bravo-San Pedro, J.M.; Stoll, G.; Kroemer, G. Oxidative phosphorylation as a potential therapeutic target for cancer therapy. *Int. J. Cancer* **2020**, *146*, 10–17. [CrossRef]
42. Li, X.; Fang, P.; Mai, J.; Choi, E.T.; Wang, H.; Yang, X.F. Targeting mitochondrial reactive oxygen species as novel therapy for inflammatory diseases and cancers. *J. Hematol. Oncol.* **2013**, *6*, 19. [CrossRef]
43. Horwich, A.; Hugosson, J.; de Reijke, T.; Wiegel, T.; Fizazi, K.; Kataja, V. Prostate cancer: ESMO consensus conference guidelines 2012. *Ann. Oncol.* **2013**, *24*, 1141–1162. [CrossRef] [PubMed]
44. Caffo, O.; De Giorgi, U.; Fratino, L.; Alesini, D.; Zagonel, V.; Facchini, G.; Gasparro, D.; Ortega, C.; Tucci, M.; Verderame, F. Clinical outcomes of castration-resistant prostate cancer treatments administered as third or fourth line following failure of docetaxel and other second-line treatment: Results of an Italian multicentre study. *Eur. Urol.* **2015**, *68*, 147–153. [CrossRef] [PubMed]
45. Armstrong, C.M.; Gao, A.C. Drug resistance in castration resistant prostate cancer: Resistance mechanisms and emerging treatment strategies. *Am. J. Clin. Exp. Urol.* **2015**, *3*, 64–76. [PubMed]
46. Sabutskii, Y.E.; Denisenko, V.A.; Popov, R.S.; Polonik, S.G. Acid-Catalyzed Heterocyclization of Trialkylnaphthazarin Thioglucosides in Angular Quinone-Carbohydrate Tetracycles. *Russ. J. Org. Chem.* **2019**, *55*, 147–151. [CrossRef]
47. Wellington, K.W. Understanding cancer and the anticancer activities of naphthoquinones—A review. *RSC Adv.* **2015**, *5*, 20309–20338. [CrossRef]

48. Lown, J.W.; Sim, S.K.; Majumdar, K.C.; Chang, R.Y. Strand scission of DNA by bound adriamycin and daunorubicin in the presence of reducing agents. *Biochem. Biophys. Res. Commun.* **1977**, *76*, 705–710. [CrossRef]
49. Leopold, W.R.; Shillis, J.L.; Mertus, A.E.; Nelson, J.M.; Roberts, B.J.; Jackson, R.C. Anticancer activity of the structurally novel antibiotic CI-920 and its analogues. *Cancer Res.* **1984**, *44*, 1928–1932.
50. Tewey, K.M.; Chen, G.L.; Nelson, E.M.; Liu, L.F. Intercalative antitumor drugs interfere with the breakage-reunion reaction of mammalian DNA topoisomerase II. *J. Biol. Chem.* **1984**, *259*, 9182–9187.
51. Chamberlain, G.R.; Tulumello, D.V.; Kelley, S.O. Targeted delivery of doxorubicin to mitochondria. *ACS Chem. Biol.* **2013**, *8*, 1389–1395. [CrossRef]
52. Battogtokh, G.; Choi, Y.S.; Kang, D.S.; Park, S.J.; Shim, M.S.; Huh, K.M.; Cho, Y.Y.; Lee, J.Y.; Lee, H.S.; Kang, H.C. Mitochondria-targeting drug conjugates for cytotoxic, anti-oxidizing and sensing purposes: Current strategies and future perspectives. *Acta Pharm. Sin. B* **2018**, *8*, 862–880. [CrossRef]
53. Ashton, T.M.; McKenna, W.G.; Kunz-Schughart, L.A.; Higgins, G.S. Oxidative phosphorylation as an emerging target in cancer therapy. *Clin. Cancer Res.* **2018**, *24*, 2482–2490. [CrossRef] [PubMed]
54. Dyshlovoy, S.A.; Fedorov, S.N.; Shubina, L.K.; Kuzmich, A.S.; Bokemeyer, C.; Keller-von Amsberg, G.; Honecker, F. Aaptamines from the marine sponge *Aaptos* sp. display anticancer activities in human cancer cell lines and modulate AP-1-, NF-kappa B-, and p53-dependent transcriptional activity in mouse JB6 Cl41 cells. *Biomed Res. Int.* **2014**, *2014*, 1–7. [CrossRef] [PubMed]
55. Dyshlovoy, S.A.; Tabakmakher, K.M.; Hauschild, J.; Shchekaleva, R.K.; Otte, K.; Guzii, A.G.; Makarieva, T.N.; Kudryashova, E.K.; Fedorov, S.N.; Shubina, L.K.; et al. Guanidine alkaloids from the marine sponge *Monanchora pulchra* show cytotoxic properties and prevent EGF-induced neoplastic transformation In Vitro. *Mar. Drugs* **2016**, *14*, 133. [CrossRef] [PubMed]
56. Dyshlovoy, S.A.; Naeth, I.; Venz, S.; Preukschas, M.; Sievert, H.; Jacobsen, C.; Shubina, L.K.; Gesell Salazar, M.; Scharf, C.; Walther, R.M.; et al. Honecker, Proteomic profiling of germ cell cancer cells treated with aaptamine, a marine alkaloid with anti proliferative activity. *J. Proteome Res.* **2012**, *11*, 2316–2330. [CrossRef] [PubMed]
57. Dyshlovoy, S.A.; Venz, S.; Shubina, L.K.; Fedorov, S.N.; Walther, R.; Jacobsen, C.; Stonik, V.A.; Bokemeyer, C.; Balabanov, S.; Honecker, F. Activity of aaptamine and two derivatives, demethyloxyaaptamine and isoaaptamine, in cisplatin-resistant germ cell cancer. *J. Proteom.* **2014**, *96*, 223–239. [CrossRef] [PubMed]
58. Dyshlovoy, S.A.; Venz, S.; Hauschild, J.; Tabakmakher, K.M.; Otte, K.; Madanchi, R.; Walther, R.; Guzii, A.G.; Makarieva, T.N.; Shubina, L.K.; et al. Amsberg, Anti-migratory activity of marine alkaloid monanchocidin A—Proteomics-based discovery and confirmation. *Proteomics* **2016**, *16*, 1590–1603. [CrossRef]
59. Dyshlovoy, S.; Rast, S.; Hauschild, J.; Otte, K.; Alsdorf, W.; Madanchi, R.; Kalinin, V.; Silchenko, A.; Avilov, S.; Dierlamm, J.; et al. Frondoside A induces AIF-associated caspase-independent apoptosis in Burkitt's lymphoma cells. *Leuk. Lymphoma* **2017**, *58*, 2905–2915. [CrossRef]

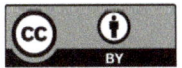 © 2020 by the authors. Licensee MDPI, Basel, Switzerland. This article is an open access article distributed under the terms and conditions of the Creative Commons Attribution (CC BY) license (http://creativecommons.org/licenses/by/4.0/).

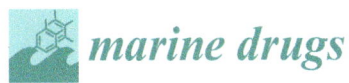

Article

Synthesis, Cytotoxic Activity Evaluation and Quantitative Structure-Activity Analysis of Substituted 5,8-Dihydroxy-1,4-Naphthoquinones and their *O*- and *S*-Glycoside Derivatives Tested against Neuro-2a Cancer Cells

Sergey Polonik [1,†], Galina Likhatskaya [1,†], Yuri Sabutski [1], Dmitry Pelageev [1,2], Vladimir Denisenko [1], Evgeny Pislyagin [1], Ekaterina Chingizova [1], Ekaterina Menchinskaya [1] and Dmitry Aminin [1,3,*]

1. G.B. Elyakov Pacific Institute of Bioorganic Chemistry of Far Eastern Branch of Russian Academy of Sciences, Prospekt 100-let Vladivostoku, 159, 690022 Vladivostok, Russia; sergpol@piboc.dvo.ru (S.P.); galin56@mail.ru (G.L.); alixar2006@gmail.com (Y.S.); pelageev@piboc.dvo.ru (D.P.); vladenis@piboc.dvo.ru (V.D.); pislyagin@hotmail.com (E.P.); martyyas@mail.ru (E.C.); ekaterinamenchinskaya@gmail.com (E.M.)
2. School of Natural Sciences, Far Eastern Federal University, Sukhanova St. 8, 690091 Vladivostok, Russia
3. Department of Biomedical Science and Environmental Biology, Kaohsiung Medical University, 100, Shih-Chuan 1st Road, Kaohsiung 80708, Taiwan
* Correspondence: daminin@piboc.dvo.ru; Tel.: +7-423-233-9932
† Equal contribution.

Received: 4 November 2020; Accepted: 24 November 2020; Published: 29 November 2020

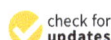

Abstract: Based on 6,7-substituted 2,5,8-trihydroxy-1,4-naphtoquinones (1,4-NQs) derived from sea urchins, five new acetyl-*O*-glucosides of NQs were prepared. A new method of conjugation of per-*O*-acetylated 1-mercaptosaccharides with 2-hydroxy-1,4-NQs through a methylene spacer was developed. Methylation of 2-hydroxy group of quinone core of acetylthiomethylglycosides by diazomethane and deacetylation of sugar moiety led to 28 new thiomethylglycosidesof 2-hydroxy- and 2-methoxy-1,4-NQs. The cytotoxic activity of starting 1,4-NQs (13 compounds) and their *O*- and *S*-glycoside derivatives (37 compounds) was determined by the MTT method against Neuro-2a mouse neuroblastoma cells. Cytotoxic compounds with EC_{50} = 2.7–87.0 µM and nontoxic compounds with EC_{50} > 100 µM were found. Acetylated *O*- and *S*-glycosides 1,4-NQs were the most potent, with EC_{50} = 2.7–16.4 µM. Methylation of the 2-OH group innaphthoquinone core led to a sharp increase in the cytotoxic activity of acetylated thioglycosidesof NQs, which was partially retained for their deacetylated derivatives. Thiomethylglycosides of 2-hydroxy-1,4-NQs with OH and MeO groups in quinone core at positions 6 and 7, respectively formed a nontoxic set of compounds with EC_{50} > 100 µM. A quantitative structure-activity relationship (QSAR) model of cytotoxic activity of 22 1,4-NQ derivatives was constructed and tested. Descriptors related to the cytotoxic activity of new 1,4-NQ derivatives were determined. The QSAR model is good at predicting the activity of 1,4-NQ derivatives which are unused for QSAR models and nontoxic derivatives.

Keywords: neuroblastoma Neuro-2a cells; 5,8-dihydroxy-1,4-naphthoquinone; *O*-glucoside; thiomethylglycoside; cytotoxic activity; QSAR

1. Introduction

Cancer is one of the leading causes of death worldwide. Brain cancer is considered one of the most insidious forms of cancer. This disease is characterized by a poor prognosis and a high rate of relapses, leading to high mortality [1]. Standard antitumor therapy procedures, including surgery, radiotherapy or chemotherapy, are ofteninineffective. The removal of tumors by surgery is often impossible or difficult due to the anatomical location of the tumor and its proximity to the vital structure of the brain. Surgical excision or radiotherapy can damage these areas and disrupt the functioning of the brain. In the case of medicamentous therapy, the patient requires large doses of antitumor drugs to overcome the blood-brain barrier [2]. This, in turn, leads to an increase in the toxicity of drugs and the appearance of undesirable side effects. In this regard, considerable attention is currently being paid to the search for new antitumor compounds that can easily penetrate into the brain tissue and purposefully suppress malignant neoplasms [3,4].

Widely distributed in nature, 1,4-Napthoquinones (1,4-NQs) occur in plants, echinodermsand microorganisms [5]. The diverse activity of 1,4-NQs, from antibacterial to antitumor [6,7], makes them a promising platform inthe search of drug-leads and the designof new medicines. In various studies, 1,4-NQs and their derivatives have been tested for activity against different cancer cell lines such as colon adenocarcinoma, breast ductal carcinoma, chronic myelogenous leukemia, human cervical cancer HeLa, acute myeloid leukemia HL60, human breast cancer MCF-7 and MDA-MB-231, nonsmall cell lung cancer H1975, nasopharyngeal carcinoma HNE1, gastric cancer SG7901, human alveolar basal epithelial adenocarcinoma A549, mouse Leydig cell tumor I-10, and others, and have been shown to exhibit relatively high cytotoxic properties at micromolar concentrations [8]. Despite a fairly large number of studies on the cytotoxic effect of 1,4-NQs on various cancer cell lines aimed at elucidating the molecular mechanisms of their antitumor action, no investigations have been undertakento date on brain cancer cells.

Neuroblastoma is a common human malignant brain tumor, especially in children, that arises from the sympathetic nervous system. It is characterized by a variety of clinical features, including rapid tumor progression with long-term survival of less than 40% in spite of surgical interventions, chemotherapy, radiotherapy and biotherapy approaches [9]. The neuro-2a cell line originates from mouse brain tumor cells, and is one of the most convenient models for studying the anticancer effects of low-molecular compounds, as well as for the search for nontoxic substances to treat neurodegenerative disorders such as Alzheimer's and Parkinson's diseases. Neuro-2a cells are really neuronal cells that have neurites, and are even able to form some kinds of neural networks in vitro [10]. Thus, murine neuroblastoma Neuro-2a was selected as a model of human neuroblastoma and studied as part of the search for effective cytotoxic compounds to treat brain cancer.

An attractive group of natural 1,4-naphthoquinones are spinochromes, i.e., the pigments of echinoderms with naphthazarin **1** (5,8-dihydroxy-1,4-naphthoquinone) core [5,11]. Natural hydroxylated naphthazarins from echinoderms and plants are presented in Figure 1.

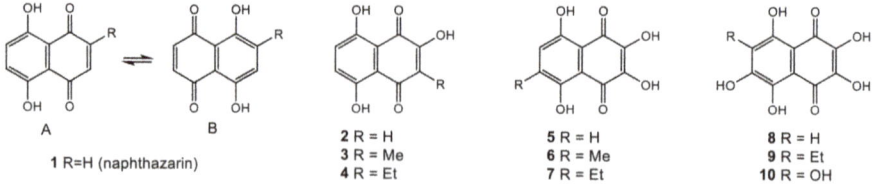

Figure 1. Natural hydroxynaphthazarins: **1,3,4**: naphthazarins from terrestrial plants; **2,5–10**: from sea urchins.

Hydroxynaphthazarins demonstrated various biological activities, such as antimicrobial [11], antialgae [12], cardioprotective [13,14] and antioxidant [15]. Methoxylated naphthazarins, as well as other polymethoxylated natural and semisynthetic compounds with aromatic cores, are an attractive model for the design of new anticancer agents [16]. For example, natural 2,3,6-trimethoxynaphthazarin (tricrozarin B) inhibited HeLa S_3 cell colony formation with an IC_{50} of 0.007 µg/mL [17]. Most available sea urchin pigment echinochrome **9** is used for the treatment of ischemia, myocardial infarction, traumas and burns tothe eyes [13], as well as intraocular hemorrhages, various degenerative processes and inflammation of the eye [18]. Additionally, 5,8-dihydroxy-1,4-naphthoquinone derivatives exist in various tautomeric forms, which react with the formation of different reaction products [19] (Figure 1). The tautomeric equilibrium in the naphthazarin core depends on the nature of the substituent in core, the pH, and the reaction medium properties [20]. Recently, the ability of echinochrome to enhance mitochondrial biogenesis in cardiac [21] and skeletal muscles [22] was revealed. Echinochrome demonstrated a potential toimprove the musculoskeletal system and lipid and protein metabolism in both types of diabetes mellitus [23]. It is assumed that echinochrome activity is due to the ability of β-hydroxyl groups to inhibit radical reactions and chelatethe transition metal anions that are responsible for the initiation of free-radical oxidation in biological systems [24,25].

To improve their solubility and achieve atargeted action, naphthoquinones can easily be converted into *O*- and *S*-glycosides [26] or nonglycoside *O*- and *S*-carbohydrate conjugates with promising cytotoxic activity and selectivity [27–29]. Well-developed methods of chemical transformation of NQs and their biological activities have led to a number of works describing quantitative structure–activity relationship (QSAR)analyses of the cytotoxicity of NQs with various structures. The effect of substituents on the bioactivity of new NQ derivatives may be predicted using the obtained QSAR models [30–36].

In this study, in continuation of our drug development project, we synthesized a batch of five new NQ *O*-glycosides derived from hydroxynaphthazarins related to sea urchin pigments. The *O*-glycosidic bond attached to the quinone ring waschemically reactive and could easily be substituted under basic conditions [37], or degraded in vivo via enzyme-catalyzed hydrolysis with the release of bioactive 1,4-naphthoquinone moiety. It is known that thioglycosides are stable to acidic and basic hydrolysis and do not undergo enzymatic degradation [38]. In order to prepare NQ-sugar derivatives which were resistant to enzyme-mediated degradation, we developed a new synthetic method and synthesized thiomethyl conjugates of 1-mercaptosaccharides with NQs. In this type of naphthoquinone-thioglycoside derivative, 1-thiosugars were attached to the quinone nucleus through a methylene spacer which blocked the conjugation of sulfur atom π-orbitals with the quinone core and, therefore, did not affects its red-ox properties. The set of new NQ thiomethylglycosides and their acetyl and 2-methoxy derivatives (28 compounds) were designed and prepared. The cytotoxic activity both newly-prepared and stocked collections of NQs was determined on a model of mouse neuroblastoma Neuro-2a cancer cells. In order to evaluate the effects of chemical modifications on the cytotoxicity of a naphthazarin skeleton, a QSAR analysis was done. A QSAR model of the cytotoxic activity of 22 1,4-NQ derivatives was constructed and tested. Descriptors were determined to be related to the cytotoxic activity of the new 1,4-NQ derivatives.

2. Results

2.1. Synthesis of the O-Glucosides of Substituted Naphthazarins

In our previous research, we converted sea urchin pigments hydroxynaphthazarin **2**, spinazarin **5** and echinochrome **9** to related acetylated *mono*-, *bis*- and *tris*O-glucosides **12**, **13** and **14** by condensation with 3,4,6-tri-*O*-acetyl-α-D-glucopyranose 1,2-(*tert*-butoxy orthoacetate) **11** [39]. It was found that *tris* acetyl-*O*-glucoside of echinochrome (U-133) **14** possessed antitumor activity in vivo [40]. Treatment of acetylglucosides **12**–**14** with MeONa/MeOH led to deacetylated polar *O*-glucosides **15**–**17**, which were moderately soluble in water. It was found that the stability of glucosides **15**–**17** decreased significantly with thenumber of glucoside moieties attached to the naphthazarin core. So, if the water solution of naphthopurpurin monoglucoside **15** was stable for several days, spinazarin *bis*-*O*-glucoside **16** was stable for a day, while echinochrome *tris*O-glucoside **17** quickly decomposed after dissolution with the loss of the glucoside portions [39] (Figure 2). Taking into account the instability of deacetylated glucosides, further studies on the biological activity of stable acetyl-*O*-glycoside derivatives were performed, mainly on acetyl tris-*O*-glucoside echinochrome **14** (U-133). It was shown that U-133 exhibited pronounced antitumor activity in vivo in the model mouse Ehrlich carcinoma cells [40], and also that it has therapeutic potential for the prevention and/or deceleration of Parkinson's-like neurodegeneration [41,42].

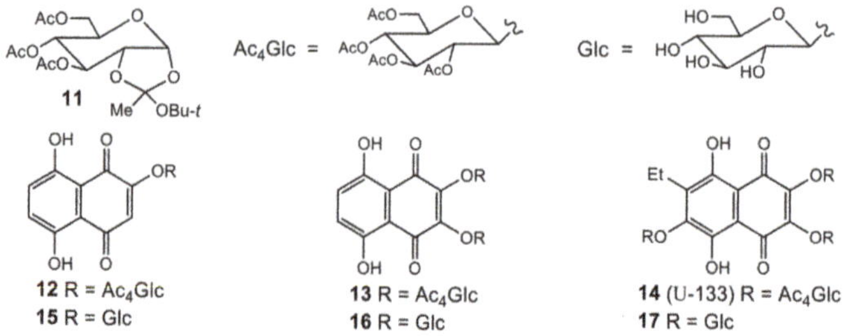

Figure 2. 3,4,6-Tri-O-acetyl-α-D-glucopyranose 1,2-(*tert*-butoxy orthoacetate) 11 and related hydroxynaphthazarin O-glucosides 12–17.

2.2. Design and Synthesis of Simplified O-Glucoside Analogues of (U-133)

In order to find more effective derivatives derived from natural naphthazarins 3, 4 and 6, 7, we created a new set of mono- and bis acetyl-O-glucoside derivatives 18–21, which were more accessible simplified analogues of echinochrome trisglucoside (U-133) 14 (Figure 3). The synthetic 2-hydroxy-6,7-dimethylnaphthazarin 22 and its O-acetylglucoside derivative 23 were added to that set for comparison with isomeric quinones 4 and 19.

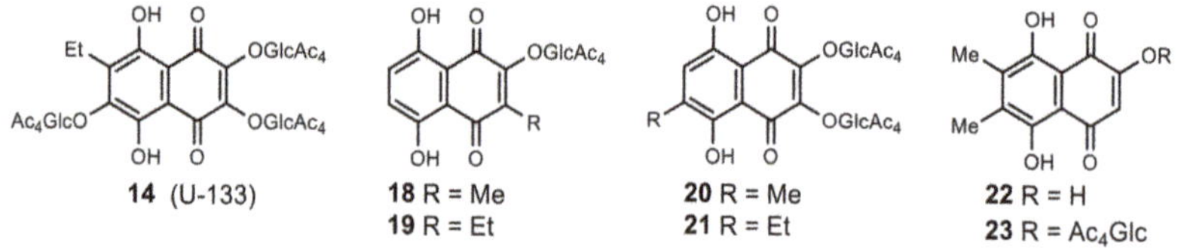

Figure 3. Acetylated tris-O-glucoside echinochrome 14 (U-133) and its simplified analogues 18–21 and 23.

The synthesis of naphthazarin O-glucosides 18–21, 23 was carried out by autocatalytic condensation of quinones 3, 4, 6, and 7 with the D-glucopyranose 1,2-(*tert*-butoxy orthoacetate) 11 in dry chlorobenzene at reflux in a ratio of 1 mol of D-glucopyranose 1,2-orthoacetate 11 per one quinone β-hydroxy group as earlier for glucosides 12, 13 and 14 [39]. In this autocatalytic variant, the activation of 1,2-orthoacetate 11 was achieved through catalysis of the acidic proton β-hydroxyl group of quinone. The reaction proceeded stereospecifically within 0.3–0.5 h and resulted in acetylated β-D-glucopyranosides 18–21, 23 in yields of 60–85%.

2.3. Design and Synthesis of Thiomethylglycoside Derivatives of 6,7-Substituted 2-Hydroxynaphthazarines

The above-mentioned instability of hydroxynaphthazarin O-glucosides 15–17 prompted us to synthesize more stable thioglycoside conjugates with a naphthazarin core. Using the tetra-O-acetyl-1-mercapto-D-glucose 27 as a thiol component, and a collection of substituted naphthazarins 2, 22, 24–26 available in our laboratory, we developed a new method for thiomethylation of 6,7-substituted 2,5,8-trihydroxy-1,4-naphthoquinones with acetylthioglucose 27 and produced the corresponding acetylated thiomethylglucosides 28–32 in 63–85% yields with bisnaphthoquinone methanes 33–37 as minor byproducts (yields 8–12%) (Scheme 1).

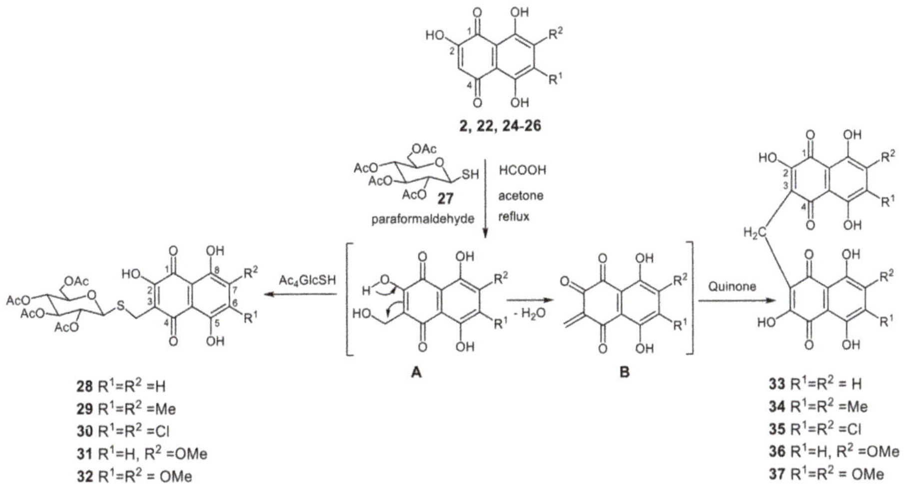

Scheme 1. Acid-catalyzed condensation of tetra-O-acetyl-1-mercapto-D-glucose **27** with 6,7-substituted 2-hydroxynaphthazarines **2, 22, 24–26** and paraformaldehyde.

The acetylthioglucosides **28–32** were readily deacetylated under treatment in MeOH/HCl solution, and resulted in polar hydrophilic thioglucosides **38–42** in good yields, i.e., 75–85% (Scheme 2). The methylation of 2-hydroxy derivatives **28–32** with diazomethane solution gave the corresponding 2-methoxyderivatives **43–47** in yields of 85–95%. The subsequent deacetylation 2-methoxyacetylderivatives **43–47** in MeOH/HCl solution led to a new set of polar 2-methoxythiomethylglucosides **48–52** (Scheme 2).

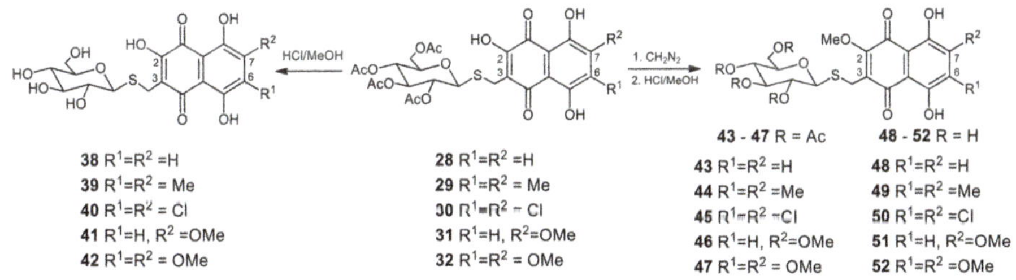

Scheme 2. Synthesis of thiomethylglucosides **38–52**.

Inspired by the unique activity of echinochrome, a set of structurally-related thiomethylglycoside derivatives was formed using sea urchin pigment spinochrome D **8** (Figure 4). The free position in the core of this quinone allowed us to introduce various thiomethyl radicals with D-glucose, D-galactose, D-mannose and D-xylose moiety and obtainnew, stable lipophilic thioglycosides **56–59**, bearing three β-hydroxyl groups in the naphthazarin core, which were responsible for the antioxidant properties (Figure 4). The deacetylation of acetylglucoside **56** in HCl/MeOH solution proceeded with the opening of the glucose ring and the formation of an unseparated impurity of isomeric furanoside derivatives. The effective deacetylation of the thioglycosides **56–59** was achieved by treatment in MeONa/MeOH solution in argon atmosphere, and resulted in hydrophilic polar thiomethylglycosides **60–63** in good yields 59–72%. The structures of the new compounds were determined by NMR, IR spectroscopy and HR mass spectrometry. The β-configuration of the glucosidic bond was confirmed by the value of the signal of anomeric carbon C-1' that variedbetween 82.4–83.8 ppm for acetylderivatives **56–59** and 85.2–86.5 ppm for glycosides **60–63**.

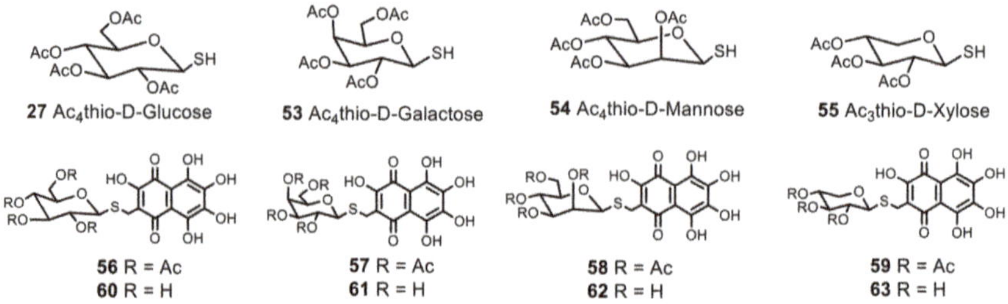

Figure 4. Per-O-acetyl-1-mercaptoderivatives of D-glucose **27**, D-galactose **53**, D-mannose **54**, D-xylose **55** and thiomethyl glycosides **56–63** derived from spinochrome D **8**.

2.4. Cytotoxic Activity of 5,8-dihydroxy-1,4-naphthoquinone Derivatives

The cytotoxic activity of naphthazarins from terrestrial plants **1,3,4**, sea urchin pigments **2,5–9**, their synthetic intermediates **22, 24–26**, O-glucoside derivatives **12–21, 23** and thiomethylglucosides of substituted nahtazarins **28–52** was assessed on mouse Neuro-2a cancer cells. The obtained results are presented in Table 1. Other thiomethylglycosidic derivatives **56–63** (Figure 4) derived from spinochrome D were also tested on Neuro-2a cancer cells. Both acetylated and free carbohydrate spinochrome D derivatives **56–63** were nontoxic at concentrations $EC_{50} > 100$ μM, and formed the group of new, nontoxic analogues of echinochrome **9**.

Table 1. Cytotoxic activity * (EC_{50}, μM) of substituted 5,8-dihydroxy-1,4-naphthoquinones and their O- and S-glycoside derivatives tested against mouse Neuro-2a cancer cells.

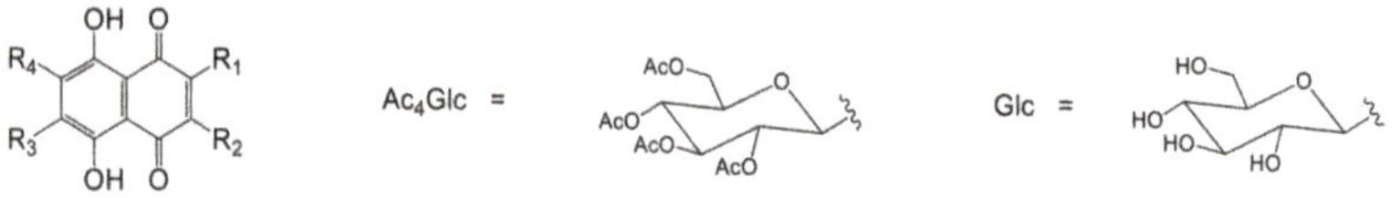

Compound	Code PIBOC	R_1	R_2	R_3	R_4	EC_{50}, μM
1	U-193	H	H	H	H	>100
2	U-139	HO	H	H	H	>100
3	U-574	HO	Me	H	H	>100
4	U-575	HO	Et	H	H	>100
5	U-134	HO	HO	H	H	>100
6	U-572	HO	HO	Me	H	>100
7	U-573	HO	HO	Et	H	>100
8	U-504	HO	HO	HO	H	>100
9	U-138	HO	HO	HO	Et	>100
12	U-127	Ac₄GlcO	H	H	H	16.43 ± 4.01
13	U-136	Ac₄GlcO	Ac₄GlcO	H	H	10.60 ± 0.63
14	U-133	Ac₄GlcO	Ac₄GlcO	Ac₄GlcO	Et	8.45 ± 1.13
15	U-132	GlcO	H	H	H	87.40 ± 2.37
18	U-444	Ac₄GlcO	Me	H	H	5.33 ± 0.73
19	U-443	Ac₄GlcO	Et	H	H	4.46 ± 0.23
20	U-420	Ac₄GlcO	Ac₄GlcO	Me	H	4.46 ± 0.56
21	U-421	Ac₄GlcO	Ac₄GlcO	Et	H	8.84 ± 0.98
22	U-434	HO	H	Me	Me	82.75 ± 4.36
23	U-330	Ac₄GlcO	H	Me	Me	9.43 ± 0.25
24	U-195	HO	H	Cl	Cl	23.10 ± 1.01
25	U-622	HO	H	H	MeO	>100
26	U-623	HO	H	MeO	MeO	>100
28	U-633	HO	Ac₄GlcSCH₂	H	H	>100
29	U-519	HO	Ac₄GlcSCH₂	Me	Me	84.00 ± 0.48

Table 1. Cont.

Compound	Code PIBOC	R_1	R_2	R_3	R_4	EC_{50}, µM
30	U-518	HO	Ac$_4$GlcSCH$_2$	Cl	Cl	32.20 ± 4.05
31	U-639	HO	Ac$_4$GlcSCH$_2$	H	MeO	>100
32	U-637	HO	Ac$_4$GlcSCH$_2$	MeO	MeO	>100
38	U-635	HO	GlcSCH$_2$	H	H	>100
39	U-520	HO	GlcSCH$_2$	Me	Me	>100
40	U-624	HO	GlcSCH$_2$	Cl	Cl	>100
41	U-644	HO	GlcSCH$_2$	H	MeO	>100
42	U-640	HO	GlcSCH$_2$	MeO	MeO	>100
43	U-634	MeO	Ac$_4$GlcSCH$_2$	H	H	2.72 ± 0.21
44	U-521	MeO	Ac$_4$GlcSCH$_2$	Me	Me	>100
45	U-523	MeO	Ac$_4$GlcSCH$_2$	Cl	Cl	3.14 ± 0.66
46	U-645	MeO	Ac$_4$GlcSCH$_2$	H	MeO	11.61 ± 2.34
47	U-638	MeO	Ac$_4$GlcSCH$_2$	MeO	MeO	11.05 ± 0.14
48	U-636	MeO	GlcSCH$_2$	H	H	19.02 ± 0.11
49	U-522	MeO	GlcSCH$_2$	Me	Me	11.47 ± 0.48
50	U-625	MeO	GlcSCH$_2$	Cl	Cl	38.02 ± 1.14
51	U-646	MeO	GlcSCH$_2$	H	MeO	80.76 ± 1.70
52	U-641	MeO	GlcSCH$_2$	MeO	MeO	61.60 ± 2.90
Cladoloside C						11.92 ± 0.45

* Cytotoxic activity evaluation with MTT reagent; data is expressed as mean ± SEM (n = 3).

To this end, Neuro-2a cells were cultured in the presence of compounds for 24 h. Determination of cell viability in the presence of various concentrations of 5,8-dihydroxy-1,4-NQs derivatives was carried out by the MTT method followed by spectrophotometry. As a result, for each of the 50 studied compounds, the values of the half-maximum effective concentration which suppressed cell viability by 50% relative to control intact cells (EC_{50}) were established (Figure 5A–F). The values of the obtained EC_{50} are presented in Table 1. Thus, for each compound, the range of cytotoxic concentrations and the EC_{50} were determined, which allowed us to further study the dependence of the biological activity of 5,8-dihydroxy-1,4-NQs derivatives on their chemical structure.

Based on the obtained EC_{50} values, all tested compounds could be conditionally divided into four groups: (a) high toxicity ($EC_{50} \leq 5$ µM); (b) moderate toxicity (EC_{50} = 5–30 µM); (c) low toxicity (EC_{50} = 30–90 µM); (d) nontoxic (EC_{50} > 100 µM). Nontoxic compounds accounted for the majority (56%) of all tested compounds; low toxicity compounds comprised 14%; moderate toxicity comprised 20% and highly toxic compounds accounted for 10% (Figure 5G, Table 1).

The results of previous studies using the QSAR method to analyze the cytotoxic activity of naphthoquinones showed that the cytotoxic activity of compounds depends on the type of cells and structural features of naphthoquinones. Thus, the effectiveness of 1,4-NQs on lung, liver and lymphocytic leukemia tumor cells depends not only on the applied concentration, but also on the type of tumor and the type of cells isolated from these tumors [8]. Currently, data on cytotoxic activity against nerve and brain cells are not available in the literature.

The aim of this study was to investigate the quantitative structure-activity relationship for naphthazarin derivative cytotoxic activity against Neuro-2a mouse neuroblastoma cells. In this study, the cytotoxic activity of 22 naphthoquinones was measured and used to build a QSAR model to determine the relationship between the naphthoquinone structure and cytotoxic activity.

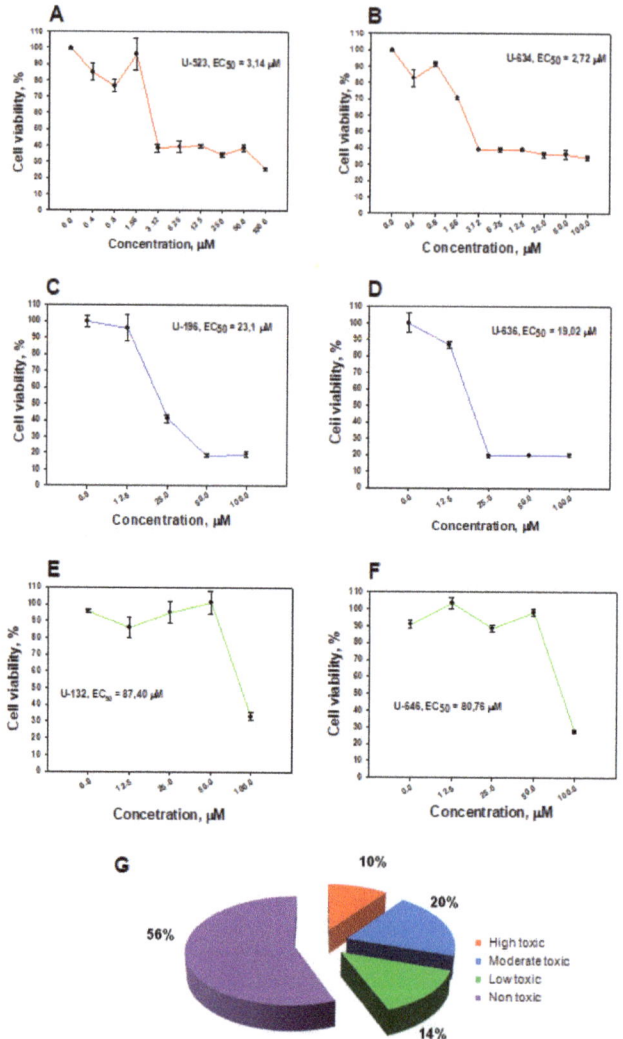

Figure 5. Cytotoxic activity of 5,8-dihydroxy-1,4-naphthoquinone derivatives on mouse Neuro-2a cells. Dose-dependent representative curves of cytotoxic action of some studied 5,8-dihydroxy-1,4-naphthoquinone derivatives on Neuro-2a mouse neuroblastoma cells: high toxic compounds (**A,B**); moderate toxic compounds (**C,D**); low toxic compounds (**E,F**). Ratio of tested cytotoxic and nontoxic 1,4-NQs (**G**).

2.4.1. Data Set Preparation and Descriptor Calculation

In the present study, a dataset of 50 1,4-NQs derivatives (Table 1, Figure 4) was used for 3D-structure modeling and optimization with Amber10:EHT force field using the Build module of the MOE 2019.01 program. The MOE database of the energy minimized 3D-structures of 50 1,4-NQs derivatives was used for descriptor calculation with the QuaSAR module of MOE 2019.01. The EC_{50} values were converted into corresponding pEC_{50} values ($-logEC_{50}$) to be included in the database. The pEC_{50} values determined in this work for 22 selected cytotoxic compounds with $4 < pEC_{50} < 6$ were added to the database with the 3D structures of the studied compounds. The dataset of the 22 1,4-NQs derivatives with $4 < pEC_{50} < 6$ was divided into training (18) and test (4) sets, which were used for the generation of a QSAR model and its validation, respectively.

2.4.2. QSAR Models Generation and Validation

A QSAR analysis was performed on a data set of 22 molecules with $4 < pEC_{50} < 6$. The data set was randomly divided into a training set and a test set. The training set was initially used to build the model, and the test set was used to evaluate the prediction. The 320 descriptors were calculated using the MOE QuaSAR-Model module for each molecule in the data sets. The calculated descriptors were initially screened using the QuaSAR-Contingency module of MOE, which is a statistical application designed to assist in the selection of descriptors for QSAR. Only 57 molecular descriptors were selected among the 320 used descriptors after analysis of the training set (18 compounds) by the QuaSAR-Contingency module. The QuaSAR-Model module in MOE was used to generate the QSAR models with the partial least square (PLS) method. An analysis of the models using the QuaSAR-Model report made it possible to select a smaller number of the most important molecular descriptors and to obtain models with a smaller number of descriptors. The descriptors having an effect on the performance of prediction of cytotoxic activity 1,4-NQs with QSAR models and used for QSAR models generation are described in Table 2.

Table 2. Description of the 12 molecular descriptors used for QSAR models generation.

Class	Code	Description
2D	SMR_VSA0	Molecular refractivity (including implicit hydrogens). This property is an atomic contribution that assumes the correct protonation state (washed structures). Sum of vi such that Ri is in [0,0.11].
2D	SlogP_VSA2	Log of the octanol/water partition coefficient (including implicit hydrogens). This property is an atomic contribution model that calculates logP from the given structure; i.e., the correct protonation state). Sum of vi such that Li is in (−0.2,0].
2D	vsa_acc	Approximation to the sum of VDW surface areas (Å2) of pure hydrogen bond acceptors (not counting atoms that are both hydrogen bond donors and acceptors such as −OH).
2D	vsa_hyd	Approximation to the sum of VDW surface areas of hydrophobic atoms (Å2).
2D	Q_VSA_HYD	Total hydrophobic van der Waals surface area. This is the sum of the v_i such that $|q_i|$ is less than or equal to 0.2. The v_i are calculated using a connection table approximation.
2D	PEOE_VSA_HYD	Total hydrophobic van der Waals surface area. This is the sum of the v_i such that $|q_i|$ is less than or equal to 0.2. The v_i are calculated using a connection table approximation.
2D	PEOE_VSA_PNEG	Total negative polar van der Waals surface area. This is the sum of the vi such that qi is less than −0.2. The vi are calculated using a connection table approximation.
2D	PEOE_VSA_POL	Total polar van der Waals surface area. This is the sum of the vi such that $|q_i|$ is greater than 0.2. The vi are calculated using a connection table approximation.
2D	PEOE_VSA_POS	Total positive van der Waals surface area. This is the sum of the vi such that qi is non-negative. The vi are calculated using a connection table approximation.
i3D	ASA	Water accessible surface area calculated using a radius of 1.4 A for the water molecule. A polyhedral representation is used for each atom in calculating the surface area.
i3D	ASA_H	Water accessible surface area of all hydrophobic ($|q_i| < 0.2$) atoms.
i3D	vsurf_S	Interaction field surface area

The QSAR models were constructed based on the 12 selected molecular descriptors using the QuaSAR-Model module in MOE 2019.01. The regression analysis of QuaSAR-Model was used to build the QSAR model using PLS for the training set (18 compounds) with a correlation coefficient ($R2$) of 0.9242 and a RMSE of 0.1285. The Z-score method was adopted for the detection of outliers; any compound with a Z-score value higher than 2.5 was considered an outlier. Compound **50** (U-625) was defined as an outlier. The QSAR model generated for the training set (17 compounds) without outlier **50** (U-625) had a correlation coefficient ($R2$) of 0.9579 and a RMSE of 0.0965 (Table 3, Figure 6). The obtained model was validated using cross-validation leave-one-out (LOO), leading to the calculation of cross-validated correlation coefficient, and used to predict the activities of the test data set in the external validation. The best QSAR model established using a training set consisting of 17 naphthoquinones and a test set of fournaphthoquinones was as follows:

$$pEC_{50} = 5.79098 \tag{1}$$
$$+0.03973 \text{ ASA} \tag{2}$$
$$-0.01013 \text{ ASA\_H} \tag{3}$$
$$-0.00227 \text{ PEOE\_VSA\_HYD} \tag{4}$$
$$-0.03175 \text{ PEOE\_VSA\_PNEG} \tag{5}$$
$$+0.02857 \text{ PEOE\_VSA\_POL} \tag{6}$$
$$-0.02663 \text{ PEOE\_VSA\_POS} \tag{7}$$
$$+0.01627 \text{ Q\_VSA\_HYD} \tag{8}$$
$$+0.01372 \text{ SlogP\_VSA2} \tag{9}$$
$$-0.03089 \text{ SMR\_VSA0} \tag{10}$$
$$+0.09770 \text{ vsa\_acc} \tag{11}$$
$$+0.03843 \text{ vsa\_hyd} \tag{12}$$
$$-0.05253 \text{ vsurf\_S} \tag{13}$$
$$R2 = 0.95786, \text{ RMSE} = 0.09650, \text{ PRED R2} = 0.9914 \tag{14}$$

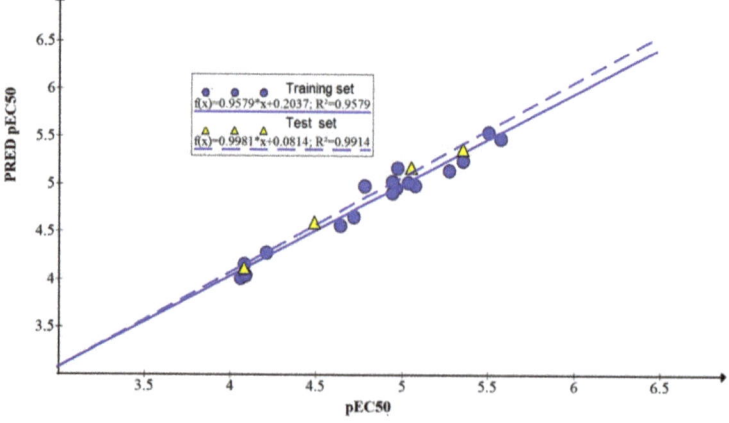

Figure 6. Predicted cytotoxic activity of 5,8-dihydroxy-1,4-naphthoquinone derivatives as a function of experimental values for Neuro-2a cell line.

Table 3. Comparison of the experimental pEC$_{50}$ values and the predicted activity values of the training and test sets of 5,8-dihydroxy-1,4-naphthoquinone derivatives according to the obtained QSAR model.

Compound	Code PIBOC	Data Set	pEC$_{50}$	PRED pEC$_{50}$	RES *
12	U-127	train	4.78	4.98	−0.20
15	U-132	train	4.06	4.01	0.05
14	U-133	train	5.07	4.98	0.09
13	U-136	train	4.97	5.16	−0.19
23	U-330	train	5.03	5.02	0.01
20	U-420	train	5.35	5.24	0.11
18	U-444	train	5.27	5.14	0.13
24	U-195	train	4.64	4.56	0.08
43	U-634	train	5.57	5.47	0.10
48	U-636	train	4.72	4.65	0.07
47	U-638	train	4.96	4.95	0.01
52	U-641	train	4.21	4.27	−0.06
46	U-645	train	4.94	4.90	0.04
51	U-646	train	4.09	4.04	0.05
29	U-519	train	4.07	4.04	−0.03
49	U-522	train	4.94	5.02	−0.08
45	U-523	train	5.50	5.54	−0.06
21	U-421	test	5.05	5.18	−0.13
19	U-443	test	5.35	5.37	−0.02
22	U-434	test	4.08	4.12	−0.04
30	U-518	test	4.49	4.59	−0.10
28	U-633	-	<4.00	4.08	-
9	U-138	-	<4.00	2.30	-
38	U-635	-	<4.00	3.39	-

*—RES = pEC$_{50}$ − PRED pEC$_{50}$.

The prediction correlation coefficient reached 0.9914, indicating that the model had better external prediction ability (Table 3, Figure 6).

An analysis of the relative importance of the 1,4-NQs QSAR model descriptors showed that the most important descriptors were the i3D descriptors vsurf_S (Interaction field surface area) and ASA (Water accessible surface area), compared to 2D descriptors (Figure 7). The activity 1,4-NQs increased with increasing of the sum of VDW surface areas of hydrophobic atoms (Å2) and of the sum of VDW surface areas (Å2) of pure hydrogen bond acceptors (not −OH). The other descriptors we used did not play such a significant role and had rather low values of relative importance of descriptors (RID) compared to ASA and vsurf_S (Figure 7). For example, in our experiments, it was found that the correlation coefficient pEC$_{50}$ from SlogP_VSA2 amounted to R2 = 0.2353 (data not shown), and the RID value for the SlogP_VSA2 descriptor, describing the octanol/water partition coefficient of the molecules, was rather low (RID = 0.154369, Figure 7).

The QSAR model was used to predict the activities of the test data set in the external validation. An analysis of the quality of the model using the QuaSAR module of the MOE 2019.01 program showed that the experimentally determined pEC$_{50}$ values of 5,8-dihydroxy-1,4-NQ derivatives correlated with those calculated by the program. The validation of the QSAR model showed that the QSAR model effectively predicted the activity of 1,4-NQs test set of **19** (U-443), **21** (U-421), **22** (U-434), **30** (U-518) (Table 3, Figure 6). The model correctly predicted the activities of compounds **9** (U-138) and **38** (U-635), for which pEC$_{50}$ < 4 (Table 3).

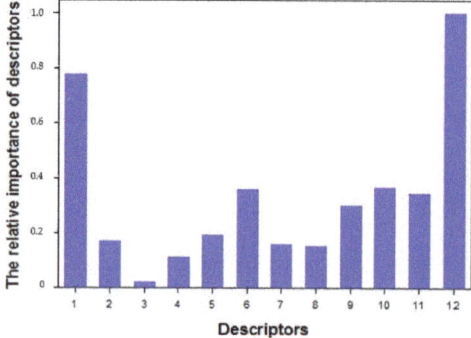

#	Descriptor	RID
1	ASA	0.778351
2	ASA_H	0.172114
3	PEOE_VSA_HYD	0.023157
4	PEOE_VSA_PNEG	0.115116
5	PEOE_VSA_POL	0.192644
6	PEOE_VSA_POS	0.360916
7	Q_VSA_HYD	0.160785
8	SlogP_VSA2	0.154369
9	SMR_VSA0	0.300893
10	vsa_acc	0.365973
11	vsa_hyd	0.345058
12	vsurf_S	1.000000

Figure 7. The relative importance of descriptors (RID) used for QSAR model of cytotoxic activity of 5,8-dihydroxy-1,4-NQ derivatives.

It was found that the introduction of acetylated O-glucose into the structure of positions C-2, (C-2 and C-3), (C-2, C-3 and C-7) led to the appearance of a moderate cytotoxic activity (5–30 µM). An increase in cytotoxicity highly correlated with an increase in the total size of molecules and the surface area of hydrophobic atoms of these molecules. The ASA_H descriptor values describing the water accessible surface area of all hydrophobic atoms in the series of compounds **2** (U-139), **12** (U-127), **13** (U-136) and **14** (U-133) varied within the range of 148.7 < 746.9 < 1083.2 < 1519.0 Å2, which corresponded to changes in cytotoxic activity (EC_{50}, µM) in the range > 100 > 16.4 > 10.6 > 8.4, respectively (Figure 8).

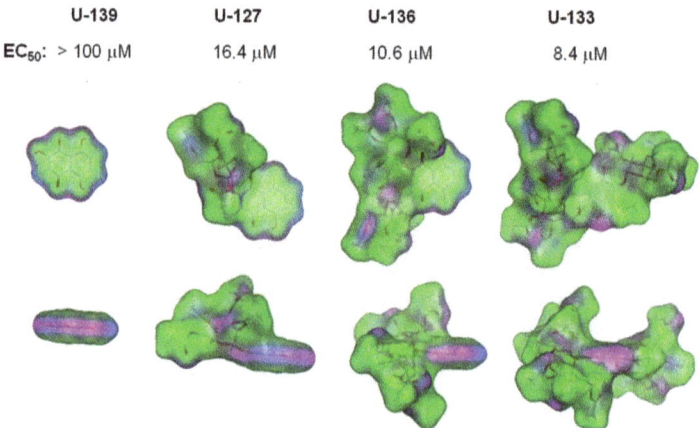

Figure 8. Molecular surface of 1,4-NQs of nontoxic **2** (U-139) and its derivatives of *mono-*, *di-* and *tris*-O-acetylglycosides: compounds **12** (U-127), **13** (U-136) and **14** (U-133), respectively. Molecular surface colors are pink (H-bonding), green (hydrophobic) and blue (mild polar).

To elucidate the structural elements of naphthoquinone molecules (pharmacophores) which determine high cytotoxic activity, a pharmacophore analysis of active 5,8-dihydroxy-1,4-NQ derivatives and their low-active analogues was carried out. An analysis of pharmacophores showed that an important role in the toxicity of naphthoquinone compounds is played by the carbohydrate component with hydrophobic functional groups (AcO-) for both O- and S-glycosides. The introduction of a hydrophilic hydroxy group at C-2, instead of hydrophobic methoxy, reduced the cytotoxic activity, even in the presence of a hydrophobic carbohydrate component (Figure 9).

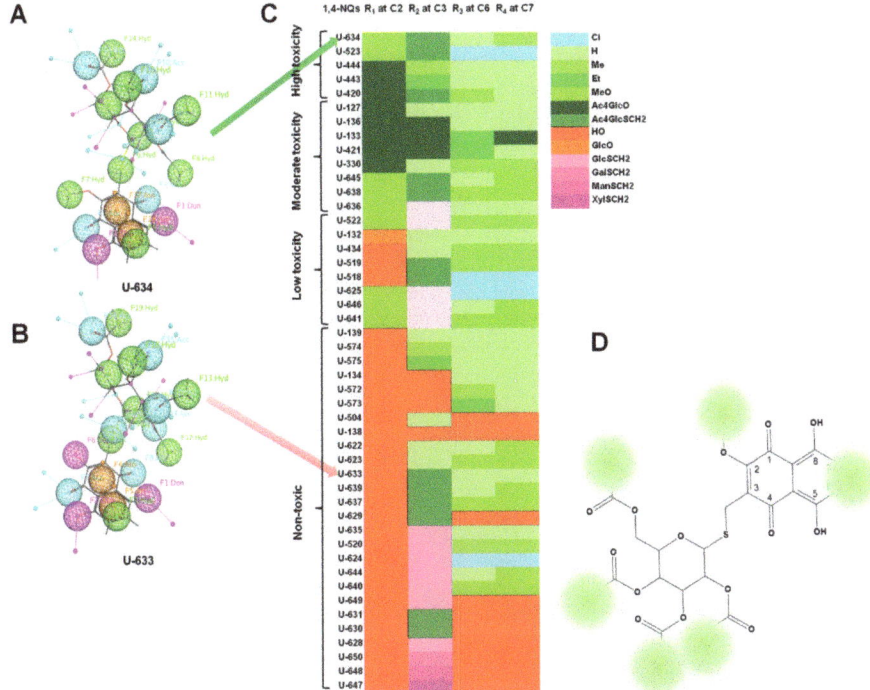

Figure 9. The structure of the pharmacophores of high toxic **43** (U-634) and nontoxic **28** (U-633) compounds. A pharmacophore annotation scheme: Hyd—hydrophobe (green), Acc—H-bond acceptor (turquoise), Don—H-bond donor (pink), Aro—aromatic (orange) (**A**,**B**); a heat map of high, moderate, low toxic and nontoxic compounds describing the contribution of substituent compositions of 1,4-NQ main core to the cytotoxic activity (**C**); structure of S-glycoside of 1,4-NQ pharmacophore where the green spots indicate hydrophobic substituent positions required for high cytotoxicity (**D**).

The substituents at C-2 played a key role in the manifestation of the cytotoxic activity of the naphthazarin derivatives. Derivatives with a 2-methoxy group or acetylated monosaccharide at the C-2 position exhibited cytotoxic activity, while all derivatives with a 2-hydroxy group were nontoxic (Figure 9).

3. Discussion

The starting naphthazarin **1** and its natural hydroxy- and methoxyderivatives **2–9,25,26** were nontoxic at concentrations > 100 µM, while synthetic 6,7-dimethyl- and 6,7-dichloro derivatives **22** and **24** showed moderate toxicity with EC_{50} of 82.75 ± 4.36 and 23.10 ± 1.01 µM, respectively. Conversion hydroxynaphthazarins **2–7,9,22** into respective O-glucosides led to cytotoxic NQ *mono*, *bis* and *tris* acetyl O-glucosides **12–14,18–21, 23** with EC_{50} = 1.46–16.43 µM. Significant differences in the cytotoxicity of *mono*, *bis* and *tris* acetyl O-glycosides were not observed. The EC_{50} values varied mainly in the range of 4.46–10.60 µM, excluding acetylglucoside **12**. Deacetylation of acetyl monoglycoside **12** (EC_{50} = 16.43 ± 4.01 µM) led to polar low toxic O-glucoside derivative **15** (EC_{50} = 87.40 ± 2.37 µM).

The instability of hydroxynaphthazarin O-glucosides prompted us to synthesize stable S-glycoside derivatives. We developed a new method of conjugation of per-O-acetyl-1-mercaptosaccharides D-glucose, D-galactose, D-mannose and D-xylose with 6,7-substituted 2,5,8-trihydroxy-1,4-naphthoquinones and paraformaldehyde through the use of a methylene spacer and produced corresponding acetylated thiomethylglycosides in 63–85% yields. Acetylated thiomethylglucosides 2,5,8-trihydroxy-1,4-NQs **28–32**, **56–59** were not toxic ($EC_{50} > 100$ µM), excluding acetylglucosides **29** ($EC_{50} = 84.00 \pm 0.48$ µM) and **30** ($EC_{50} = 32.20 \pm 4.05$ µM) bearing Me groups and chlorine atoms at positions 6 and 7. After deacetylation of quinones **28–32** and **56–59**, we obtained nontoxic thiomethyl glycosides **38–42** and **60–63**, including compounds bearing methyl groups and chlorine atoms in the quinoid nucleus. The conversion of the 2-hydroxy group of the quinone core to methoxyl led to asharp increase in the cytotoxicity of acetylatedthioglucosides of 2-MeO-1,4-NQs **43**, **45–47** with $EC_{50} = 2.72–11.61$ µM, excluding acetylglucoside **44** ($EC_{50} > 100$ µM), which was partially retained for their deacetylated derivatives **47–52**. All acetylated and deacetylated 2-hydroxy-1,4-NQ thioglycoside conjugates **31–32**, **41–42**, **56–63** with OH and MeO groups at positions 6 and 7 of the naphthoquinone core formed a nontoxic set of compounds with $EC_{50} > 100$ µM.

In our previous study, a series of new, tetracyclic oxathiine-fused quinone-thioglycoside conjugates based on biologically active 1,4-naphthoquinones (chloro-, hydroxy-, and methoxysubstituted) was synthesized and characterized. These compounds showed relatively high cytotoxic activity toward various types of cancer cells such as HeLa, Neuro-2a and mouse ascites Ehrlich carcinoma, and mouse normal epithelial cell line Jb6 Cl 41-5a without pronounced selectivity for a certain type of tumor cells [29]. The positive effect of heterocyclization with mercaptosugars on cytotoxic activity for a group of 1,4-naphthoquinones was observed. The effect of chloro-, hydroxy-, and metoxysubstituents on teracycles activity was also studied, and a significant effect of the hydroxy group on activity was shown. The results of the presented work concerning the effects of substituents on biological activity are also in agreement with our early research.

A number of studies have been carried out to establish the cytotoxic activity of 1,4-NQs against various cell types and the relationship with the features of the chemical structure by the different QSAR method. Thus, it was shown that the antiproliferative and cytotoxic activity of a series of 1,4-naphthoquinone derivatives against different types of tumor cells largely depends on their hydrophobicity/polarity, partial atomic charge and total dipole moment [30–36].

The calculation of the molecular properties from 3D molecular fields of interaction energies is a relatively novel approach to correlate 3D molecular structures with pharmacokinetic and physicochemical properties [43]. In our investigation of 5,8-dihydroxy-1,4-naphthoquinone derivatives, the vsurf_S (Interaction field surface area) descriptor turned out to be the most important in describing the cytotoxic properties of naphthoquinones. This descriptor is included in the equation for pEC_{50} with a minus sign, which indicates that substituent increases in the interaction field, such as OH-, will lead to a decrease in pEC_{50} and a loss of toxic activity. The ASA and ASA_H descriptors for the studied naphthoquinones positively correlated with their cytotoxic activity. With an increase in the surface area of hydrophobic atoms available to water molecules, the cytotoxic activity of naphthoquinones increased. These compounds interacted more strongly with cell membranes. A comparative analysis of the descriptor valuesof highly active U-634 and nontoxic U-633 is shown in Table 4. It can be noted that the values of almost all of the model descriptors selected by QSAR decreased for U-633 compared to U-634. This change in descriptor's values means that the nontoxic naphthoquinone derivative has low water accessible surface area, total hydrophobic and positive van der Waals surface area, octanol/water partition coefficient, i.e., hydrophobicity, molecular refractivity, surface areas of pure hydrogen bond acceptors and hydrophobic atoms, and low interaction field surface area.

It is currently known that 1,4-NQs inhibit cancer cell proliferation and growth due to: the induction of semiquinone radicals and super oxide formation followed by DNA strand breaks; the increase in intracellular ROS amount; the effect on DNA topoisomerase II, Itch protein and GPR55; and the induction of cell apoptosis and cell cycle arrest via regulation of caspase-3/7, p53, Mdm-2, Bcl-2 and Bax gene expression and MAPK, Akt and STAT3 signaling pathways [44–52]. To date, with the exception of GLUT1 glucose transporter, no specialized channels, pores, receptors or carriers have been found for these compounds specifically interacting with some glucose-conjugated 1,4-NQs due to the Warburg effect [28,53].

Table 4. Analysis of descriptors of high cytotoxic compound U-634 and nontoxic U-633.

Descriptor	43 (U-634)	28 (U-633)	Alteration *
pEC_{50}	5.57	<4	↓
ASA	846.8	805.7	↓
ASA_H	589	504.2	↓
PEOE_VSA_HYD	347.7	309	↓
PEOE_VSA_NEG	156.2	161.1	↑
PEOE_VSA_POL	199.9	215.2	↑
PEOE_VSA_POS	391.4	363.4	↓
Q_VSA_HYD	302	269	↓
SlogP_VSA2	192.2	181	↓
SMR_VSA0	209.2	198	↓
vsa_acc	86.4	70	↓
vsa_hyd	320.8	285	↓
vsurf_S	776.5	745	↓

* decrease (↓) andincrease (↑) indescriptor's value for **43** (U-633) compare to **28** (U-634).

In our investigation, we showed that the cytotoxic activity of the studied 1,4-NQs is determined primarily by their hydrophobic properties. It turned out that the greater the hydrophobicity of the naphthoquinone molecule, the greater the cytotoxic effect of the compound on tumor neuronal cells. In all likelihood, it is precisely the hydrophobic properties that allow relatively small molecules of the most hydrophobic 1,4-NQs to easily penetrate biomembranes and accessthe intracellular compartment of cancer cells, where they exert a toxic effect. Probably, the compounds studied by us can penetrate biomembranes into cells along a concentration gradient due to their hydrophobicity. This is what the results of our 3D-QSAR analysis indicated. The most cytotoxic compounds were the highly hydrophobic O- and S-glycosides of 5,8-dihydroxy-1,4-naphthoquinone. Perhaps S-glycosides will turn out to be the preferred molecules rather than O-glycosides, since they are not subject to the action of various glycosidases and will retain the integrity of their chemical structure for longer in biological tissues. Theoretically, an increase in the hydrophobicity of such derivatives by replacing key substituents with more hydrophobic ones could lead to a significant increase in cytotoxic properties. In future, we plan to investigate their ability to penetrate the blood-brain barrier and enter the cells and tissues of the brain in vivo. It is possible that these properties of the selected S-glycosides of 1,4-NQs may be useful in the therapy of malignant neoplasm of the brain.

4. MaterialsandMethods

4.1. Chemistry

4.1.1. General Chemistry (Reagents, Solvents and Equipment)

Reagents and solvents were purchased from Fluka (Taufkirchen, Germany) and Vekton (St. Peterburg, Russia). The initial quinones were purchased from Fluka or synthesized as described elsewhere. Moisture sensitive reactions were performed under calcium chloride tube protection. Chlorobenzene was preliminarily treated with concentrated sulfuric acid, washed by water, dried with calcium chloride, and distilled over phosphorous pentoxide. Acetone, benzene, ethylacetate, hexane, methanol, and toluene were distilled.The melting points were determined on a Boetius melting-point apparatus (Dresden, Germany) and are uncorrected. The ^{1}H and ^{13}C NMR spectra were recorded using Bruker Avance-300 (300 MHz), Bruker Avance III-500 HD (500 MHz), and Bruker Avance III-700 (700 MHz) spectrometers (Bruker Corporation, Bremen, Germany) using CDCl$_3$ and DMSO-d_6 as the solvents with the signal of the residual nondeuterated solvent as the internal reference. In assigning NMR spectra, 2D NMR experiments {^{1}H–^{1}H} COSY, {^{1}H–^{13}C} HMBC-qs, and {^{1}H–^{13}C} HSQC were used where necessary. Spin–spin coupling constants (J) were reported in hertz (Hz). Multiplicity was tabulated using standard abbreviations: s for singlet, d for doublet, dd for doublet of doublets, t for triplet and m for multiplet (br means broad). ESI mass spectra and ESI high resolution mass spectra were recorded on a Bruker Maxis Impact II instrument. The progress of the reaction was monitored by thin-layer chromatography (TLC) on Sorbfil plates (IMID, Krasnodar, Russia) using the following solvent systems as eluents: hexane/benzene/acetone, 3:1:1 (v/v) (System A), hexane/benzene/acetone, 2:1:1 (v/v) (System B), hexane/benzene/acetone, 2:1:2 (v/v) (System C), benzene/ethylacetate/methanol, 2:1:1 (v/v) (System D), and benzene/ethyl acetate/methanol, 7:4:2 (v/v) (System E). TLC plates were preliminary deactivated by immersion in 0.5%acetone solution of tartaric acid and drying in air. Individual substances were isolated and purified using crystallization, column chromatography, as well as preparative TLC on silica gel (Silicagel 60, 0.040–0.063 mm, Alfa Aesar, Karlsruhe, Germany). In order to reduce a residual adsorption of quinones, silica gel was preliminarily treated for 1 h with a boiling mixture of concentrated hydrochloric and nitric acids (3:1 v/v), washed with water to achievepH~ 7, and activated at 120 °C.

Naphthazarin (Fluka) (1) was recrystallized from ethanol, while 2-hydroxynaphthazarin (naphthopurpurin) (2), 2-hydroxy-3-methylnaphthazarin (3) and 2-hydroxy-3-ethylnaphthazarin (4) were prepared according with Anufriev's paper [54]; 2,3-Dihydroxynaphthazarin (5), 2,3-dihydroxy-6-methynaphthazarin (6), 6-ethyl-2,3-dihydroxynaphthazarin (7) and spinochrome D (8) were obtained according the the method described in our previous papers [55,56]; 2,3,6-Trihydroxy-7-ethylnaphthazarin (echinochrome A) (9) was isolated from sea urchins *Scaphechinus mirabilis*; 3,4,6-Tri-O-acetyl-α-D-glucopyranose 1,2-(*tert*-butoxy orthoacetate) 11 was prepared according to a method described in [57]; 2-Hydroxy-6,7-dimethylnaphthazarin (22) and 6,7-dichloro-2-hydroxynaphthazarin (23) were prepared according to a method described in [14]; 2-Hydroxy-7-methoxynaphthazarin (24) and 2-hydroxy-6,7-dimethoxynaphthazarin (25) were prepared as described in our previous work [58]. Tetra-O-acetyl-1-thio-β-D-glucopyranose (27), tetra-O-acetyl-1-thio-β-D-galactopyranose (53), tetra-O-acetyl-1-thio-β-D-mannopyranose (54), tri-O-acetyl-1-thio-β-D-xylopyranose (55) were prepared as described in [59].

4.1.2. General Procedure for Synthesis of the Acetylated O-Glucosides 18–21, 23 by Autocatalytic Condensation of Hydroxynaphthoquinones 3, 4, 6, 7 and 22 with 3,4,6-Tri-O-acetyl-α-D-glucopyranose 1,2-(*tert*-butoxy orthoacetate) 11 in Chlorobenzene (Figure 2)

Hydroxynaphthoquinone 3, 4, 6, 7 or 22 (0.50 mM) and 1,2-(*tert*-butoxy orthoacetate) D-glucopyranose 11 202 mg (0.50 mM) per one β-OH group were stirred in dry PhCl (7 mL) at reflux (20–30 min) [39]. The chlorobenzene was evaporated in vacuo and the red residue was subjected to column chromatography on silica gel, eluting with system hexane:acetone 4:1 → 2:1 v/v, to give red polar orange fraction with R_f = 0.24–0.56 (A). Crystallization from hexane-acetone yielded acetylglucosides 18, 19, 23. The bisglucosides 20 and 21 were isolated as amorphous red powder.

2-(Tetra-O-acetyl-β-D-glucopyranosyl-1-oxy)-5,8-dihydroxy-3-methylnaphthalene-1,4-dione 18 (U-444). Red solid; yield 199 mg (73%); R_f= 0.32 (A); m.p. 192–193 °C. IR (CHCl$_3$): 3104, 2960, 1756, 1609, 1573, 1456, 1410, 1368 $^{-1}$. ^{1}H NMR (500 MHz, CDCl$_3$): δ 1.99 (s, 3H, COCH$_3$), 2.03 (s, 3H, COCH$_3$), 2.04 (s, 3H, COCH$_3$), 2.12 (s, 3H, COCH$_3$), 2.13 (s, 3H, ArCH$_3$), 3.75 (ddd, 1H, H-5′, J = 2.3, 5.0, 10.1 Hz), 4.10 (dd, 1H, H-6′, J = 2.5, 12.4 Hz), 4.19 (dd, 1H, H-6′, J = 5.0, 12.4 Hz), 5.15 (dd, 1H, H-4′, J = 9.1, 10.1 Hz), 5.27 (dd, 1H, H-2′, J = 7.5, 9.5 Hz), 5.32 (dd, 1H, H-3′, J = 9.1, 9.5 Hz), 5.69 (d, 1H, H-1′, J = 7.5 Hz), 7.20 (d, 1H, J = 6.0 Hz), 7.22 (d, 1H, J = 6.0 Hz), 12.26 (s, 1H, α-OH), 12.63 (s, 1H, α-OH). ^{13}C NMR (125 MHz, CDCl$_3$):δ 9.6 (ArCH$_3$), 20.50 (COCH$_3$), 20.55 (COCH$_3$), 20.57 (COCH$_3$),

20.74 (CO$\underline{C}$H$_3$), 61.6 (C-6′), 68.3 (C-4′),71.6 (C-2′), 72.3 (C-5′), 72.5 C-3′), 99.7 (C-1′), 111.1, 111.2, 129.2, 130.4, 137.1, 153.3, 158.3, 158.9, 169.4 ($\underline{C}$OCH$_3$), 169.5 ($\underline{C}$OCH$_3$), 170.1 ($\underline{C}$OCH$_3$), 170.4 ($\underline{C}$OCH$_3$), 182.2 (C=O), 187.4 (C=O). HRMS (ESI): m/z [M + Na]$^+$ calcd. for C$_{25}$H$_{26}$O$_{14}$Na: 573.1209; found 573.1215.

2-(Tetra-O-acetyl-β-D-glucopyranosyl-1-oxy)-3-ethyl-5,8-dihydroxynaphthalene-1,4-dione **19** (U-443). Red solid; yield 239 mg (85%); R_f= 0.34 (A); m.p. 200–201 °C. IR (CHCl$_3$): 1756, 1609, 1574, 1456, 1409, 1369, 1323, 1288, 1180, 1068, 1043 cm^{-1}. ^{1}H NMR (500 MHz, CDCl$_3$):δ 1.11 (t, 3H, CH$_2$C$\underline{H}_3$,J = 7.4 Hz). 1.99 (s, 3H, COC$\underline{H}_3$), 2.03 (s, 3H, COC$\underline{H}_3$), 2.04 (s, 3H, COC$\underline{H}_3$), 2.12 (s, 3H, COC$\underline{H}_3$), 2.65 (m, 2H, C$\underline{H}_2$CH$_3$), 3.76 (ddd, 1H, H-5′, J = 2.5, 5.0, 10.2 Hz), 4.08 (dd, 1H, H-6′a, J = 2.5, 12.4 Hz), 4.17 (dd, 1H, H-6′b, J = 5.0, 12.4 Hz), 5.14 (dd, 1H, H-4′, J = 9.4, 10.2 Hz), 5.26 (dd, 1H, H-2′, J = 7.8, 9.4 Hz), 5.33 (dd, 1H, H-3′, J = 9.4 Hz), 5.80 (d, 1H, H-1′, J = 7.8 Hz), 7.20 (d, 1H, Ar$\underline{H}$, J = 9.4 Hz), 7.25 (d, 1H, Ar$\underline{H}$, J = 9.4 Hz), 12.26 (s, 1H, α-O$\underline{H}$), 12.69 (s, 1H, α-O$\underline{H}$). ^{13}C NMR (125 MHz, CDCl$_3$): δ 12.8 (ArCH$_2$$\underline{C}H_3$), 17.3 (Ar$\underline{C}H_2CH_3$), 20.4 (CO$\underline{C}H_3$), 20.5 (CO$\underline{C}H_3$), 20.6 (CO$\underline{C}H_3$), 20.7 (CO$\underline{C}H_3$), 61.6 (C-6′), 68.3 (C-4′),71.7 (C-2′), 72.3 (C-5′), 72.5 C-3′), 99.2 (C-1′), 111.2, 111.3, 129.1, 130.4, 141.9, 152.8, 158.3, 158.8, 169.4 ($\underline{C}$OCH$_3$), 169.5 ($\underline{C}$OCH$_3$), 170.1 ($\underline{C}$OCH$_3$), 170.4 ($\underline{C}$OCH$_3$), 182.6 (C=O), 187.2 (C=O). HRMS (ESI): m/z [M + Na]$^+$ calcd. for C$_{26}$H$_{28}$O$_{14}$Na: 587.1351; found 587.1361.

2,3-Bis(tetra-O-acetyl-β-D-glucopyranosyl-1-oxy)-5,8-dihydroxy-6-methylnaphthalene-1,4-dione**20** (U-420). Red amorphous solid; 291 mg (65%); R_f = 0.24 (A). IR (CHCl$_3$): 1756, 1612, 1579, 1445, 1369, 1248, 1187, 1066, 1043 cm^{-1}. ^{1}H NMR (500 MHz, CDCl$_3$):δ 2.02 (s, 3H, COC$\underline{H}_3$), 2.03 (s, 9H, 3 × COC$\underline{H}_3$), 2.04 (s, 6H, 2 × COC$\underline{H}_3$), 2.08 (s, 3H, COC$\underline{H}_3$), 2.09 (s, 3H, COC$\underline{H}_3$), 2.32 (s, 3H, ArC$\underline{H}_3$), 3.82 (m, 2H, 2H-5′), 4.11 (dd, 2H, 2H-6′, J = 2.7, 12.5 Hz), 4.27 (m, 1H, H-6′), 4.30 (m, 1H, H-6′), 5.24–5.32 (m, 6H, 2H-2′, 2H-3′, 2H-4′), 5.81 (d, 1H, H-1′, J = 6.9 Hz), 5.87 (d, 1H, H-1′, J = 6.9 Hz), 7.08 (s, 1H, Ar$\underline{H}$), 12.39 (s, 1H, α-O$\underline{H}$), 12.78 (s, 1H, α-O$\underline{H}$). ^{13}C NMR (125 MHz, CDCl$_3$): δ 16.4 (Ar$\underline{C}$H$_3$), 20.54 (CO$\underline{C}$H$_3$), 20.56 (3 × CO$\underline{C}$H$_3$), 20.62 (2×CO$\underline{C}$H$_3$), 20.69 (CO$\underline{C}$H$_3$), 61.70 (C-6′), 61.74 (C-6′), 68.09 (C-4′), 68.15 (C-4′), 71.8 (2 × C-2′), 72.44 (C-5′), 72.49 (C-5′), 72.6 (2 × C-3′), 99.5 (C-1′), 99.6 (C-1′), 108.7, 109.4, 129.7, 142.5, 145,5, 145.8, 160.1, 160.4, 169.2 ($\underline{C}$OCH$_3$), 169.3 ($\underline{C}$OCH$_3$), 169.4 (2 × $\underline{C}$OCH$_3$), 170.2 (2 × $\underline{C}$OCH$_3$), 170.5 (2 × $\underline{C}$OCH$_3$), 180.5 (C=O), 181.3 (C=O). HRMS (ESI): m/z [M + Na]$^+$ calcd. for C$_{39}$H$_{44}$O$_{24}$Na: 919.2108; found 919.2115.

2,3-Bis(tetra-O-acetyl-β-D-glucopyranosyl-1-oxy)-6-ethyl-5,8-dihydroxynaphthalene-1,4-dione **21** (U-421). Red amorphous solid; 355 mg (78%); R_f=0.30 (A). IR (CHCl$_3$): 17554, 1611, 1578, 1434, 1369, 1254, 1215, 1184, 1086, 1041 cm^{-1}. ^{1}H NMR (500 MHz, CDCl$_3$):δ 1.25 (t, 3H, CH$_2$C$\underline{H}_3$,J = 7.5 Hz), 2.02 (s, 3H, COC$\underline{H}_3$), 2.03 (s, 6H, 2 × COC$\underline{H}_3$), 2.04 (s, 3H, COC$\underline{H}_3$), 2.05 (s, 6H, 2 × COC$\underline{H}_3$), 2.08 (s, 3H, COC$\underline{H}_3$), 2.09 (s, 3H, COC$\underline{H}_3$), 2.73 (q, 2H, ArC$\underline{H}_2$CH$_3$, J = 7.5 Hz), 3.82 (m, 2H, 2H-5′), 4.11 (dd, 2H, 2H-6′, J = 2.5, 12.5 Hz), 4.27 (m, 1H, H-6′), 4.29 (m, 1H, H-6′), 5.22–5.32 (m, 6H, 2H-2′, 2H-3′, 2H-4′), 5.81 (d, 1H, H-1′, J = 7.0 Hz), 5.86 (d, 1H, H-1′, J = 6.8 Hz), 7.07 (s, 1H, Ar$\underline{H}$),12.43 (s, 1H, α-O$\underline{H}$), 12.85 (s, 1H, α-O$\underline{H}$). ^{13}C NMR (125 MHz, CDCl$_3$): δ 12.7 (ArCH$_2$$\underline{C}H_3$), 20.54 (CO$\underline{C}H_3$), 20.57 (3 × CO$\underline{C}H_3$), 20.61 (2 × CO$\underline{C}H_3$), 20.69 (2 × CO$\underline{C}H_3$), 23.1 (Ar$\underline{C}H_2CH_3$), 61.7 (C-6′), 61.8 (C-6′), 68.1 (C-4′), 68.2 (C-4′), 71.8 (2 × C-2′), 72.4 (C-5′), 72.5 (C-5′), 72.6 (2×C-3′), 99.5 (C-1′), 99.6 (C-1′), 108.6, 109.5, 128.2, 145.5, 145,8, 148.1, 160.2, 161.0, 169.2 ($\underline{C}$OCH$_3$), 169.3 ($\underline{C}$OCH$_3$), 169.4 (2 × $\underline{C}$OCH$_3$), 170.2 (2 × $\underline{C}$OCH$_3$), 170.5 (2 × $\underline{C}$OCH$_3$), 180.2 (C=O), 181.1 (C=O). HRMS (ESI): m/z [M + Na]$^+$ calcd. for C$_{40}$H$_{46}$O$_{24}$Na: 933.2270; found 933.2271.

2-(Tetra-O-acetyl-β-D-glucopyranosyl-1-oxy)-5,8-dihydroxy-6,7-dimethylnaphthalene-1,4-dione **23** (U-330). Red solid; 440 mg (78%); R_f= 0.60 (A); m.p. 221–222 °C. IR (CHCl$_3$): 1758, 1604, 1456, 1416, 1375, 1279, 1166, 1070, 1037 cm^{-1}. ^{1}H NMR (500 MHz, CDCl$_3$):δ 2.05 (s, 3H, COC$\underline{H}_3$), 2.06 (s, 3H, COC$\underline{H}_3$), 2.08 (s, 3H, COC$\underline{H}_3$), 2.12 (s, 3H, COC$\underline{H}_3$), 2.22 (s, 3H, ArC$\underline{H}_3$), 2.23 (s, 3H, ArC$\underline{H}_3$), 3.92 (ddd, 1H, H-5′, J = 2.4, 6.0, 8.5 Hz), 4.20 (dd, 1H, H-6′a, J = 3.4, 12.0 Hz), 4.26 (dd, 1H, H-6′b, J = 6.0, 12.0 Hz), 5.15 (m, 1H, H-4′), 5.17 (d, 1H, H-1′, J = 7.0 Hz), 5.33 (m, 1H, H-3′), 5.37 (m, 1H, H-2′), 6.63 (s, 1H, Ar$\underline{H}$), 12.88 (s, 1H. α-O$\underline{H}$), 13.03 (s, 1H, α-O$\underline{H}$). ^{13}C NMR (125 MHz, CDCl$_3$): δ 12.3 (Ar$\underline{C}$H$_3$), 12.5 (Ar$\underline{C}$H$_3$), 20.54 (CO$\underline{C}$H$_3$), 20.57 (2 × CO$\underline{C}$H$_3$), 20.62 (CO$\underline{C}$H$_3$), 61.8 (C-6′), 68.1 (C-4′),70.6 (C-2′), 72.2 (C-3′), 72.8 C-5′), 98.6 (C-1′), 107.7, 110.7, 114.0, 141.1, 142.7, 155.6, 164.7, 169.2, 169.3 ($\underline{C}$OCH$_3$), 170.1

(COCH$_3$), 170.6 (COCH$_3$), 172.3 (COCH$_3$), 172.4 (C=O), 173.8 (C=O). HRMS (ESI): m/z [M + Na]$^+$ calcd. forC$_{26}$H$_{28}$O$_{14}$Na: 587.1351; found 587.1355.

4.1.3. General Procedure for the Synthesis of Acetylated Thiomethylglucosides **28–32** by Acid-Catalytic Condensation of Hydroxynaphthoquinones **2, 22, 24–26** with Tetra-O-acetyl-1-thio-D-glucose **27** and Paraformaldehyde in Acetone (Scheme 1)

First, 2-Hydroxy-1,4-napthoquinones **2, 22, 24–26** (0.50 mmol) was dissolved in acetone (13 mL), to which tetra-O-acetyl-1-mercapto-β-D-glucopyranose **27** (273 mg, 0.75 mmol), aq HCOOH 85% (0.20 mL), and paraformaldehydepowder (90 mg, 3.00 mmol) were added. The mixture gently refluxed with mixing (2 h) until TLC indicated that the reaction was complete. The mixture was evaporated invacuowith tolueneand the solid was subjected tocolumn or preparative TLC to give two colored fractions. The polar colored fraction with R_f = 0.39–0.65 was tetra-O-acetyl-β-D-glucopyranosyltiomethyl conjugate **28–32**, and the second colored fraction with R_f = 0.82–0.92 was 3,3′-bis(2-hydroxynaphthalene-1,4-dione)methane **33–37** (Scheme 1).

3-(Tetra-O-acetyl-β-D-glucopyranosyl-1-thiomethyl)-2,5,8-trihydroxynaphthalene-1,4-dione **28** (U-633).Red solid; 234 mg (80%); R_f = 0.43 (B); m.p. 152–154 °C. IR (CHCl$_3$): 3400, 1755, 1637, 1606, 1571, 1458, 1414, 1375, 1329, 1240, 1193, 1040 cm^{-1}. ^{1}H NMR ^{1}H (500 MHz, CDCl$_3$): δ 1.99 (s, 3H, COCH$_3$), 2.00 (s, 3H, COCH$_3$), 2.02 (s, 3H, COCH$_3$), 2.03 (s, 3H, COCH$_3$), 3.67 (m, 1H, H-5), 3.74 (d, 1H, CH$_2$-S, J = 13.7 Hz), 3.93 (d, 1H, CH$_2$-S, J = 13.7 Hz), 3.97 (dd, 1H, H-6′, J = 2.8, 4.6, 12.3 Hz), 4.18 (dd, 1H, H-6′, J = 4.6, 12.3 Hz), 4.68 (d, 1H, H-1′, J = 10.7 Hz), 5.05 (m, 1H, H-2′), 5.08 (m, 1H, H-4′), 5.21 (m, 1H, H-3′), 7.22 (d, 1H, ArH, J = 9.3 Hz), 7.32 (d, 1H, ArH, J = 9.3 Hz), 7.67 (s, 1H, β-OH), 11.48 (s, 1H, α-OH), 12.69 (s, 1H, α-OH). ^{13}C NMR (125 MHz, CDCl$_3$): δ 20.55 (COCH$_3$), 20.58 (COCH$_3$), 20.65 (COCH$_3$), 20.66 (COCH$_3$), 21.7 (CH$_2$S), 62.1 (C-6′), 68.5 (C-4′), 70.0 (C-2′), 73.9 (C-3′), 75.8 (C-5′), 83.9 (C-1′), 110.3, 110.5, 122.4, 128.0, 132.0, 153.8, 157.4, 158.1, 169.3(COCH$_3$), 169.4(COCH$_3$), 170.2(COCH$_3$), 170.6(COCH$_3$), 181.8 (C=O), 187.4 (C=O). HRMS (ESI): m/z [M − H]$^-$ calcd. for C$_{25}$H$_{25}$O$_{14}$S:581.0971; found 581.0967.

3-(Tetra-O-acetyl-β-D-glucopyranosyl-1-thiomethyl)-2,5,8-trihydroxy-6,7-dimethylnaphthalene-1,4-dione **29** (U-519). Red solid;244 mg(82%). R_f = 0.40 (B); m.p. 104–106 °C. IR (CHCl$_3$): 3395, 3023, 2954, 1755, 1624, 1598, 1450, 1394, 1376, 1335, 1249, 1192, 1096, 1038 cm^{-1}. ^{1}H NMR ^{1}H (500 MHz, CDCl$_3$): δ 1.99 (s, 6H, 2 × COCH$_3$), 2.01 (s, 3H, COCH$_3$), 2.03 (s, 3H, COCH$_3$), 2.27 (s, 3H, ArCH$_3$), 2.30 (s, 3H, ArCH$_3$),3.67(m, 1H, H-5′), 3.74 (d, 1H, CH$_2$-S, J = 13.4 Hz), 3.93 (d, 1H, CH$_2$-S, J = 13.4 Hz), 3.96 (dd, 1H, H-6′, J = 2.4, 12.0 Hz), 4.19 (dd, 1H, H-6′, J = 4.3, 12.0 Hz), 4.70 (d, 1H, H-1′, J = 10.0 Hz), 5.04 (m, 1H, H-2′), 5.08 (m, 1H, H-4′), 5.21 (m, 1H, H-3′), 7.68 (s, 1H, β-OH), 12.15 (s, 1H, α-OH), 13.42 (s, 1H, α-OH). ^{13}C NMR ^{1}H (125 MHz, CDCl$_3$): δ 12.15 (CH$_3$), 12.8 (CH$_3$), 20.5 (COCH$_3$), 20.6 (COCH$_3$), 20.7 (COCH$_3$), 21.9, 62.1 (C-6′), 68.5 (C-4′), 70.1 (C-2′), 74.0 (C-3′), 75.8 (C-5′), 84.0 C-1′), 107.5, 107.8, 121.7, 136.6, 141.5, 153.9, 157.8, 158.6, 169.3 (COCH$_3$), 169.4(COCH$_3$), 170.2(COCH$_3$), 170.6 (COCH$_3$), 180.1 (C=O), 186.4 (C=O). HRMS (ESI): m/z [M −H]$^-$ calcd. for C$_{27}$H$_{29}$O$_{14}$S: 609.1284; found 609.1286.

3-(Tetra-O-acetyl-β-D-glucopyranosyl-1-thiomethyl)-6,7-dichloro-2,5,8-trihydroxynaphthalene-1,4-dione **30** (U-518). Red solid; 224 mg (69%); R_f = 0.39 (B); m.p. 106–108 °C. IR (CHCl$_3$): 3407, 3021, 2956, 2360, 1755, 1630, 1610, 1553, 1432, 1402, 1379, 1323, 1246, 1221, 1182, 1117, 1040 cm^{-1}. ^{1}H NMR ^{1}H (300 MHz, CDCl$_3$): δ 2.01 (s, 6H, 2 × COCH$_3$), 2.03 (s, 3H, COCH$_3$), 2.04 (s, 3H, COCH$_3$), 3.67 (, 1H, H-5′), 3.76 (d, 1H, CH$_2$-S, J = 14.0 Hz), 3.93 (d, 1H, CH$_2$-S, J = 14.0 Hz), 4.01 (dd, 1H, H-6′a, J = 3.0, 12.5 Hz), 4.19 (dd, 1H, H = 6′b, J = 4.3, 12.5 Hz), 4.65 (d, 1H, H-1′, J = 10.3 Hz), 5.06 (m, 1H, H-2′), 5.08 (m, 1H, H-4′), 5.22 (m, 1H, H-3′), 7.95 (s, 1H, β-OH), 12.06 (s, 1H, α-OH), 13.37 (s, 1H, α-OH). ^{13}C NMR ^{1}H (75 MHz, CDCl$_3$): δ 20.5 (2 × COCH$_3$), 20.58 (COCH$_3$), 20.60 (COCH$_3$), 21.4 (CH$_2$S), 61.9 (C-6′), 68.4 (C-2′), 69.8 (C-2′), 73.6 (C-3′), 75.7 (C-5′), 83.6(C-1′), 108.8 (2), 122.6, 131.5, 135.3, 153.8, 154.4, 154.5, 169.3 (COCH$_3$), 169.4 (COCH$_3$), 170.1 (COCH$_3$), 170.5 (COCH$_3$), 180.9 (C=O), 186.5 (C=O). HRMS (ESI): m/z [M − H]$^-$ calcd. for C$_{25}$H$_{23}$HCl$_2$O$_{14}$S: 649.0191; found 649.0191.

3-(Tetra-O-acetyl-β-D-glucopyranosyl-1-thiomethyl)-2,5,8-trihydroxy-7-methoxynaphthalene-1, 4-dione **31** (U-639). Red solid; 220 mg (72%); R_f = 0.53 (C), m.p. 117–120 °C. IR (CHCl$_3$): 3510, 3397,

3085, 2948, 1755, 1599, 1466, 1415, 1403, 1376, 1339, 1298, 1258, 1218, 1180, 1137, 1040 cm^{-1}. ^{1}H NMR (500 MHz, CDCl$_3$):δ1.997 (s, 3H, COC$\underline{H}_3$), 2.00 (s, 3H, COC$\underline{H}_3$), 2.02 (s, 3H, COC$\underline{H}_3$), 2.04 (s, 3H, COC$\underline{H}_3$), 3.67 (ddd, 1H, H-5′, J = 9.5, 4.5, 2.7 Hz), 3.76 (d, 1H, C$\underline{H}_2$S, J = 13.5 Hz), 3.95 (d, 1H, C$\underline{H}_2$S, J = 13.5 Hz), 3.97 (dd, 1H, H-6′a, J = 12.3, 2.7 Hz), 3.98 (s, 3H, OC$\underline{H}_3$), 4.20 (dd, 1H, H-6′b, J = 12.7, 4.5 Hz), 4.72 (d,1H, H-1′J = 10.2 Hz), 5.05 (dd,1 -2′, J = 10.2, 9.5 Hz), 5.08 (t, 1H, H-4′, J = 9.5 Hz), 5.21 (t, 1H, H-3′, J = 9.5 Hz), 6.59 (s, 1H, H-6), 7.61 (br s, 1H, β-O$\underline{H}$), 12.03 (s, 1H, α-O$\underline{H}$), 13.19 (s, 1H, α-O$\underline{H}$). ^{13}C NMR (125 MHz, CDCl$_3$):δ 20.5 (2 × CO$\underline{C}$H$_3$), 20.6 (2 × CO$\underline{C}$H$_3$), 21.8, 56.7 (O$\underline{C}$H$_3$), 62.0 (C-6′), 68.5 (C-4′), 70.0 (C-2′), 73.9 (C-3′), 75.7 (C-5′), 83.9 (C-1′), 103.9, 108.6, 110.3, 123.2, 153.1, 154.9, 157.0, 163.4, 169.3 (2 × $\underline{C}$OCH$_3$), 170.2 ($\underline{C}$OCH$_3$), 170.6 ($\underline{C}$OCH$_3$), 177.7 (C=O), 181.9 (C=O). HRMS (ESI): m/z [M − H]$^-$ calcd. for C$_{26}$H$_{27}$O$_{15}$S: 611.1076; found: 611.1077.

3-(Tetra-O-acetyl-β-D-glucopyranosyl-1-thiomethyl)-2,5,8-trihydroxy-6,7-dimethoxynaphthalene-1,4-dione **32** (U-637). Red solid; 244 mg (76%); R_f = 0.60(C), m.p. 83–85 °C. IR (CHCl$_3$): 3410, 3083, 2944, 1755, 1601, 1478, 1435, 1412, 1396, 1367, 1324, 1304, 1273, 1254, 1236, 1179, 1150, 1040 cm^{-1}. ^{1}H NMR (500 MHz, CDCl$_3$):δ1.99 (s, 3H, COC$\underline{H}_3$), 2.00 (s, 3H, COC$\underline{H}_3$), 2.02 (s, 3H, COC$\underline{H}_3$), 2.04 (s, 3H, COC$\underline{H}_3$), 3.66 (ddd, 1H, H-5′, J = 9.5, 4.5, 2.7 Hz), 3.75 (d, 1H, C$\underline{H}_2$S, J = 13.5 Hz), 3.95 (d,1H, C$\underline{H}_2$S, J = 13.5 Hz), 3.99 (dd, 1H, H-6′a, J = 12.3, 2.7 Hz), 4.06 (s, 3H, OC$\underline{H}_3$), 4.15 (s, 3H, OC$\underline{H}_3$), 4.18 (dd, 1H, H-6′b, J = 12.7, 4.5 Hz), 4.68 (d,1H, H-1′, J = 10.2 Hz), 5.04 (dd, 1H, H-2′, J = 10.2, 9.5 Hz), 5.08 (t, 1H, H-4′, J = 9.5 Hz), 5.21 (t, 1H, H-3′, J = 9.5 Hz), 7.62 (br s, 1H, β-O$\underline{H}$), 12.15 (s, 1H,α-O$\underline{H}$), 13.34 (s, 1H, α-O$\underline{H}$). ^{13}C NMR (125 MHz, CDCl$_3$):δ 20.5 (2 × CO$\underline{C}$H$_3$), 20.6 (2 × CO$\underline{C}$H$_3$), 21.8, 61.6 (O$\underline{C}$H$_3$), 61.7 (O$\underline{C}$H$_3$), 62.1 (C-6′), 68.5 (C-4′), 70.0 (C-2′), 73.9 (C-3′), 75.7 (C-5′), 83.9 (C-1′), 106.1, 106.8, 121.7, 146.4, 150.4, 153.8, 159.6, 160.8, 169.3 ($\underline{C}$OCH$_3$), 169.4 ($\underline{C}$OCH$_3$), 170.2 ($\underline{C}$OCH$_3$), 170.6 ($\underline{C}$OCH$_3$), 173.9 (C=O), 181.5 (C=O). HRMS (ESI): m/z [M − H]$^-$ calcd. for C$_{27}$H$_{29}$O$_{16}$S: 641.1182; found: 641.1182.

4.1.4. General Procedure for Synthesis of Thiomethylglucosides **38–42** and **48–52** by Acid-Catalytic Deacetylation Acetylthiomethylglucosides **28–32** and **43–47** in Methanol (Scheme 2)

To a partially dissolved suspension of (tetra-O-acetyl-β-D-glucopyranosyl-1-thiomethyl)naphthalene-1,4-dione **28–32** or **43–47** (0.20mmol) in dry methanol (15 mL) was added acetylchloride (1.0 mL) dropwise under vigorous stirring; then, the flask was carefully closed. The obtained reaction mixture was stirred for 48 h at room temperature, and then toluene (15 mL) was added; the resulting red solution evaporated under reduced pressure. The residue was subjected topreparative TLC (system B), yielding a polar red colored solid. The solid was crystallized with MeOH to give **38–42** or **48–52** as red crystals.

3-(β-D-Glucopyranosyl-1-thiomethyl)-2,5,8-trihydroxynaphthalene-1,4-dione **38** (U-635). Red solid; 71 mg (86%); R_f = 0.26 (D); m.p. 169–170 °C. IR (KBr): 3422, 1600, 1561, 1453, 1410, 1385, 1296, 1181, 1108, 1077, 1031, 970 cm^{-1}. ^{1}H NMR ^{1}H (500 MHz, DMSO-d_6): δ 2.96 (m, 1H, H-2′), 3.02 (m, 1H, H-5′), 3.10 (m, 2H, H-3′, H-4′), 3.40 (dd, 1H, H-6a′, J = 5.1, 11.9 Hz), 3.50 (dd, 1H, H-6b′, J = 2.1, 11.9 Hz), 3.63 (d, 1H, C$\underline{H}_2$-S-, J = 13.2 Hz), 3.75 (d, 1H, C$\underline{H}_2$-S-, J = 13.2 Hz), 4.38 (d, 1H, H-1′, J = 9.7 Hz), 7.31 (d, 1H, Ar$\underline{H}$, J = 9.5 Hz), 7.37 (d, 1H, Ar$\underline{H}$, J = 9.5 Hz), 11.71 (s, 1H, α-O$\underline{H}$), 12.79 (s, 1H, α-O$\underline{H}$). ^{13}C NMR ^{1}H (125 MHz, DMSO-d_6): δ 21.2 ($\underline{C}$H$_2$-S), 60.8 (C-6′), 69.6 (C-4′), 73.0 (C-2′), 78.4 (C-3′), 80.7 (C-5′), 86.1 (C-1′), 110.8, 111.1, 122.7, 127.6, 130.2, 155.5, 156.2, 156.6, 182.9 (C=O), 188.0 (C=O). HRMS (ESI): m/z [M − H]$^-$ calcd. for C$_{17}$H$_{18}$O$_{10}$S: 413.0548; found 413.0551.

3-(β-D-Glucopyranosyl-1-thiomethyl)-2,5,8-trihydroxy-6,7-dimethylnaphthalene-1,4-dione **39** (U-520). Red solid; 84 mg (95%); R_f = 0.44 (D); m.p. 179–181 °C. IR (KBr): 3426, 2920, 2360, 1592, 1423, 1384, 1312, 1287, 1183, 1149, 1089, 1031 cm^{-1}. ^{1}H NMR ^{1}H (500 MHz, DMSO-d_6): δ 2.21 (s, 3H, ArC$\underline{H}_3$), 2.22 (s, 3H, ArC$\underline{H}_3$), 2.95 (m, 1H, H-2′), 3.02 (m, 1H, H-5′), 3.10 (m, 1H, H-3′), 3.13 (m, 1H, H-4′), 3.40 (dd, 1H, H-6a′, J = 5.0, 12.2 Hz), 3.50 (dd, 1H, H-6b′, J = 2.4, 12.2 Hz), 3.63 (d, 1H, C$\underline{H}_2$-S, J = 13.0 Hz), 3.75 (d, 1H, C$\underline{H}_2$-S, J = 13.0 Hz), 4.37 (d, 1H, H-1′, J = 10.0 Hz), 12.52 (s, 1H, α-O$\underline{H}$), 13.53 (s, 1H, α-O$\underline{H}$). ^{13}C NMR ^{1}H (125 MHz, DMSO-d_6): δ 11.9 (Ar$\underline{C}$H$_3$), 12.4 (Ar$\underline{C}$H$_3$), 21.3 ($\underline{C}$H$_2$-S), 60.8 (C-6′), 69.6(C-4′), 73.1 (C-2′), 78.5 (C-3′), 80.7 (C-5′), 86.1 (C-1′), 107.5, 108.2, 122.6, 135.7, 1 39.3,

156.2, 156.4, 157.2, 181.3 (C=O), 186.5 (C=O). HRMS (ESI): m/z [M −H]⁻ calcd. for $C_{19}H_{22}O_{10}S$: 441.0861; found 441.0864.

6,7-Dichloro-3-(β-D-glucopyranosyl-1-thiomethyl)-2,5,8-trihydroxynaphthalene-1,4-dione 40 (U-624). Red solid 83 mg (86%); R_f = 0.38 (D); m.p. 184–186 °C. IR (KBr): 3433, 2361, 1597, 1549, 1385, 1298, 1270, 1178, 1114, 1034, 996 cm⁻¹. ¹H NMR ¹H (500 MHz, DMSO-d_6): δ 2.96 (m, 1H, H-2′), 3.03 (m, 1H, H-5′), 3.09 (m, 2H, H-3′, H-4′), 3.37 (dd, 1H, H-6′a, J = 5.3, 11.9 Hz), 3.52 (dd, 1H, H-6′b, J = 2.1, 11.9 Hz), 3.65 (d, 1H, C$\underline{H}_2$-S, J = 12.9 Hz), 3.74 (d, 1H, C$\underline{H}_2$-S, J = 12.9 Hz), 4.38 (d, 1H, H-1′, J = 9.8 Hz), 12.30 (s, 1H, α-O$\underline{H}$), 14.04 (s, 1H, α-O$\underline{H}$). ¹³C NMR ¹H (125 MHz, DMSO-d_6): δ 21.5 (C$\underline{H}_2$S), 60.9 (C-6′), 69.8 (C-4′), 73.0 (C-2′), 78,4 (C-3′), 80.7 (C-5′), 86.1 (C-1′), 110.3, 110.8, 121.5, 128.5, 131.4, 152.4, 152.5, 159.0, 182.6(C=O), 185.8 (C=O). HRMS (ESI): m/z [M −H]⁻ calcd. for $C_{17}H_{15}Cl_2O_{10}S$: 480.9768; found 480.9770.

3-(β-D-Glucopyranosyl-1-thiomethyl)-2,5,8-trihydroxy-7-methoxynaphthalene-1,4-dione 41 (U-644). Red solid; 61 mg (69%); R_f = 0.38 (E); m.p. 211–213 °C. IR (KBr):3412, 2360, 1590, 1477, 1424, 1385, 1312, 1200, 1164, 1111, 1064, 1029, 984, 953 cm⁻¹.¹H NMR (700 MHz, DMSO-d_6):δ2.95 (dd, 1H, H-2′, J = 9.8, 8.5 Hz), 3.03 (ddd,1H, H-5′,J = 8.5, 5.0, 2.0 Hz), 3.10 (t, 1H, H-3′, J = 8.5 Hz), 3.13 (t, 1H, H-4′, J = 8.5 Hz), 3.41 (dd, 1H, H-6′a, J = 11.8, 5.0 Hz), 3.51 (dd, 1H, H-6′b, J = 11.8, 2.0 Hz), 3.63 (d, 1H, ArC$\underline{H}_2$, J = 13.0 Hz), 3.77 (d, 1H, ArC$\underline{H}_2$, J = 13.0 Hz), 3.91 (s, 3H, OC$\underline{H}_3$), 4.39 (d,1H, H-1′, J = 9.8 Hz), 6.77 (s, 1H, H-6), 11.42 (br s, 1H, β-O$\underline{H}$), 12.22 (s, 1H, α-O$\underline{H}$), 13.37 (s, 1H, α-O$\underline{H}$). ¹³C NMR (175 MHz, DMSO-d_6):δ 21.3(C$\underline{H}_2$S), 56.8 (OC$\underline{H}_3$), 60.8 (C-6′), 69.7 (C-4′), 73.1 (C-2′), 78.4 (C-3′), 80.7 (C-5′), 86.0 (C-1′), 103.4, 108.3, 110.6, 123.4, 155.1, 155.2, 156.9, 163.4, 176.9 (C=O), 181.0 (C=O). HRMS (ESI): m/z [M − H]⁻ calcd. for $C_{18}H_{19}O_{11}S$: 443.0654; found: 443.0654.

3-(β-D-Glucopyranosyl-1-thiomethyl)-2,5,8-trihydroxy-6,7-dimethoxynaphthalene-1,4-dione 42 (U-640). Red solid; 71 mg (75%); R_f = 0.42 (E); m.p. 193–195 °C. IR (KBr):3354, 2957, 2854, 1604, 1461, 1423, 1384, 1330, 1276, 1215, 1180, 1161, 1123, 1100, 1060, 1029, 986 cm⁻¹. ¹H NMR (500 MHz, DMSO-d_6):δ2.95 (dd, 1H, H-2′, J = 9.8, 8.5 Hz), 3.03 (ddd, 1H, H-5′, J = 8.5, 5.0, 2.0 Hz), 3.09 (t, 1H, H-3′,J = 8.5 Hz), 3.13 (t, 1H, H-4′, J = 8.5 Hz), 3.42 (dd,1H, H-6′a,J = 11.8, 5.0 Hz), 3.53 (dd, 1H, H-6′b, J = 11.8, 2.0 Hz), 3.64 (d, 1H, ArC$\underline{H}_2$,J = 13.0 Hz), 3.79 (d, 1H ArC$\underline{H}_2$S, J = 13.0 Hz), 3.96 (s, 3H, OC$\underline{H}_3$), 4.01 (s, 3H, OC$\underline{H}_3$), 4.37 (d, 1H, H-1′, J = 9.8 Hz), 11.47 (br s, 1H, β-O$\underline{H}$), 12.43 (s, 1H, α-O$\underline{H}$), 13.43 (s, 1H, α-O$\underline{H}$).¹³C NMR (125 MHz, DMSO-d_6):δ 21.2, 60.8 (C-6′), 61.3 (2 × OC$\underline{H}_3$), 69.7 (C-4′), 73.1 (C-2′), 78.4 (C-3′), 80.7 (C-5′), 86.0 (C-1′), 105.7, 107.5, 122.3, 146.4, 149.1, 156.0, 160.5, 161.8, 172.7 (C=O), 179.4 (C=O). HRMS (ESI): m/z [M − H]⁻ calcd. for $C_{19}H_{21}O_{12}S$: 473.0759; found: 473.0760.

4.1.5. General Procedure of Methylation of 2-Hydroxy 3-(Tetra-O-acetyl-β-D-glucopyranosyl-1-thiomethyl)-1,4-naphthoquinone 28–32 to 2-Methoxy Derivatives 43–47 Using Diazomethane (Scheme 2)

To solution of 2-hydroxy-3-(tetra-O-acetyl-β-D-glucopyranosyl-1-thiomethyl)-1,4-naphthoquinone 28–32 (0.50 mmol) in ethylacetate (20 mL) was added dropwise an ethereal solution of diazomethane until TLC (system A) indicated the disappearance of the starting quinone. The reaction mixture was evaporated in vacuo and the residue was crystallized with MeOH, yielding 2-methoxyderivatives 43–47 as a red crystals.

3-(Tetra-O-acetyl-β-D-glucopyranosyl-1-thiomethyl)-5,8-dihydroxy-2-methoxynaphthalene-1,4-dione 43 (U-634). Red solid; yield 286 mg (96%); R_f = 0.59(B); m.p. 66–67 °C. IR (CHCl₃): 1755, 1606, 1571, 1456, 1410, 1375, 1293, 1255, 1181, 1141, 1080, 1039 cm⁻¹. ¹H NMR ¹H (500 MHz, CDCl₃): δ 1.99 (s, 3H, COC$\underline{H}_3$), 2.02 (s, 6H, 2 × COC$\underline{H}_3$), 2.01 (s, 3H, COC$\underline{H}_3$), 3.65 (ddd, 1H, H-5, J = 2.5, 4.5, 10.0 Hz), 3.74 (d, 1H, C$\underline{H}_2$-S, J = 13.1 Hz), 3.88 (d, 1H, C$\underline{H}_2$-S, J = 13.1 Hz), 3.95 (dd, 1H, H-6′a, J = 2.5, 12.1 Hz), 4.14 (dd, 1H, H-6′b, J = 4.5, 12.1 Hz), 4.27 (s, 3H, C$\underline{H}_3$O), 4.68 (d, 1H, H-1′, J = 10.1 Hz), 5.04 (m, 1H, H-2′), 5.08 (m, 1H, H-4′), 5.21 (m, 1H, H-3′), 7.22 (d, 1H, Ar$\underline{H}$, J = 9.1 Hz), 7.26 (d, 1H, Ar$\underline{H}$, J = 9.1 Hz), 12.30 (s, 1H, α-O$\underline{H}$), 12.65 (s, 1H, α-O$\underline{H}$).¹³C NMR ¹H (125 MHz, CDCl₃): δ 20.54 (COC$\underline{H}_3$), 20.58 (COC$\underline{H}_3$), 20.62 (COC$\underline{H}_3$), 20.65 (COC$\underline{H}_3$), 22.2 (C$\underline{H}_2$S), 61.8 (C-6′) 62.0 (C$\underline{H}_3$O), 68.3 (C-4′), 70.0 (C-2′), 73.9 (C-3′), 75.8 (C-5′), 84.0 (C-1′), 110.8, 111.7, 129.2, 130.5, 133.0, 157.8, 159.0, 169.3

(2 × CH$_3$$\underline{C}$O), 170.2 (CH$_3$$\underline{C}$O), 170.4 (CH$_3$$\underline{C}$O), 183.2 (C=O), 186.8 (C=O). HRMS (ESI): *m/z* [M − H]$^-$ calcd. for C$_{26}$H$_{27}$O$_{14}$S:595.1127; found 595.1126.

3-(Tetra-*O*-acetyl-β-D-glucopyranosyl-1-thiomethyl)-5,8-dihydroxy-2-methoxy-6,7-dimethylnaphthalene-1,4-dione **44**. (U-521) Red solid; yield 299 mg (97%); *R$_f$* = 0.55 (B); m.p. 105–107 °C. IR (CHCl$_3$): 1755, 1598, 1453, 1425, 1397, 1376, 1298, 1243, 1194, 1096, 1042 cm^{-1}. ^{1}H NMR (500 MHz, CDCl$_3$): δ 2.00 (s, 6H, 2 × COC$\underline{H}$$_3$), 2.01 (s, 3H, COC$\underline{H}$$_3$), 2.03 (s, 3H, COC$\underline{H}$$_3$), 2.25 (s, 3H, ArC$\underline{H}$$_3$), 2.26 (s, 3H, ArC$\underline{H}$$_3$), 3.66 (ddd, 1H, H-5′, *J* = 2.6, 4.5, 10.1 Hz), 3.77 (d, 1H, C$\underline{H}$$_2$-S, *J* = 13.0 Hz), 3.96 (d, 1H, C$\underline{H}$$_2$-S, *J* = 13.0 Hz), 3.97 (dd, 1H, H-6′a, *J* = 2.6, 12.3 Hz), 4.17 (dd, 1H, H-6′b, *J* = 4.5, 12.3 Hz), 4.20 (s, 3H, C$\underline{H}$$_3$O), 4.68 (d, 1H, H-1′, *J* = 10.2 Hz), 5.02 (m, 1H, H-2′), 5.08 (m, 1H, H-4′), 5.20 (m, 1H, H-3′), 13.11 (s, 1H, α-O$\underline{H}$), 13.39 (s, 1H, α-O$\underline{H}$).^{13}C NMR ^{1}H (125 MHz, CDCl$_3$): δ 12.3 (ArC$\underline{H}$$_3$), 12.5 (ArC$\underline{H}$$_3$), 20.5 (C$\underline{H}$$_3$CO), 20.6 (2×C$\underline{H}$$_3$CO), 20.7 (C$\underline{H}$$_3$CO), 22.4 (C$\underline{H}$$_2$S), 61.8 (C$\underline{H}$$_3$O), 61.9 (C-6′), 68.4 (C-4′), 70.1 (C-2′), 74.0 (C-3′), 75.8 (C-5′), 83.9 (C-1′), 107.9, 110.0, 131.8, 140.0, 141.5, 156.9, 167.6, 169.0, 169.3 (CH$_3$$\underline{C}$O), 169.4 (CH$_3$$\underline{C}$O), 170.2 (CH$_3$$\underline{C}$O), 170.5 (CH$_3$$\underline{C}$O), 172.0 (C=O), 176.3 (C=O). HRMS (ESI): *m/z* [M − H]$^-$ calcd. for C$_{28}$H$_{31}$O$_{14}$S: 623.1440; found 623.1446.

3-(Tetra-*O*-acetyl-β-D-glucopyranosyl-1-thiomethyl)-6,7-dichloro-5,8-dihydroxy-2-methoxynaphthalene-1,4-dione **45** (U-523). Red solid; yield 304 mg (92%); *R$_f$* = 0.53 (B); m.p. 126–127 °C. IR (CHCl$_3$): 1755, 1608, 1562, 1450, 1404, 1375, 1296, 1250, 1187, 1111, 1040 cm^{-1}. ^{1}H NMR (500 MHz, CDCl$_3$): δ 1.99 (s, 3H, COC$\underline{H}$$_3$), 2.00 (s, 3H, COC$\underline{H}$$_3$), 2.01 (s, 3H, COC$\underline{H}$$_3$), 2.02 (s, 3H, COC$\underline{H}$$_3$), 3.64 (ddd, 1H, H-5′, *J* = 2.7, 4.5, 10.0 Hz), 3.77 (d, 1H, C$\underline{H}$$_2$-S, *J* = 13.4 Hz), 3.96 (d, 1H, C$\underline{H}$$_2$-S, *J* = 13.4 Hz), 3.99 (dd, 1H, H-6a′, *J* = 2.7, 12.5 Hz), 4.14 (dd, 1H, H-6b′, *J* = 4.5, 12.5 Hz), 4.27 (s, 3H, C$\underline{H}$$_3$O), 4.64 (d, 1H, H-1′, *J* = 10.2 Hz), 5.03 (m, 1H, H-2′), 5.07 (m, 1H, H-4′), 5.20 (m, 1H, H-3′), 12.85 (s, 1H, α-O$\underline{H}$), 13.24 (s, 1H, α-O$\underline{H}$).^{13}C NMR ^{1}H (125 MHz, CDCl$_3$): δ 20.5 (2 × C$\underline{H}$$_3$CO), 20.6 (2 × C$\underline{H}$$_3$CO), 22.0 (C$\underline{H}$$_2$S), 61.7 (C-6′), 62.3 (C$\underline{H}$$_3$O), 68.3 (C-4′), 70.0 (C-2′), 73.8 (C-3′), 75.9 (C-5′), 83.8 (C-1′), 108.6, 110.3, 132.5, 134.8, 136.1, 157.4, 159.4, 160.4, 169.3 (CH$_3$$\underline{C}$O), 169.4 (CH$_3$$\underline{C}$O), 170.1 (CH$_3$$\underline{C}$O), 170.4 (CH$_3$$\underline{C}$O), 176.5 (C=O), 180.5 (C=O). HRMS (ESI): *m/z* [M − H]$^-$ calcd. for C$_{26}$H$_{25}$Cl$_2$O$_{14}$S: 663.0348; found 663.0346.

3-(Tetra-*O*-acetyl-β-D-glucopyranosyl-1-thiomethyl)-5,8-dihydroxy-2,7-dimethoxynaphthalene-1,4-dione **46** (U-645).Red solid; yield 303 mg(97%); *R$_f$* = 0.62 (C); m.p. 127–129 °C. IR (CHCl$_3$):3083, 2946, 1755, 1606, 1475, 1457, 1436, 1408, 1368, 1302, 1284, 1257, 1180, 1153, 1099, 1039 cm^{-1}. ^{1}H NMR (700 MHz, CDCl$_3$):δ1.99 (s, 6H, 2 × COC$\underline{H}$$_3$), 2.01 (s, 3H, COC$\underline{H}$$_3$), 2.04 (s, 3H, COC$\underline{H}$$_3$), 3.66 (ddd, *J* = 9.5, 4.5, 2.5 Hz, 1H, H-5′), 3.81 (d, *J* = 13.1 Hz, 1H, C$\underline{H}$$_2$-S), 3.95 (s, 3H, OC$\underline{H}$$_3$), 3.99 (dd, *J* = 12.4, 2.5 Hz, 1H, H-6′a), 4.02 (d, *J* = 13.1 Hz, 1H, C$\underline{H}$$_2$-S), 4.15 (s, 3H, OC$\underline{H}$$_3$), 4.19 (dd, *J* = 12.4, 4.5 Hz, 1H, H-6′b), 4.69 (d, *J* = 10.2 Hz, 1H, H-1′), 5.03 (dd, *J* = 10.2, 9.5 Hz, 1H, H-2′), 5.09 (t, *J* = 9.5 Hz, 1H, H-4′), 5.20 (t, *J* = 9.5 Hz, 1H, H-3′), 6.29 (s, 1H, H-3), 12.73 (s, 1H, α-OH), 13.33 (s, 1H, α-O$\underline{H}$).^{13}C NMR (175 MHz, CDCl$_3$):δ20.6 (2 × COC$\underline{H}$$_3$), 20.7 (2 × COC$\underline{H}$$_3$), 22.5 (C$\underline{H}$$_2$-S), 56.8 (OC$\underline{H}$$_3$), 61.7 (OC$\underline{H}$$_3$), 61.9 (C-6′), 68.3 (C-4′), 70.1 (C-2′), 74.0 (C-3′), 75.8 (C-5′), 83.9 (C-1′), 105.9, 109.4, 111.6, 132.8, 155.0, 159.9, 162.2, 165.2, 169.3 (2 × $\underline{C}$OCH$_3$), 170.2 ($\underline{C}$OCH$_3$), 170.5 ($\underline{C}$OCH$_3$), 173.6 (C=O), 179.4 (C=O). HRMS (ESI): *m/z* [M − H]$^-$ calcd. for C$_{17}$H$_{29}$O$_{15}$S: 625.1233; found: 625.1226.

3-(Tetra-*O*-acetyl-β-D-glucopyranosyl-1-thiomethyl)-5,8-dihydroxy-2,6,7-trimethoxynaphthalene-1,4-dione **47** (U-638). Red solid; yield 311 mg (95%); *R$_f$* = 0.65 (C); m.p. 135–137 °C. IR (CHCl$_3$):3083, 2950, 1755, 1602, 1458, 1408, 1376, 1287, 1257, 1151, 1045 cm^{-1}. ^{1}H NMR (500 MHz, CDCl$_3$):δ1.99 (s, 6H, 2 × COC$\underline{H}$$_3$), 2.01 (s, 3H, COC$\underline{H}$$_3$), 2.04 (s, 3H, COC$\underline{H}$$_3$), 3.66 (ddd, 1H, H-5′, *J* = 9.5, 4.5, 2.5 Hz), 3.81 (d, 1H, C$\underline{H}$$_2$-S, *J* = 13.1 Hz), 4.01 (dd, 1H, H-6′a, *J* = 12.4, 2.5 Hz), 4.03 (d, 1H, C$\underline{H}$$_2$-S, *J* = 13.1 Hz), 4.10 (s, 3H, OC$\underline{H}$$_3$), 4.14 (s, 3H, OC$\underline{H}$$_3$), 4.15 (s, 3H, OC$\underline{H}$$_3$), 4.18 (dd, 1H, H-6′b, *J* = 12.4, 4.5 Hz), 4.66 (d, 1H, H-1′,*J* = 10.2 Hz), 5.02 (dd, 1H, H-2′, *J* = 10.2, 9.5 Hz), 5.09 (t, 1H, H-4′, *J* = 9.5 Hz), 5.19 (t, 1H, H-3′, *J* = 9.5 Hz), 12.91 (s, 1H, α-O$\underline{H}$), 13.12 (s, 1H, α-O$\underline{H}$).^{13}C NMR (125 MHz, CDCl$_3$):δ 20.5 (2 × COC$\underline{H}$$_3$), 20.6 (2 × COC$\underline{H}$$_3$), 22.4 (C$\underline{H}$$_2$-S), 61.6 (OC$\underline{H}$$_3$), 61.7 (2×OC$\underline{H}$$_3$), 61.9 (C-6′), 68.4 (C-4′), 70.0 (C-2′), 74.0 (C-3′), 75.8 (C-5′), 83.8 (C-1′), 106.3, 109.8, 130.6, 147.5, 148.6, 155.7, 157.9, 163.0, 169.3 (2 × $\underline{C}$OCH$_3$), 170.2 ($\underline{C}$OCH$_3$), 170.5 ($\underline{C}$OCH$_3$), 178.2 (C=O), 179.6 (C=O). HRMS (ESI): *m/z* [M − H]$^-$ calcd. for C$_{28}$H$_{31}$O$_{16}$S: 655.1338; found: 655.1332.

Deacetylation of 3-(tetra-O-acetyl-β-D-glucopyranosyl-1-thiomethyl)-5,8-dihydroxy-2-methoxynaphthalene-1,4-diones **43–47** was done according Section 4.1.4 General Procedure and led to thiomethyl glucosides **48–52** (Scheme 2)

3-(β-D-Glucopyranosyl-1-thiomethyl)-5,8-dihydroxy-3-methoxynaphthalene-1,4-dione **48** (U-636). Red solid; yield 62 mg (72%); R_f = 0.37 (D); m.p. 103–105 °C. IR (KBr): 3417, 2922, 1608, 1455, 1409, 1385, 1283, 1181, 1110, 1077, 1029, 789 cm^{-1}. ^{1}H NMR ^{1}H (500 MHz, DMSO-d_6): δ 2.96 (m, 1H, H-2′), 3.05 (m, 1H, H-5′), 3.08 (m, 1H, H-4′), 3.11 (m, 1H, H-3′), 3.39 (dd, 1H, H-6′a, J = 5.4, 12.0 Hz), 3.55 (dd, 1H, H-6′b, J = 1.7, 12.0 Hz), 3.60 (d, 1H, C$\underline{H}_2$-S, J = 13.2 Hz), 3.83 (d, 1H, C$\underline{H}_2$-S, J = 13.2 Hz), 4.15 (s, 3H, OC$\underline{H}_3$), 4.32 (d, 1H, H-1′, J = 9.9 Hz), 7.35 (d, 1H, Ar$\underline{H}$, J = 9.4 Hz), 7.38 (d, 1H, Ar$\underline{H}$, J = 9.4 Hz), 12.00 (s, 1H, α-O$\underline{H}$), 12.50 (s, 1H, α-O$\underline{H}$). ^{13}C NMR ^{1}H (125 MHz, DMSO-d_6): δ 21.0 ($\underline{C}H_2$-S), 61.0 (C-6′), 61.8 (O$\underline{C}H_3$), 69.9 (C-4′), 73.0 (C-2′), 78.4(C-3′), 81.0 (C-5′), 85.4 (C-1′), 111.0, 111.8, 128.8, 129.7, 133.0, 156.2, 156.9, 157.7, 183.4 (C=O), 187.3 (C=O). HRMS (ESI): m/z [M − H]$^-$ calcd. for C$_{18}$H$_{19}$O$_{10}$S: 427.0704; found 427.0700.

3-(β-D-Glucopyranosyl-1-thiomethyl)-5,8-dihydroxy-2-methoxy-6,7-dimethylnaphthalene-1,4-dione **49** (U-522). Red solid; yield 74 mg (81%); R_f = 0.53 (D); m.p. 209–211 °C. IR (KBr): 3391, 2923, 1605, 1582, 1454, 1421, 1384, 1334, 1300, 1281, 1191, 1137, 1086, 1047, 809 cm^{-1}. ^{1}H NMR ^{1}H (700 MHz, DMSO-d_6): δ 2.20 (s, 3H, ArC$\underline{H}_3$), 2.21 (s, 3H, ArC$\underline{H}_3$), 2.96 (m, 1H, H-2′), 3.06 (m, 1H, H-5′), 3.09 (m, 2H, H-2′, H-4′), 3.41 (m, 1H, H-6′a), 3.57 (m, 1H, H-6′b), 3.64 (d, 1H, C$\underline{H}_2$-S, J = 13.2 Hz), 3.88 (d, 1H, C$\underline{H}_2$-S, J = 13.2 Hz), 4.11 (c, 3H, C$\underline{H}_3$O), 4.33 (d, 1H, H-1′, J = 10.0 Hz), 4.41 (t, 1H, CH$_2$O$\underline{H}$, J = 5.9 Hz), 4.86 (d, 1H, CH-O$\underline{H}$, J = 4.5 Hz), 4.97 (d, 1H, CH-O$\underline{H}$, J = 3.9 Hz), 5.02 (d, 1H, CH-O$\underline{H}$, J = 6.1 Hz), 12.91 (s, 1H, α-O$\underline{H}$), 13.29 (s, 1H, α-O$\underline{H}$). ^{13}C NMR ^{1}H (175 MHz, DMSO-d_6): δ 12.1 (Ar$\underline{C}H_3$), 12.3(Ar$\underline{C}H_3$), 21.1 ($\underline{C}H_2$-S), 61.0 (C-6′), 61.8 (MeO), 69.9 (C-4′), 73.0 (C-2′), 78.4 (C-3′), 81.0 (C-5′), 85.3 (C-1′), 107.9, 109.5, 132.6, 138.8, 140.1, 156.7, 164.0, 165.0, 174.5 (C=O), 178.8 (C=O). HRMS (ESI): m/z [M − H]$^-$ calcd. for C$_{20}$H$_{23}$O$_{10}$S: 455.1017; found 455.1018.

6,7-Dichloro-3-(β-D-glucopyranosyl-1-thiomethyl)-5,8-dihydroxy-2-methoxynaphthalene-1,4-dione **50** (U-625) Red solid; yield 66 mg (67%); R_f = 0.48 (D); m.p. 180–182 °C. IR (KBr): 3417, 2895, 1611, 1587, 1452, 1402, 1333, 1279, 1227, 1180, 1115, 1043, 1017, 906, 855 cm^{-1}. ^{1}H NMR ^{1}H (500 MHz, DMSO-d_6): δ 2.96 (dd, 1H, H-2′, J = 8,3, 9.7 Hz), 3.05 (m, 2H, H-4′, H-5′), 3.11 (m, 1H, H-3′), 3.37 (dd, 1H, H-6′a, J = 4.4, 12.1 Hz), 3.57 (d,1H, H-6′b, J = 12.1 Hz), 3.66 (d, 1H, C$\underline{H}_2$-S, J = 13.1), 3.86 (d, 1H, C$\underline{H}_2$-S, J = 13.1), 4.16 (s, 3H, OC$\underline{H}_3$), 4.33 (d, 1H, H-1′, J = 9.7 Hz), 12.43 (s, 1H, α-O$\underline{H}$), 13.01 (s, 1H, α-O$\underline{H}$). ^{13}C NMR ^{1}H (125 MHz, DMSO-d_6): δ 21.2 ($\underline{C}H_2$-S), 61.1 (C-6′), 62.0 (O$\underline{C}H_3$), 70.0 (C-4′), 73.0 (C-2′), 78.3 (C-3′), 81.0 (C-5′), 85.4 (C-1′), 109.8, 111.3, 132.4, 132.5, 133.1, 156.9, 157.1, 157.5, 177.2 (C=O), 181.6 (C =O). HRMS (ESI): m/z [M − H]$^-$ calcd. for C$_{18}$H$_{17}$Cl$_2$O$_{10}$S: 494.9925; found 494.9922.

3-(β-D-Glucopyranosyl-1-thiomethyl)-5,8-dihydroxy-2,7-dimethoxynaphthalene-1,4-dione **51** (U-646). Red solid; yield 62 mg (67%); R_f = 0.44 (E); m.p. 141–143 °C. IR (KBr):3402, 2936, 2361, 1603, 1451, 1430, 1403, 1385, 1291, 1223, 1192, 1180, 1142, 1100, 1074, 1032, 955 cm^{-1}. ^{1}H NMR (500 MHz, DMSO-d_6):δ2.96 (m, 1H, H-2′), 3.06-3.12 (m, 3H, H-3′,H-4′, H-5′), 3.43 (dd, J = 11.8, 4.8 Hz, 1H, H-6′a), 3.60 (dd, J = 11.8, 2.0 Hz, 1H, H-6′b), 3.69 (d, J = 13.0 Hz, 1H, C$\underline{H}_2$-S), 3.92 (s, 3H, OC$\underline{H}_3$), 3.94 (d, 1H, C$\underline{H}_2$-S, J = 13.0 Hz), 4.03 (s, 3H, OC$\underline{H}_3$), 4.34 (d, 1H, H-1′, J = 9.8 Hz), 4.42 (br s, 1H, O$\underline{H}$′), 4.87 (br s, 1H, O$\underline{H}$′), 4.98 (br s, 1H, O$\underline{H}$′), 5.03 (br s, 1H, O$\underline{H}$′), 6.58 (s, 1H, H-6), 12.48 (s, 1H, α-O$\underline{H}$), 13.32 (s, 1H, α-O$\underline{H}$). ^{13}C NMR (125 MHz, DMSO-d_6):δ 21.2 ($\underline{C}H_2$-S), 57.1 (O$\underline{C}H_3$), 61.1 (C-6′), 61.5 (O$\underline{C}H_3$), 70.0 (C-4′), 73.1 (C-2′), 78.4 (C-3′), 81.1 (C-5′), 85.3 (C-1′), 105.7, 109.3, 111.4, 133.3, 154.6, 159.7, 163.3, 166.5, 170.9 (C=O), 177.7 (C=O). HRMS (ESI): m/z [M − H]$^-$ calcd. for C$_{19}$H$_{21}$O$_{11}$S: 457.0810; found: 457.0812.

3-(β-D-Glucopyranosyl-1-thiomethyl)-5,8-dihydroxy-2,6,7-trimethoxynaphthalene-1,4-dione **52** (U-641). Red solid; 74 mg (76%); R_f = 0.51 (E); m.p. 155–157 °C. IR (KBr):3415, 2950, 1601, 1455, 1403, 1385, 1275, 1211, 1180, 1142, 1102, 1068, 1049, 1023, 943, 876 cm^{-1}. ^{1}H NMR (700 MHz, DMSO-d_6):δ2.96 (m, 1H, H-2′), 3.06-3.12 (m, 3H, H-3′,H-4′, H-5′), 3.44 (dd, 1H, H-6′a, J = 11.8, 2.0 Hz), 3.62 (dd, 1H, H-6′b, J = 11.8, 2.0 Hz), 3.68 (d, J = 13.0 Hz, 1H, C$\underline{H}_2$-S), 3.95 (d, J = 13.0 Hz, 1H, C$\underline{H}_2$-S), 3.99 (s, 3H, OC$\underline{H}_3$), 4.02 (s, 3H, OC$\underline{H}_3$), 4.03 (s, 3H, OC$\underline{H}_3$), 4.32 (d, 1H, H-1′, J = 9.8 Hz), 4.46 (br s, 1H, O$\underline{H}$′), 4.88 (br s, 1H, O$\underline{H}$′), 4.98 (br s, 1H, O$\underline{H}$′), 5.04 (br s, 1H, O$\underline{H}$′), 12.71 (br s, 1H, α-O$\underline{H}$), 12.97 (s, 1H, α-O$\underline{H}$).

^{13}C NMR (175 MHz, DMSO-d_6): δ 21.2 (CH$_2$-S), 61.2 (C-6′), 61.4 (2×OCH$_3$), 61.6 (OCH$_3$), 70.1 (C-4′), 73.1 (C-2′), 78.5 (C-3′), 81.1 (C-5′), 85.3 (C-1′), 106.5, 109.6, 131.6, 147.6, 148.4, 155.1, 158.4, 163.5, 176.7 (C=O), 177.8 (C=O). HRMS (ESI): m/z [M − H]$^-$ calcd. for C$_{20}$H$_{23}$O$_{12}$S: 487.0916; found: 487.0918.

4.1.6. General Procedure for Synthesis of Spinochrome D Acetylated Thiomethylglycosides 56–59 by Acid-Catalytic Condensation of Spinochrome D 8 with per-O-acetyl-1-thiomercapto Derivatives of d-Glucopyranose 27, d-Galactopyranose 53, d-Mannopyranose 54, d-Xylopyranose 55 and Paraformaldehyde in Dioxane (Figure 4)

Spinochrome D 8 (119 mg, 0.50 mmol) was dissolved in a warm mixture of 1,4-dioxane (20 mL), water (3 mL), and acetic acid (0.2 mL), to which powdered paraformaldehyde (60 mg, 2.00 mmol) and corresponding per-O-acetylated 1-mercaptoshugar 27, 53–55 (0.65 mmol) were added. The reaction mixture was gently refluxed with mixing for 3h, concentrated in vacuo, and the resulting solid was purified by preparative TLC (silica gel, system C, two developments), yielding a red-colored fraction of thiomethylated product 56–59 with R_f = 0.55–0.57 (Figure 4).

3-(Tetra-O-acetyl-β-d-glucopyranosyl-1-thiomethyl)-2,5,6,7,8-pentahydroxynaphthalene-1,4-dione 56 (U-629). Red solid; 212 mg (69.0%); R_f = 0.55 (C); m.p. 127–129 °C. IR (CHCl$_3$): 3524, 3421, 3053, 3007, 1748, 1715, 1601, 1458, 1428, 1367, 1294, 1247, 1229, 1221, 1200, 1187, 1090, 1044 cm^{-1}. ^{1}H NMR (700 MHz, CDCl$_3$): δ 2.00 (s, 6H, 2 × COCH$_3$), 2.02 (s, 3H, COCH$_3$), 2.06 (s, 3H, COCH$_3$), 3.69 (m, 1H, H-5′), 3.82 (d, 1H, J = 13.6 Hz, CH$_2$S), 4.04 (dd, 1H, H-6′a, J = 12.3, 2.9 Hz), 4.06 (d, 1H, CH$_2$S, J = 13.6 Hz), 4.22 (dd, 1H, J = 12.3, 4.6 Hz), 4.68 (d, 1H, J = 10.2 Hz, H-1′), 5.05 (t, 1H, J = 9.7 Hz, H-2′), 5.09 (t, 1H, H-4′, J = 9.7 Hz), 5.22 (t, 1H, H-3′, J = 9.2 Hz), 6.55 (s, 1H, β-OH), 6.91 (s, 1H, β-OH), 7.19 (s, 1H, β-OH), 12.02 (brs, 1H, α-OH), 12.36 (s, 1H, α-OH). ^{13}C NMR (176 MHz, CDCl$_3$): δ20.6 (3 × COCH$_3$), 20.7 (COCH$_3$), 21.8 (CH$_2$-S), 62.3 (C-6′), 68.7 (C-4′), 70.1 (C-2′), 73.8 (C-3′), 75.7 (C-5′), 83.8 (C-1′), 102.4, 107.6, 121.1, 137.2, 139.2, 150.1, 152.4, 161.4, 169.4 (2 × COCH$_3$), 170.2 (COCH$_3$), 170.8 (COCH$_3$), 177.8 (C=O), 179.5 (C=O). HRMS (ESI): m/z [M − H]$^-$ calcd. for C$_{25}$H$_{25}$O$_{16}$S 613.0869; found 613.0865.

3-(Tetra-O-acetyl-β-d-galactopyranosyl-1-thiomethyl)-2,5,6,7,8-pentahydroxynaphthalene-1,4-dione 57 (U-631). Red solid; 204 mg (66.5%); R_f = 0.55 (C); m.p. 135–137 °C. IR (CHCl$_3$): 3523, 3432, 3054, 3007, 1750, 1687, 1590, 1465, 1429, 1371, 1294, 1248, 1188, 1150, 1084, 1055 cm^{-1}. ^{1}H NMR (700 MHz, DMSO-d_6): δ 1.90 (s, 3H, COCH$_3$), 1.95 (s, 3H, COCH$_3$), 1.97 (s, 3H, COCH$_3$), 2.11 (s, 3H, COCH$_3$), 3.72 (d, 1H, CH$_2$S, J = 12.9 Hz), 3.88 (d, 1H, CH$_2$S, J = 12.9 Hz), 3.90 (dd, 1H, H-6′a, J = 11.1, 6.5 Hz), 3.97 (dd, 1H, H-6′b, J = 11.1, 6.3 Hz), 4.14 (m, 1H, H-5′), 4.91 (d, 1H, H-1′, J = 10.2 Hz), 4.94 (t, 1H, H-2′, J = 9.8 Hz), 5.20 (dd, 1H, H-3′, J = 9.5, 3.6 Hz), 5.29 (dd, 1H, H-4′, J = 3.6, 0.9 Hz), 10.31 (s, 3H, 3 × β-OH), 12.60 (brs, 1H, α-OH), 13.29 (s, 1H, α-OH). ^{13}C NMR (176 MHz, DMSO-d_6): δ20.3 (COCH$_3$), 20.4 (2 × COCH$_3$), 20.5 (COCH$_3$), 21.8 (CH$_2$-S), 61.1 (C-6′), 67.5 (C-4′), 67.6 (C-2′), 71.1 (C-3′), 73.4 (C-5′), 83.0 (C-1′), 102.1, 107.0, 119.7, 139.8, 142.4, 155.3, 157.7, 166.1, 169.3 (COCH$_3$), 169.4 (COCH$_3$), 169.8 (COCH$_3$), 170.0 (COCH$_3$), 172.1 (C=O), 173.8 (C=O). HRMS (ESI): m/z [M − H]$^-$ calcd. for C$_{25}$H$_{25}$O$_{16}$S 613.0869; found 613.0858.

3-(Tetra-O-acetyl-β-d-mannopyranosyl-1-thiomethyl)-2,5,6,7,8-pentahydroxynaphthalene-1,4-dione 58 (U-630). Red solid; 200 mg (65.0%); R_f = 0.55 (C); m.p. 160–162 °C. IR (CHCl$_3$): 3524, 3446, 3054, 3007, 1749, 1686, 1637, 1600, 1541, 1508, 1458, 1430, 1369, 1293, 1247, 1187, 1104, 1052 cm^{-1}. ^{1}H NMR (500 MHz, CDCl$_3$): δ 1.96 (s, 3H, COCH$_3$), 2.04 (s, 3H, COCH$_3$), 2.09 (s, 3H, COCH$_3$), 2.16 (s, 3H, COCH$_3$), 3.68 (m, 1H, H-5′), 3.83 (d, 1H, CH$_2$S, J = 13.7 Hz), 4.07 (d, 1H, CH$_2$S, J = 13.7 Hz), 4.10 (dd, 1H, H-6′a, J = 12.2, 2.2 Hz), 4.30 (dd, 1H, H-6′b, J = 12.2, 5.2 Hz), 4.90 (d, 1H, H-1′, J = 1.0 Hz), 5.05 (d.d, 1H, H-3′, J = 10.0, 3.5 Hz), 5.27 (t, 1H, H-4′, J = 10.0 Hz), 5.46 (dd, 1H, H-2′, J = 3.6, 1.0 Hz), 6.50 (s, 1H, β-OH), 6.87 (s, 1H, β-OH), 7.12 (s, 1H, β-OH), 12.01 (brs, 1H, α-OH), 12.33 (s, 1H, α-OH). ^{13}C NMR (125 MHz, CDCl$_3$): δ20.5 (2 × COCH$_3$), 20.7 (COCH$_3$), 20.8 (COCH$_3$), 22.4 (CH$_2$-S), 63.0 (C-6′), 66.4 (C-4′), 70.3 (C-2′), 71.9 (C-3′), 76.3 (C-5′), 82.4 (C-1′), 102.6, 107.7, 121.1, 137.1, 139.1, 149.8, 152.4, 161.0, 169.6 (COCH$_3$), 170.1 (COCH$_3$), 170.2 (COCH$_3$), 170.9 (COCH$_3$), 178.0 (C=O), 179.7 (C=O). HRMS (ESI): m/z [M − H]$^-$ calcd. for C$_{25}$H$_{25}$O$_{16}$S 613.0869; found 613.0866.

3-(Tri-O-acetyl-β-d-xylopyranosyl-1-thiomethyl)-2,5,6,7,8-pentahydroxynaphthalene-1,4-dione 59 (U-628). Red solid; 171 mg (63.0%); R_f = 0.57 (C); m.p. 235–237 °C. IR (CHCl$_3$): 3467, 3342, 3046, 3009,

1732, 1592, 1422, 1376, 1330, 1287, 1267, 1241, 1220, 1208, 1200 cm^{-1}. ^{1}H NMR (500 MHz, DMSO-d_6): δ 1.94 (s, 3H, COC$\underline{H}_3$), 1.97 (s, 3H, COC$\underline{H}_3$), 1.99 (s, 3H, COC$\underline{H}_3$), 3.45 (d.d, 1H, H-5′a, J = 11.4, 9.8 Hz), 3.71 (d, 1H, C$\underline{H}_2$S, J = 12.7 Hz), 3.85 (d, 1H, C$\underline{H}_2$S, J = 12.7 Hz), 3.98 (dd, 1H, H-5′b, J = 11.4, 5.3 Hz), 4.81 (t, 1H, H-2′, J = 9.0), 4.84 (m, 1H, H-4′), 4.88 (d, 1H, H-1′, J = 9.2 Hz), 5.16 (t, 1H, H-3′, J = 8.8 Hz), 10.46 (brs, 3H, 3 × β-O$\underline{H}$), 12.48 (brs, 1H, α-O$\underline{H}$),13.35 (s, 1H, α-O$\underline{H}$). ^{13}C NMR (125 MHz, DMSO-d_6): δ20.4 (2 × CO$\underline{C}$H$_3$), 20.5 (CO$\underline{C}$H$_3$), 21.7 ($\underline{C}$H$_2$-S), 64.9 (C-5′), 68.5 (C-4′), 69.9 (C-2′), 72.2 (C-3′), 83.1(C-1′), 102.2, 107.0, 119.5, 139.7, 142.4, 155.5, 158.5, 166.7, 169.1 ($\underline{C}$OCH$_3$), 169.5 (2 × $\underline{C}$OCH$_3$), 171.3 (C=O), 173.0 (C=O). HRMS (ESI): m/z [M − H]$^-$ calcd. for C$_{22}$H$_{21}$O$_{14}$S 541.0657; found 541.0651.

4.1.7. General Procedure for Base-Catalytic Deacetylation of Acetylated Thiomethylglycosides Spinochrome D **56–59** in MeONa/Methanol Solution (Figure 4)

Acetylated thiomethylglycosides of spinochrome D **56–59** (0.25 mmol) were suspended in dry MeOH (10 mL) and (2.0 mL, 1.0 mM) of 0.5 N MeONa/MeOH solution was added under argon atmosphere. The reaction mixture was kept at room temperature for 1 h and then acidified with 2N HCl to give a clear red solution. The reaction mixture was concentrated in vacuoand the resulting solid was purified by preparative TLC (system E), yielding a red-colored fraction of desacetylated glycosides **60–63** with R_f = 0.30–0.40 (Figure 4).

3-(β-D-Glucopyranosyl-1-thiomethyl)-2,5,6,7,8-pentahydroxynaphthalene-1,4-dione **60** (U-649). Red solid; 81 mg (72.6%); R_f = 0.33 (E); m.p. 177–180 °C. IR (KBr): 3402, 2923, 1588, 1468, 1427, 1385, 1285, 1097, 1046, 983, 876, 786, 766, 719 cm^{-1}. ^{1}H NMR (700 MHz, DMSO-d_6): δ 2.96 (dd, 1H, H-2′, J = 9.7, 8.5 Hz), 3.05 (m, 1H, H-5′), 3.10 (t, 1H, H-3′, J = 8.5 Hz), 3.13 (m, 1H, H-4′), 3.45 (dd, 1H, H-6′a, J = 11.8, 5.0 Hz), 3.57 (dd, 1H, H-6′b, J = 11.9, 2.0 Hz), 3.68 (d, 1H, C$\underline{H}_2$S, J = 13.0 Hz), 3.86 (d, 1H, C$\underline{H}_2$S, J = 13.0 Hz), 4.39 (d, 1H, H-1′, J = 9.8 Hz), 4.90 (br s, 4H, carbohydr. hydroxyls), 10.39 (br s, 3H, 3 × β-O$\underline{H}$), 12.50 (br s, 1H, α-O$\underline{H}$), 13.29 (br s, 1H, α-O$\underline{H}$). ^{13}C NMR (176 MHz, DMSO-d_6): δ21.2 ($\underline{C}$H$_2$-S), 60.8 (C-6′), 69.7 (C-4′), 73.2 (C-2′), 78.5 (C-3′), 80.7 (C-5′), 85.9 (C-1′), 102.2, 106.8, 121.2, 139.9, 142.4, 154.9, 158.0, 166.5, 172.0 (C=O), 173.6 (C=O). HRMS (ESI): m/z [M − H]$^-$ calcd. for C$_{17}$H$_{17}$O$_{12}$S 445.0450; found 445.0451.

3-(β-D-Galactopyranosyl-1-thiomethyl)-2,5,6,7,8-pentahydroxynaphthalene-1,4-dione **61** (U-650). Red solid; 75 mg (67.3%); R_f = 0.30 (E); m.p. 186–189 °C. IR (KBr): 3345, 2925, 1587, 1469, 1425, 1385, 1285, 1140, 1083, 1052, 980, 865, 768 cm^{-1}. ^{1}H NMR (500 MHz, DMSO-d_6): δ 3.23 (dd, 1H, H-3′, J = 9.0, 3.2 Hz), 3.27 (t, 1H, H-2′, J = 9.2 Hz), 3.31 (m, 1H, H-5′), 3.38 (dd, 1H, H-6′a, J = 10.5, 5.8 Hz), 3.48 (dd, 1H, H-6′b, J = 10.5, 7.0 Hz), 3.70 (m, 1H, H-4′), 3.70 (d, 1H, C$\underline{H}_2$S, J = 12.8 Hz), 3.83 (d, 1H, C$\underline{H}_2$S, J = 12.8 Hz), 4.37 (d, 1H, H-1′, J = 9.5 Hz), 4.71 (br s, 4H, carbohydr. hydroxyls), 10.37 (br.s, 3H, 3 × β-O$\underline{H}$), 12.34 (br s, 1H, α-O$\underline{H}$), 13.30 (br s, 1H, α-O$\underline{H}$). ^{13}C NMR (125 MHz, DMSO-d_6): δ21.3 ($\underline{C}$H$_2$-S), 60.0 (C-6′), 68.1 (C-4′), 70.2 (C-2′), 74.9 (C-3′), 78.9 (C-5′), 86.5 (C-1′), 102.2, 106.8, 121.1, 128.4, 139.8, 142.4, 154.9, 157.8, 166.3, 172.2 (C=O), 173.9 (C=O). HRMS (ESI): m/z [M − H]$^-$ calcd. for C$_{17}$H$_{17}$O$_{12}$S 445.0450, found 445.0446.

3-(β-D-Mannopyranosyl-1-thiomethyl)-2,5,6,7,8-pentahydroxynaphthalene-1,4-dione **62** (U-648). Red solid; 77 mg (69.0%); R_f = 0.30 (E); m.p. 185–187 °C. IR (KBr): 3394, 2936, 1704, 1591, 1463, 1426, 1385, 1293, 1054, 985, 881, 772 cm^{-1}. ^{1}H NMR (500 MHz, DMSO-d_6): δ 3.00 (m, 1H, H-5′), 3.26 (dd, 1H, H-3′, J = 9.3, 3.4 Hz), 3.36 (t, 1H, H-4′, J = 9.3 Hz), 3.44 (dd, 1H, H-6′a, J = 11.5, 5.1 Hz), 3.51 (dd, 1H, H-6′b, J = 11.5, 2.4 Hz), 3.62 (m, 1H, H-2′), 3.76 (s, 2H, C$\underline{H}_2$S), 4.15 (br s, 4H, carbohydr. hydroxyls), 4.75 (d, 1H, H-1′, J = 1.2 Hz), 10.14 (br s, 1H, β-O$\underline{H}$), 10.48 (br s, 1H, β-O$\underline{H}$), 11.19 (br s, 1H, β-O$\underline{H}$), 12.72 (br s, 1H, α-O$\underline{H}$), 13.22 (br s, 1H, α-O$\underline{H}$). ^{13}C NMR (DMSO-d_6, 125 MHz): δ22.5 ($\underline{C}$H$_2$-S), 61.1 (C-6′), 66.6 (C-4′), 72.2 (C-2′), 74.7 (C-3′), 81.2 (C-5′), 85.2 (C-1′), 102.3, 106.8, 121.5, 140.0, 142.3, 154.3, 157.7, 166.4, 172.3 (C=O), 173.8 (C=O). HRMS (ESI): m/z [M − H]$^-$ calcd. for C$_{17}$H$_{17}$O$_{12}$S 445.0450; found 445.0446.

3-(β-D-Xylopyranosyl-1-thiomethyl)-2,5,6,7,8-pentahydroxynaphthalene-1,4-dione **63** (U-647). Red solid; 62 mg (59.6%); R_f = 0.40 (E); m.p. 177–179 °C. IR (KBr): 3380, 2921, 1588, 1464, 1426, 1286, 1157, 1136, 1092, 1041, 980, 926, 769, 717, 630 cm^{-1}. ^{1}H NMR (500 MHz, DMSO-d_6): δ 2.96 (dd, 1H,

H-2′, J = 9.4, 8.3 Hz), 3.02 (dd, 1H, H-5′a, J = 11.3, 10.2 Hz), 3.07 (t, 1H, H-3′, J = 8.3 Hz), 3.29 (m, 1H, H-4′), 3.65 (d, 1H, C$\underline{H}_2$S, J = 13.0 Hz), 3.74 (dd, 1H, H-5′b, J = 11.3, 5.3 Hz), 3.83 (d, 1H, C$\underline{H}_2$S, J = 13.0 Hz), 4.35 (d, 1H, H-1′, J = 9.4 Hz), 4.91 (br s, 3H, carbohydr. hydroxyls), 10.15 (br s, 1H, β-O$\underline{H}$), 10.49 (br s, 1H, β-O$\underline{H}$), 11.20 (br s, 1H, β-O$\underline{H}$), 12.73 (br s, 1H, α-O$\underline{H}$), 13.23 (br s, 1H, α-O$\underline{H}$). ^{13}C NMR (176 MHz, DMSO-d_6): δ21.0 ($\underline{C}H_2$-S), 69.2 (C-5′), 69.5 (C-4′), 73.0 (C-2′), 78.0 (C-3′), 86.3 (C-1′), 102.2, 106.9, 121.2, 140.0, 142.3, 154.4, 157.4, 166.2, 172.5 (C=O), 174.1 (C=O). HRMS (ESI): m/z [M − H]$^-$ calcd. for $C_{16}H_5O_{11}S$ 415.0341, found 415.0343.

4.2. Cell Culture

The cells of the mouse Neuro-2a neuroblastoma (ATCC®CCL-131™; American Type Culture Collection, Manassas, USA) were cultured in DMEM medium containing 10% fetal bovine serum (Biolot, St. Petersburg, Russia) and 1% penicillin/streptomycin (Biolot, St. Petersburg, Russia). The cells were placed in 96-well plates in a concentration of 3×10^4 cells per well and incubated at 37 °C in a humidified atmosphere containing 5% (v/v) CO_2.

4.3. Cytotoxic Activity Assay

Neuro-2a cells (3×10^4 cells/well) were incubated with different concentrations of 5,8-dihydroxy-1,4-naphthoquinone derivatives in a CO_2-incubator for 24 h at 37 °C. After incubation, the medium with tested substances was replaced with 100 μL of pure medium. Cell viability was determined using the MTT (3-(4,5-dimethylthiazol-2-yl)-2,5-diphenyltetrazolium bromide) method, according to the manufacturer's instructions (Sigma-Aldrich, St. Louis, USA). For this purpose, 10 μL of MTT stock solution (5 mg/mL) was added to each well and the microplate was incubated for 4 h at 37 °C. After that, 100 μL of SDS-HCl (1 g SDS/10 ml dH_2O/17 μL 6 N HCl) was added to each well, followed by incubation for 4–18 h. The absorbance of the converted dye formazan was measured using a Multiskan FC microplate photometer (Thermo Scientific, Waltham, USA) at a wavelength of 570 nm. The results were presented as percent of control data, and the concentration required for 50% inhibition of cell viability (EC_{50}) was calculatedusing SigmaPlot 3.02 (Jandel Scientific, San Rafael, CA, USA). All data were obtained in three independent replicates and expressed as mean ± SEM.

Stocks of substances were prepared in DMSO at a concentration of 10 mM. All studied 1,4-NQ derivatives were tested in a concentration range from 0.4 μM to 100 μM with two-fold dilution. All tested compounds were added in a volume of 20 μL dissolved in PBS to 180 μL of cell culture with the cells in each of the wells (final DMSO concentration < 1%). Triterpene glycoside cladoloside C isolated from the sea cucumber *Cladolabes schmeltzii* [60] was used as a reference cytotoxic compound.

4.4. Computer Modeling and Quantitative Structure-Activity Relationship (QSAR)

In the present study, a dataset of 50 1,4-NQs derivatives (Table 1) was used for 3D-structure modeling and optimization with Amber 10:EHT force field using the Build module of the MOE 2019.01 program [61]. The dataset was used for descriptor calculations with the QuaSAR module of MOE 2019.01. The EC_{50} values were converted into corresponding pEC_{50} values ($-\log EC_{50}$) to be included in the database. The pEC50 values determined in this work for 22 compounds with 4 < pEC_{50} < 6 were added to the database with the structures of the studied compounds. The dataset of the 22 1,4-NQs derivatives with 4 < pEC_{50} < 6 was divided into training (18) and test (4) sets (Table 3), which were used for the generation of a QSAR model and its validation, respectively. The MOE Pharmacophore editor for pharmacophore modeling was used, which consisted of standard pharmacophoric features including hydrogen bond acceptor (Acc), hydrogen bond donor (Don), hydrophobic (Hyd), and aromatic ring (Aro). The energy-optimized molecules with high toxicity U-634 and nontoxic U-633 were used for the development of the pharmacophore models.

5. Conclusions

Based on 6,7-substituted 2,5,8-trihydroxy-1,4-naphtoquinones (1,4-NQs) derived from sea urchins, five new acetyl-O-glucosides of NQ were prepared. A new method of conjugation of per-O-acetylated 1-mercaptosaccharides with 2-hydroxy-1,4-NQs through a methylene spacer was developed. Methylation of the 2-hydroxy group of the quinone core of acetylthiomethylglycosides by diazamethane and deacetylation of sugar moiety led to the synthesis 28 new thiomethylglycosides of 2-hydroxy- and 2-methoxy-1,4-NQs. The cytotoxic activity of starting 1,4-NQs (13 compounds) and their O- and S-glycoside derivatives (37 compounds) was determined by the MTT method against Neuro-2a mouse neuroblastoma cells. A computer model of the effect on cancer cells of the chemical structure–activity relationship (QSAR) of 5,8-dihydroxy-1,4-NQ derivatives was constructed. The structural elements of the naphthoquinone molecules (pharmacophores) which determined the high cytotoxic activity were revealed. These results can be taken into account during the directed modification of the quinone structure to obtain new, highly selective compounds which are toxic to tumor cells. QSAR analysis can be used to predict cytotoxic activity and targeted modification of the quinone structure in the preparation of new neuroprotectors for the treatment of brain tumors.

Author Contributions: Conceptualization, planning and designing of the research, D.A., S.P. and G.L.; synthesis and purification of 1,4-naphthoquinones, S.P., Y.S. and D.P.; NMR study, V.D.; cell cultivation and cytotoxicity assay, E.C., E.M. and E.P.; computer modeling and QSAR analysis, G.L. All authors have read and agreed to the published version of the manuscript.

Funding: This work was supported by the Russian Science Foundation, Grant No. 19-14-00047.

Acknowledgments: We thank R. S. Popov for MS measurements and V. P. Glazunov for recording IR spectra. We are grateful for the NMR study performed at the Collective Facilities Center "The Far Eastern Center for Structural Molecular Research (NMR/MS) PIBOC FEB RAS".

Conflicts of Interest: The authors declare no conflict of interest.

References

1. Gould, J. Breaking down the epidemiology of brain cancer. *Nat. Cell Biol.* **2018**, *561*, S40–S41. [CrossRef]
2. Vargo, M. Brain Tumors and Metastases. *Phys. Med. Rehabil. Clin. N. Am.* **2017**, *28*, 115–141. [CrossRef]
3. El-Habashy, S.E.; Nazief, A.M.; Adkins, C.E.; Wen, M.M.; El-Kamel, A.H.; Hamdan, A.M.; Hanafy, A.S.; Terrell, T.O.; Mohammad, A.S.; Lockman, P.R.; et al. Novel treatment strategies for brain tumors and metastases. *Pharm. Pat. Anal.* **2014**, *3*, 279–296. [CrossRef] [PubMed]
4. Shah, V. Brain Cancer: Implication to Disease, Therapeutic Strategies and Tumor Targeted Drug Delivery Approaches. *Recent Patents Anti-Cancer Drug Discov.* **2018**, *13*, 70–85. [CrossRef] [PubMed]
5. Thomson, R.H. *Naturally Occurring Quinones IV*; Blackie Chapman and Hall: London, UK, 1997.
6. Sánchez-Calvo, J.M.; Barbero, G.R.; Guerrero-Vásquez, G.; Durán, A.G.; Macías, M.; Rodríguez-Iglesias, M.; Molinillo, J.M.G.; Macías, F.A. Synthesis, antibacterial and antifungal activities of naphthoquinone derivatives: A structure–activity relationship study. *Med. Chem. Res.* **2016**, *25*, 1274–1285. [CrossRef]
7. Wellington, K.W. Understanding cancer and the anticancer activities of naphthoquinones—A review. *RSC Adv.* **2015**, *5*, 20309–20338. [CrossRef]
8. Aminin, D.; Polonik, S. 1,4-Naphthoquinones: Some Biological Properties and Application. *Chem. Pharm. Bull.* **2020**, *68*, 46–57. [CrossRef]
9. Maris, J.M.; Hogarty, M.D.; Bagatell, R.; Cohn, S.L. Neuroblastoma. *Lancet* **2007**, *369*, 2106–2120. [CrossRef]
10. Kobayashi, T.; Haruta, M.; Sasagawa, K.; Matsumata, M.; Eizumi, K.; Kitsumoto, C.; Motoyama, M.; Maezawa, Y.; Ohta, Y.; Noda, T.; et al. Optical communication with brain cells by means of an implanted duplex micro-device with optogenetics and Ca2+ fluoroimaging. *Sci. Rep.* **2016**, *6*. [CrossRef]
11. Hou, Y.; Vasileva, E.A.; Carne, A.; McConnell, M.; Bekhit, A.E.-D.A.; Hou, Y. Naphthoquinones of the spinochrome class: Occurrence, isolation, biosynthesis and biomedical applications. *RSC Adv.* **2018**, *8*, 32637–32650. [CrossRef]
12. Sime, A.A.T. Biocidal Compositions Comprising Polyhydroxynaphthoquinones. GB Patent 2159056, 27 November 1985.

13. Mishchenko, N.P.; Fedoreev, S.A.; Bagirova, V.L. Histochrome: A New Original Domestic Drug. *Pharm. Chem. J.* **2003**, *37*, 48–52. [CrossRef]
14. Anufriev, V.P.; Novikov, V.L.; Maximov, O.B.; Elyakov, G.B.; Levitsky, D.O.; Lebedev, A.V.; Sadretdinov, S.M.; Shvilkin, A.; Afonskaya, N.I.; Ruda, M.Y.; et al. Synthesis of some hydroxynaphthazarins and their cardioprotective effects under ischemia-reperfusion in vivo. *Bioorg. Med. Chem. Lett.* **1998**, *8*, 587–592. [CrossRef]
15. Boguslavskaya, L.V.; Khrapova, N.G.; Maksimov, O.B. Polyhydroxynaphthoquinones? A new class of natural antioxidants. *Russ. Chem. Bull.* **1985**, *34*, 1345–1350. [CrossRef]
16. Acharya, B.R.; Bhattacharyya, S.; Choudhury, D.; Chakrabarti, G. The microtubule depolymerizing agent naphthazarin induces both apoptosis and autophagy in A549 lung cancer cells. *Apoptosis* **2011**, *16*, 924–939. [CrossRef] [PubMed]
17. Masuda, K.; Funayama, S.; Komiyama, K.; Umezawa, I.; Ito, K. Constituents of Tritonia crocosmaeflora, II. Tricrozarin B, an Antitumor Naphthazarin Derivative. *J. Nat. Prod.* **1987**, *50*, 958–960. [CrossRef]
18. Lennikov, A.; Kitaichi, N.; Noda, K.; Mizuuchi, K.; Ando, R.; Dong, Z.; Fukuhara, J.; Kinoshita, S.; Namba, K.; Ohno, S.; et al. Amelioration of endotoxin-induced uveitis treated with the sea urchin pigment echinochrome in rats. *Mol. Vis.* **2014**, *20*, 171–177.
19. Huot, R.; Brassard, P. Friedel—Crafts condensation with maleic anhydrides. III. The synthesis of polyhydroxylated naphthoquinones. *Can. J. Chem.* **1974**, *54*, 838–842. [CrossRef]
20. Moore, R.E.; Singh, H.; Chang, C.W.J.; Scheuer, P.J. Polyhydroxynaphthoquinones: Preparation and hydrolysis of methoxyl derivatives. *Tetrahedron* **1967**, *23*, 3271–3305. [CrossRef]
21. Jeong, S.H.; Kim, H.K.; Song, I.-S.; Noh, S.J.; Marquez, J.; Ko, K.S.; Rhee, B.D.; Kim, N.; Mishchenko, N.; Fedoreyev, S.; et al. Echinochrome A Increases Mitochondrial Mass and Function by Modulating Mitochondrial Biogenesis Regulatory Genes. *Mar. Drugs* **2014**, *12*, 4602–4615. [CrossRef]
22. Seo, D.Y.; McGregor, R.A.; Noh, S.J.; Choi, S.-J.; Mishchenko, N.; Fedoreyev, S.; Stonik, V.A.; Han, J. Echinochrome A Improves Exercise Capacity during Short-Term Endurance Training in Rats. *Mar. Drugs* **2015**, *13*, 5722–5731. [CrossRef]
23. Soliman, A.M.; Mohamed, A.S.; Marie, M.-A.S. Echinochrome pigment attenuates diabetic nephropathy in the models of type 1 and type 2 diabetes. *Diabetes Mellit.* **2016**, *19*, 464–470. [CrossRef]
24. Lebedev, A.V.; Ivanova, M.V.; Levitsky, D.O. Echinochrome, a naturally occurring iron chelator and free radical scavenger in artificial and natural membrane systems. *Life Sci.* **2005**, *76*, 863–875. [CrossRef] [PubMed]
25. Lebedev, A.V.; Ivanova, M.V.; Levitsky, D.O. Iron Chelators and Free Radical Scavengers in Naturally Occurring Polyhydroxylated 1,4-Naphthoquinones. *Hemoglobin* **2008**, *32*, 165–179. [CrossRef] [PubMed]
26. Polonik, S.G.; Prokof'eva, N.G.; Agafonova, I.G.; Uvarova, N.I. Antitumor and immunostimulating activity of 5-hydroxy-1,4-naphthoquinone (juglone) O- and S-acetylglycosides. *Pharm. Chem. J.* **2003**, *37*, 397–398. [CrossRef]
27. Pelageev, D.N.; Dyshlovoy, S.A.; Pokhilo, N.D.; Denisenko, V.A.; Borisova, K.L.; Amsberg, G.K.-V.; Bokemeyer, C.; Fedorov, S.N.; Honecker, F.; Anufriev, V.P. Quinone–carbohydrate nonglucoside conjugates as a new type of cytotoxic agents: Synthesis and determination of in vitro activity. *Eur. J. Med. Chem.* **2014**, *77*, 139–144. [CrossRef]
28. Dyshlovoy, S.A.; Pelageev, D.N.; Hauschild, J.; Sabutski, Y.E.; Khmelevskaya, E.A.; Krisp, C.; Kaune, M.; Venz, S.; Borisova, K.L.; Busenbender, T.; et al. Inspired by Sea Urchins: Warburg Effect Mediated Selectivity of Novel Synthetic Non-Glycoside 1,4-Naphthoquinone-6S-Glucose Conjugates in Prostate Cancer. *Mar. Drugs* **2020**, *18*, 251. [CrossRef]
29. Sabutski, Y.E.; Menchinskaya, E.S.; Shevchenko, L.S.; Chingizova, E.; Chingizov, A.R.; Popov, R.; Denisenko, V.A.; Mikhailov, V.V.; Aminin, D.L.; Polonik, S.G. Synthesis and Evaluation of Antimicrobial and Cytotoxic Activity of Oxathiine-Fused Quinone-Thioglucoside Conjugates of Substituted 1,4-Naphthoquinones. *Molecules* **2020**, *25*, 3577. [CrossRef]
30. Verma, R.P. Anti-Cancer Activities of 1,4-Naphthoquinones: A QSAR Study. *Anti-Cancer Agent. Med. Chem.* **2006**, *6*, 489–499. [CrossRef]
31. Pérez-Sacau, E.; Díaz-Peñate, R.G.; Estévez-Braun, A.; Ravelo, A.G.; García-Castellano, J.M.; Pardo, A.L.; Campillo, M. Synthesis and Pharmacophore Modeling of Naphthoquinone Derivatives with Cytotoxic Activity in Human Promyelocytic Leukemia HL-60 Cell Line. *J. Med. Chem.* **2007**, *50*, 696–706. [CrossRef]

32. Takano, A.; Hashimoto, K.; Ogawa, M.; Koyanagi, J.; Kurihara, T.; Wakabayashi, H.; Kikuchi, H.; Nakamura, Y.; Motohashi, N.; Sakagami, H.; et al. Tumor-specific cytotoxicity and type of cell death induced by naphtho[2,3-b]furan-4,9-diones and related compounds in human tumor cell lines: Relationship to electronic structure. *Anticancer. Res.* **2009**, *29*, 455–464.
33. Prachayasittikul, V.; Pingaew, R.; Worachartcheewan, A.; Nantasenamat, C.; Prachayasittikul, S.; Ruchirawat, S.; Prachayasittikul, V. Synthesis, anticancer activity and QSAR study of 1,4-naphthoquinone derivatives. *Eur. J. Med. Chem.* **2014**, *84*, 247–263. [CrossRef] [PubMed]
34. Costa, M.C.A.; Ferreira, M.M.C. Two-dimensional quantitative structure–activity relationship study of 1,4-naphthoquinone derivatives tested against HL-60 human promyelocytic leukaemia cells. *SAR QSAR Environ. Res.* **2017**, *28*, 325–339. [CrossRef]
35. Acuña, J.; Piermattey, J.; Caro, D.; Bannwitz, S.; Barrios, L.; López, J.; Ocampo, Y.; Vivas-Reyes, R.; Aristizábal, F.; Gaitán, R.; et al. Synthesis, Anti-Proliferative Activity Evaluation and 3D-QSAR Study of Naphthoquinone Derivatives as Potential Anti-Colorectal Cancer Agents. *Molecules* **2018**, *23*, 186. [CrossRef] [PubMed]
36. Costa, M.C.A.; Carvalho, P.O.M.; Ferreira, M.M.C. Four-dimensional quantitative structure-activity analysis of 1,4-naphthoquinone derivatives tested against HL-60 human promyelocytic leukemia cells. *J. Chemometr.* **2019**, *34*, e3131. [CrossRef]
37. Polonik, S.G.; Tolkach, A.M.; Denisenko, V.A.; Uvarova, N.I. Synthesis of glucosudes of 3-alk[en]yl-2-hydroxy-1,4-naphthoquinones. *Chem. Nat. Compd.* **1983**, *19*, 310–313. [CrossRef]
38. Driguez, H. Thiooligosaccharides as Tools for Structural Biology. *ChemBioChem* **2001**, *2*, 311–318. [CrossRef]
39. Polonik, S.G.; Tolkach, A.M.; Uvarova, N.I. Glycosidation of echinochrome and related hydroxynaphthazarins by orthoester method. *Rus. J. Org. Chem.* **1994**, *30*, 248–253. (In Russian)
40. Yurchenko, E.A.; Menchinskaya, E.S.; Polonik, S.G.; Agafonova, I.G.; Guzhova, I.V.; Aminin, B.A.M.A.D.L. Hsp70 Induction and Anticancer Activity of U-133, the Acetylated Trisglucosydic Derivative of Echinochrome. *Med. Chem.* **2015**, *5*, 263–271. [CrossRef]
41. Guzhova, I.V.; Plaksina, D.V.; Pastukhov, Y.F.; Lapshina, K.V.; Lazarev, V.F.; Mikhaylova, E.R.; Polonik, S.G.; Pani, B.; Margulis, B.A.; Guzhova, I.V.; et al. New HSF1 inducer as a therapeutic agent in a rodent model of Parkinson's disease. *Exp. Neurol.* **2018**, *306*, 199–208. [CrossRef]
42. Belan, D.V.; Polonik, S.G.; Ekimova, I.V. Efficiency of Preventive Therapy with Chaperon Inducer U133 in the Model of Preclinical Stage of Parkinson's Disease in Elderly Rats. *Rus. J. Physiol.* **2020**, *106*, 1251–1265. (In Russian) [CrossRef]
43. Cruciani, G.; Crivori, P.; Carrupt, P.-A.; Testa, B. Molecular fields in quantitative structure–permeation relationships: The VolSurf approach. *J. Mol. Struct. THEOCHEM* **2000**, *503*, 17–30. [CrossRef]
44. McClendon, A.K.; Osheroff, N. DNA topoisomerase II, genotoxicity, and cancer. *Mutat. Res. Fundam. Mol. Mech. Mutagen.* **2007**, *623*, 83–97. [CrossRef] [PubMed]
45. Liu, Y.-M.; Huangfu, W.-C.; Huang, H.-L.; Wu, W.-C.; Chen, Y.-L.; Yen, Y.; Huang, H.-L.; Nien, C.-Y.; Lai, M.-J.; Pan, S.-L.; et al. 1,4-Naphthoquinones as inhibitors of Itch, a HECT domain-E3 ligase, and tumor growth suppressors in multiple myeloma. *Eur. J. Med. Chem.* **2017**, *140*, 84–91. [CrossRef] [PubMed]
46. Prachayasittikul, V.; Pingaew, R.; Worachartcheewan, A.; Sitthimonchai, S.; Nantasenamat, C.; Prachayasittikul, S.; Ruchirawat, S.; Prachayasittikul, V. Aromatase inhibitory activity of 1,4-naphthoquinone derivatives and QSAR study. *EXCLI J.* **2017**, *16*, 714–726.
47. Wang, J.-R.; Shen, G.-N.; Luo, Y.-H.; Piao, X.-J.; Shen, M.; Liu, C.; Wang, Y.; Meng, L.-Q.; Zhang, Y.; Wang, H.; et al. The compound 2-(naphthalene-2-thio)-5,8-dimethoxy-1,4-naphthoquinone induces apoptosis via reactive oxygen species-regulated mitogen-activated protein kinase, protein kinase B, and signal transducer and activator of transcription 3 signaling in human gast. *Drug Dev. Res.* **2018**, *79*, 295–306. [CrossRef] [PubMed]
48. Ravichandiran, P.; Masłyk, M.; Sheet, S.; Janeczko, M.; Premnath, D.; Kim, A.R.; Park, B.H.; Han, M.K.; Yoo, D.J. Synthesis and Antimicrobial Evaluation of 1,4-Naphthoquinone Derivatives as Potential Antibacterial Agents. *Chemistryopen* **2019**, *8*, 589–600. [CrossRef]
49. Rozanov, D.V.; Cheltsov, A.; Nilsen, A.; Boniface, C.; Forquer, I.; Korkola, J.; Gray, J.; Tyner, J.; Tognon, C.E.; Mills, G.B.; et al. Targeting mitochondria in cancer therapy could provide a basis for the selective anti-cancer activity. *PLoS ONE* **2019**, *14*, e0205623. [CrossRef]

50. Wellington, K.W.; Kolesnikova, N.I.; Hlatshwayo, V.; Saha, S.T.; Kaur, M.; Motadi, L.R. Anticancer activity, apoptosis and a structure–activity analysis of a series of 1,4-naphthoquinone-2,3-bis-sulfides. *Investig. New Drugs* **2019**, *38*, 274–286. [CrossRef]
51. Aly, A.A.; El-Sheref, E.M.; Bakheet, M.E.M.; Mourad, M.A.E.; Brown, A.B.; Bräse, S.; Nieger, M.; Ibrahim, M.A.A. Synthesis of novel 1,2-bis-quinolinyl-1,4-naphthoquinones: ERK2 inhibition, cytotoxicity and molecular docking studies. *Bioorg. Chem.* **2018**, *81*, 700–712. [CrossRef]
52. Badolato, M.; Carullo, G.; Caroleo, M.C.; Cione, E.; Aiello, F.; Manetti, F. Discovery of 1,4-Naphthoquinones as a New Class of Antiproliferative Agents Targeting GPR55. *ACS Med. Chem. Lett.* **2019**, *10*, 402–406. [CrossRef]
53. Dyshlovoy, S.A.; Pelageev, D.N.; Hauschild, J.; Borisova, K.L.; Kaune, M.; Krisp, C.; Venz, S.; Sabutski, Y.E.; Khmelevskaya, E.A.; Busenbender, T.; et al. Successful Targeting of the Warburg Effect in Prostate Cancer by Glucose-Conjugated 1,4-Naphthoquinones. *Cancers* **2019**, *11*, 1690. [CrossRef] [PubMed]
54. Anufriev, V.P.; Malinovskaya, G.V.; Novikov, V.L.; Balanyova, N.N.; Polonik, S.G. The Reductive Dehalogenation of Halo-Substituted Naphthazarins and Quinizarins as a Simple Route to Parent Compounds. *Synth. Commun.* **1998**, *28*, 2149–2157. [CrossRef]
55. Polonik, N.S.; Polonik, S.G. DMSO-mediated transformation of 3-amino-2-hydroxynaphthazarins to natural 2,3-dihydroxy-naphthazarins and related compounds. *Tetrahedron Lett.* **2016**, *57*, 3303–3306. [CrossRef]
56. Polonik, S.G.; Sabutskii, Y.E.; Denisenko, V.A. The Acid-Catalyzed 2-O-Alkylation of Substituted 2-Hydroxy-1,4-naphthoquinones by Alcohols: Versatile Preparative Synthesis of Spinochrome D and Its 6-Alkoxy Derivatives. *Synthesis* **2018**, *50*, 3738–3748. [CrossRef]
57. Kochetkov, N.K.; Bochkov, A.F. The synthesis of oligosaccharides by orthoester method. In *Methods in Carbohydrate Chemistry*; Whistler, R.L., Bemiller, J.N., Eds.; Academic Press: New York, NY, USA, 1972; Volume 6, p. 239.
58. Pelageev, D.N.; Panchenko, M.N.; Pokhilo, N.D.; Anufriev, V.F. Synthesis of 2,2′-(ethane-l,l-diyl)bis(3,5,6,7,8-pentahydroxy-l,4-naphthoquinone), a metabolite of the sea urchins Spatangus purpureus, Strongylocentrotus intermedius, and S. droebachiensis. *Russ. Chem. Bull.* **2010**, *59*, 1472–1476. [CrossRef]
59. Fujihira, T.; Chida, M.; Kamijo, H.; Takido, T.; Seno, M. Novel synthesis of 1-thioglycopyranoses via thioiminium salts. *J. Carbohyd. Chem.* **2002**, *21*, 287–292. [CrossRef]
60. Silchenko, A.S.; Kalinovsky, A.I.; Avilov, S.A.; Andryjaschenko, P.V.; Dmitrenok, P.; Yurchenko, E.A.; Dolmatov, I.Y.; Kalinin, V.I.; Stonik, V.A. Structure and biological action of cladolosides B1, B2, C, C1, C2 and D, six new triterpene glycosides from the sea cucumber Cladolabes schmeltzii. *Nat. Prod. Commun.* **2013**, *8*, 1527–1534. [CrossRef] [PubMed]
61. *Molecular Operating Environment (MOE), 2019.01*; Chemical Computing Group ULC: Montreal, QC, Canada, 2019.

Publisher's Note: MDPI stays neutral with regard to jurisdictional claims in published maps and institutional affiliations.

© 2020 by the authors. Licensee MDPI, Basel, Switzerland. This article is an open access article distributed under the terms and conditions of the Creative Commons Attribution (CC BY) license (http://creativecommons.org/licenses/by/4.0/).

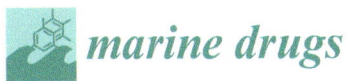

Article

Structures and Bioactivities of Quadrangularisosides A, A_1, B, B_1, B_2, C, C_1, D, D_1–D_4, and E from the Sea Cucumber *Colochirus quadrangularis*: The First Discovery of the Glycosides, Sulfated by C-4 of the Terminal 3-*O*-Methylglucose Residue. Synergetic Effect on Colony Formation of Tumor HT-29 Cells of these Glycosides with Radioactive Irradiation

Alexandra S. Silchenko [1,*], Anatoly I. Kalinovsky [1], Sergey A. Avilov [1], Pelageya V. Andrijaschenko [1], Roman S. Popov [1], Pavel S. Dmitrenok [1], Ekaterina A. Chingizova [1], Svetlana P. Ermakova [1], Olesya S. Malyarenko [1], Salim Sh. Dautov [2] and Vladimir I. Kalinin [1]

[1] G.B. Elyakov Pacific Institute of Bioorganic Chemistry, Far Eastern Branch of the Russian Academy of Sciences, Pr. 100-letya Vladivostoka 159, Vladivostok 690022, Russia; kaaniv@piboc.dvo.ru (A.I.K.); avilov-1957@mail.ru (S.A.A.); pandrijashchenko@mail.ru (P.V.A.); prs_90@mail.ru (R.S.P.); paveldmt@piboc.dvo.ru (P.S.D.); martyyas@mail.ru (E.A.C.); swetlana_e@mail.ru (S.P.E.); vishchuk@mail.ru (O.S.M.); kalininv@piboc.dvo.ru (V.I.K.)

[2] A.V. Zhirmunsky National Scientific Center of Marine Biology, Far Eastern Branch, Russian Academy of Sciences, 17 Palchevskogo Street, Vladivostok 690041, Russia; daut49shakir@mail.ru

* Correspondence: sialexandra@mail.ru; Tel.: +7(423)2-31-40-50

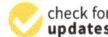

Received: 2 July 2020; Accepted: 25 July 2020; Published: 28 July 2020

Abstract: Thirteen new mono-, di-, and trisulfated triterpene glycosides, quadrangularisosides A–D_4 (**1**–**13**) have been isolated from the sea cucumber *Colochirus quadrangularis*, which was collected in Vietnamese waters. The structures of these glycosides were established by 2D NMR spectroscopy and HR-ESI (High Resolution Electrospray Ionization) mass spectrometry. The novel carbohydrate moieties of quadrangularisosides D–D_4 (**8**–**12**), belonging to the group D, and quadrangularisoside E (**13**) contain three sulfate groups, with one of them occupying an unusual position—at C(4) of terminal 3-*O*-methylglucose residue. Quadrangularisosides A (**1**) and D_3 (**11**) as well as quadrangularisosides A_1 (**2**) and D_4 (**12**) are characterized by the new aglycones having 25-hydroperoxyl or 24-hydroperoxyl groups in their side chains, respectively. The cytotoxic activities of compounds **1**–**13** against mouse neuroblastoma Neuro 2a, normal epithelial JB-6 cells, erythrocytes, and human colorectal adenocarcinoma HT-29 cells were studied. All the compounds were rather strong hemolytics. The structural features that most affect the bioactivity of the glycosides are the presence of hydroperoxy groups in the side chains and the quantity of sulfate groups. The membranolytic activity of monosulfated quadrangularisosides of group A (**1**, **2**) against Neuro 2a, JB-6 cells, and erythrocytes was relatively weak due to the availability of the hydroperoxyl group, whereas trisulfated quadrangularisosides D_3 (**11**) and D_4 (**12**) with the same aglycones as **1**, **2** were the least active compounds in the series due to the combination of these two structural peculiarities. The erythrocytes were more sensitive to the action of the glycosides than Neuro 2a or JB-6 cells, but the structure–activity relationships observed for glycosides **1**–**13** were similar in the three cell lines investigated. The compounds **3**–**5**, **8**, and **9** effectively suppressed the cell viability of HT-29 cells. Quadrangularisosides A_1 (**2**), C (**6**), C_1 (**7**), and E (**13**) possessed strong inhibitory activity on colony formation in HT-29 cells. Due to the synergic effects of these glycosides (0.02 µM) and radioactive irradiation (1 Gy), a decreasing of number of colonies was detected. Glycosides **1**, **3**, and **9** enhanced the effect of radiation by about 30%.

Keywords: *Colochirus quadrangularis*; triterpene glycosides; quadrangularisosides; sea cucumber; cytotoxic activity

1. Introduction

Triterpene glycosides, biosynthesized by the sea cucumbers, are well-known secondary metabolites that are characterized by tremendous structural diversity [1–4], different kinds of biological activities [5,6], and taxonomic specificity [7–10]. Hence, the studies on this class of metabolites are still relevant.

The chemical investigation of the sea cucumber *Colochirus quadrangularis* was started earlier and the structures of some aglycones and glycosides were established [11–15].

Hence, it seemed very interesting to reinvestigate the composition of triterpene glycosides in the sea cucumber *Colochirus quadrangularis* to compare structural data reported earlier with those obtained by us. The animals were collected near the Vietnamese sea shore. Herein, we report the isolation and structure elucidation of 13 new glycosides having holostane-type aglycones and tetrasaccharide carbohydrate chains with one, two, and three sulfate groups. The structures of compounds named quadrangularisosides A (**1**), A_1 (**2**), B (**3**), B_1 (**4**), B_2 (**5**), C (**6**), C_1 (**7**), D (**8**), D_1–D_4 (**9–12**), and E (**13**) were established by the analyses of the ^{1}H, ^{13}C NMR, 1D TOCSY (Total Correlation Spectroscopy), and 2D NMR (^{1}H,^{1}H-COSY, HMBC, HSQC, ROESY—^{1}H,^{1}H-Correlated Spectroscopy, Heteronuclear Multiple Bond Correlation, Heteronuclear Single Quantum Correlation, Rotating-Frame Overhauser Effect Spectroscopy) spectra as well as HR-ESI ((High Resolution Electrospray Ionization)) mass spectra. The original spectra are presented in Supplementary Materials. The hemolytic activities against mouse erythrocytes, cytotoxic activities against mouse neuroblastoma Neuro 2a, and normal epithelial JB-6 cells as well as the influence of **1–13** on the cell viability and colony formation of HT-29 cells have been studied.

2. Results and Discussion

2.1. Structures of the Earlier Published Glycosides from C. quadrangularis

In 2004, the group of Chinese researches reported the structure elucidation of the aglycones obtained by an acid hydrolysis from the sum of glycosides of this species of sea cucumbers [11]. However, the paper contained some inaccuracies. Firstly, the specific name of the sea cucumber was written erroneously (*quadrangulaSis* instead of *quadrangulaRis*). Moreover, the assignment to genus *Pentacta* was also incorrect, since the actual specific name of this sea cucumber indexed by the "WoRMS" database is *Colochirus quadrangularis*. Secondly, thorough analysis of the NMR data provided in this paper for philinopgenin B possessing, according to the authors, 18(16)-lactone and unique 20(25)-epoxy-fragment, has raised many questions. If an 18(16)-lactone ring was present in the genin, the signals of H-16 and H-17 would be observed as the broad singlets due to the very small value of coupling constant $J_{17/16}$ [16,17]. However, in the ^{1}H NMR spectrum of philinopgenin B, the signal of H-16 was observed as a triplet, but its *J* value was not provided, and the signal of H-17 was observed as a multiplet. Moreover, the signals of carbons adjacent to the oxygen in the epoxy fragment should be deshielded to δ_C approximately 80–85 [17,18] whenever in the paper [11] the signals assigned to C-20 and C-25 were observed at δ_C 73.0 and 71.8, correspondingly. Finally, it is inadmissible to provide only integer values of *m/z* without any decimals as HR-ESI-MS data. Considering all these errors, the structure of philinopgenin B looks doubtful.

More recently, the structures of four glycosides, philinopsides A, B [12], E, and F [13], isolated from *Pentacta* (=*Colochirus*) *quadrangularis* were discussed by the same researchers. Philinopside B was described as a disulfated tetraoside with an uncommon position of the second sulfate group at C-2 of the xylose (the third residue in the carbohydrate chain) [12]. However, the comparison of the ^{13}C NMR spectra of this glycoside and its desulfated derivative showed the absence of any differences in the δ_C values assigned to the xylose, occupying the third position in the carbohydrate chain, and therefore, the presence of the only sulfate group in the sugar chain of philinopside B—at C-4 of the first (xylose) residue. Moreover, the HR mass-spectrometric data have not been provided in the paper. The m/z of fragment ions observed in the ESI MS did not prove the presence of two sulfate groups in the compound.

Afterwards, the structures of pentacasides B and C were established as disulfated tetraosides with one of sulfate groups attached to C-2 of the quinovose residue [14], pentacasides I, II—as triosides lacking a 3-O-methylglucose unit, thus having terminal xylose residue [15] and, finally, pentacaside III—as a bioside with the carbohydrate chain identical to that of holothurins of group B [15,19]. The trisaccharide chains of pentacasides I and II are first found in the sea cucumber glycosides. The authors stated that additional studies are required for the final proving of their structures [15]. Actually, the analysis of the ^{13}C NMR spectrum of pentacaside I showed that the signal of C-3 of the terminal (xylose) residue was deshielded (δ_C 87.3) and the signals of C-2 and C-4 of the same residue were shielded (δ_C 73.7 and 69.2, correspondingly) as compared with the spectrum of pentacaside II, which is characteristic for the glycosylation effects. So, doubts arise concerning the correctness of the structure of the glycoside.

2.2. Structural Elucidation of the Glycosides

The concentrated ethanolic extract of the sea cucumber *Colochirus quadrangularis* was chromatographed on a Polychrom-1 column (powdered Teflon, Biolar, Latvia). The glycosides were eluted with 50% EtOH and separated by chromatography on a Si gel column using CHCl$_3$/EtOH/H$_2$O (100:100:17) and (100:125:25) as mobile phases. The obtained fractions were subsequently subjected to HPLC on a silica-based Supelcosil LC-Si (4.6 × 150 mm) column and on a reversed-phase semipreparative Supelco Discovery HS F5-5 (10 × 250 mm) column to yield compounds **1–13** (Figure 1) along with nine known earlier glycosides: colochirosides B$_1$, B$_2$, and B$_3$ [20], lefevreosides A$_2$ and C [21], neothyonidioside [22], hemoiedemoside A [23], and philinopsides A [12] and F [13], which were isolated earlier from different species of sea cucumbers. The known compounds were identified by the comparison of their ^{1}H and ^{13}C NMR spectra with those reported in the literature.

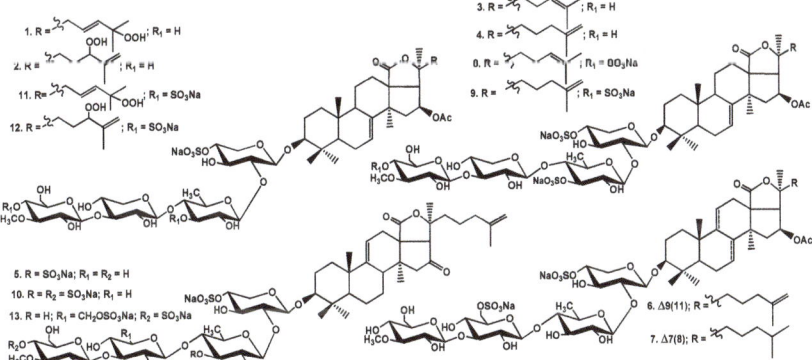

Figure 1. Chemical structures of glycosides isolated from *Colochirus quadrangularis*: **1**—quadrangularisoside A; **2**—quadrangularisoside A$_1$; **3**—quadrangularisoside B; **4**—quadrangularisoside B$_1$; **5**—quadrangularisoside B$_2$; **6**—quadrangularisoside C; **7**—quadrangularisoside C$_1$; **8**—quadrangularisoside D; **9**—quadrangularisoside D$_1$, **10**—quadrangularisoside D$_2$; **11**—quadrangularisoside D$_3$; **12**—quadrangularisoside D$_4$; **13**—quadrangularisoside E.

The ^{1}H and ^{13}C NMR spectra corresponding to the carbohydrate chains of quadrangularisosides A (**1**) and A$_1$ (**2**) (Table 1) were identical to each other and to those of known compounds isolated from this species: colochirosides B$_1$, B$_2$, and B$_3$, lefevreosides A$_2$ and C, neothyonidioside and philinopside A, having linear tetrasaccharide monosulfated carbohydrate moieties with the xylose residue as the third unit. Such a sugar chain is common in the glycosides of sea cucumbers of different taxa [2].

Table 1. ^{13}C and ^{1}H NMR chemical shifts and HMBC and ROESY correlations of the carbohydrate moiety of quadrangularisosides A (**1**) and A$_1$ (**2**). ^{a} Recorded at 176.03 MHz in C$_5$D$_5$N/D$_2$O (4/1). ^{b} Bold = interglycosidic positions. ^{c} Italic = sulfate position. ^{d} Recorded at 700.00 MHz in C$_5$D$_5$N/D$_2$O (4/1). Multiplicity by 1D TOCSY.

Atom.	δ_C mult. ^{a,b,c}	δ_H mult. ^{d} (J in Hz)	HMBC	ROESY
		Xyl1 (1→C-3)		
1	104.8 CH	4.67 d (6.9)	C-3; C: 5 Xyl1	H-3; H-3, 5 Xyl1
2	82.2 CH	3.99 t (8.9)	C: 1 Qui2; C: 1, 3 Xyl1	H-1 Qui2
3	75.0 CH	4.24 t (8.9)	C: 2, 4 Xyl1	H-1, 5 Xyl1
4	76.2 CH	4.98 m	C: 3, 5 Xyl1	-
5	63.9 CH$_2$	4.77 dd (5.4; 11.8)	C: 1, 3, 4 Xyl1	-
		3.73 dd (9.7; 11.5)	C: 1, 3, 4 Xyl1	H-1 Xyl1
		Qui2 (1→2Xyl1)		
1	104.7 CH	4.99 d (7.8)	C: 2 Xyl1; C: 5 Qui2	H-2 Xyl1; H-3, 5 Qui2
2	75.8 CH	3.86 t (9.5)	C: 1, 3 Qui2	H-4 Qui2
3	74.8 CH	3.95 t (9.5)	C: 2, 4 Qui2	H-1, 5 Qui2
4	85.6 CH	3.50 t (9.5)	C: 3, 5 Qui2, 1 Xyl3	H-1 Xyl3
5	71.4 CH	3.64 dd (6.1; 9.5)	-	H-1, 3 Qui2
6	17.8 CH$_3$	1.60 d (6.1)	C: 4, 5 Qui2	H-4, 5 Qui2
		Xyl3 (1→4Qui2)		
1	104.5 CH	4.77 d (7.8)	C: 4 Qui2	H-4 Qui2; H-3,5 Xyl3
2	73.4 CH	3.88 t (9.5)	C: 1, 3 Xyl3	-
3	86.4 CH	4.11 m	C: 2, 4 Xyl3; 1 MeGlc4	H-1 MeGlc4; H-1, 5 Xyl3
4	68.7 CH	3.93 m	C: 5 Xyl3	-
5	65.9 CH$_2$	4.11 dd (5.2; 10.4)	C: 3 Xyl3	-
		3.59 t (11.2)	C: 1, 3, 4 Xyl3	H-1, 3 Xyl3
		MeGlc4 (1→3Xyl3)		
1	104.5 CH	5.20 d (8.0)	C: 3 Xyl3; C: 5 MeGlc4	H-3 Xyl3; H-3, 5 MeGlc4
2	74.5 CH	3.87 t (8.8)	-	-
3	87.0 CH	3.67 t (8.8)	C: 2, 4 MeGlc4, OMe	H-1, 5 MeGlc4; OMe
4	70.4 CH	3.88 t (8.8)	C: 5, 6 MeGlc4	-
5	77.5 CH	3.91 m	-	H-1 MeGlc4
6	61.8 CH$_2$	4.36 dd (2.1; 11.7)	C: 4 MeGlc4	-
		4.04 dd (6.4; 11.9)	-	-
OMe	60.6 CH$_3$	3.80 s	C: 3 MeGlc4	-

The molecular formula of quadrangularisoside A (**1**) was determined to be C$_{55}$H$_{85}$O$_{27}$SNa from the [M$_{Na}$ − Na]$^-$ ion peak at m/z 1209.5004 (calc. 1209.5004) in the (−)HR-ESI-MS and [M$_{Na}$ + Na]$^+$ ion peak at m/z 1255.4779 (calc. 1255.4789) in the (+)HR-ESI-MS. The analysis of the ^{13}C and ^{1}H NMR spectra of the aglycone part of **1** suggested the presence of an 18(20)-lactone [from the signals of C(18) at δ_C 180.0 and C(20) at δ_C 84.8], a 7(8)-double bond [from the signal of secondary carbon C(7) at δ_C 120.3 and the corresponding proton signal at δ_H 5.61 (m, H(7)), the signal of quaternary carbon C(8) at δ_C 145.5] as well as the β-OAc group at C(16) [from the signal of carbon at δ_C 74.8 (C(16)) and the corresponding proton signal at δ_H 5.92 (H(16), q, J = 8.5 Hz) along with the signals of two carbons of the O-acetic group at δ_C 170.7 and 21.1 and a signal of protons of the methyl group at δ_H 1.97(s)] (Table 2). All these data indicated the presence of a holostane-type nucleus in 1. The signals of olefinic carbons at δ_C 124.2 (C(23)) and 139.5 (C(24)) indicated the presence of a double bond in the side chain of quadrangularisoside A (1). The δ_C values of the olefinic carbons were close to those in the ^{13}C NMR spectrum of psolusoside D$_3$ [24] that allowed supposing the 23(24)-position of the double bond. The HMBC correlations from methyl groups H(26) and H(27) to the olefinic carbons C(23) and C(24) corroborated the position of the double bond. The coupling pattern of olefinic protons H(23) (δ_H 5.71, dt, J = 6.6; 15.5 Hz) and H(24) (δ_H 5.97, d, J = 15.8 Hz) indicated a 23E-configuration of the double bond in 1. The signal of the tertiary bearing oxygen carbon C(25) was deduced from the HMBC correlations between the signals of methyl groups H(26) (δ_H 1.46, s) and H(27) (δ_H 1.48, s) and the signal at δ_C 81.3. This chemical shift was also close to that of the corresponding carbon (δ_C 80.8, C(25)) in the spectrum of psolusoside D$_3$ [24]. So, the NMR and HR-ESI-MS data indicated the presence of a 25-hydroperoxy-23E-ene fragment in the side chain of 1. This is the third finding of a hydroperoxyl group in the triterpene glycosides aglycones of sea cucumbers [24,25].

The (+)ESI-MS/MS of 1 demonstrated the fragmentation of the [M$_{Na}$ + Na]$^+$ ion at m/z 1255.5. The peaks of fragment ions were observed at m/z 1223.5 [M$_{Na}$ + Na − OOH + H]$^+$, 1103.5 [M$_{Na}$ + Na − OOH − NaSO$_4$ + H]$^+$, 927.5 [M$_{Na}$ + Na − OOH − NaSO$_4$ − C$_7$H$_{12}$O$_5$ (MeGlc) + H]$^+$, 795.4 [M$_{Na}$ + Na − OOH − NaSO$_4$ − C$_7$H$_{12}$O$_5$ (MeGlc) − C$_5$H$_8$O$_4$ (Xyl) + H]$^+$, 729.2 [M$_{Na}$ + Na − C$_{32}$H$_{47}$O$_6$ (Agl) + H]$^+$, 649.3 [M$_{Na}$ + Na− OOH − NaSO$_4$ − C$_7$H$_{12}$O$_5$ (MeGlc) − C$_5$H$_8$O$_4$ (Xyl) − C$_6$H$_{10}$O$_4$ (Qui) + H]$^+$, 609.2 [M$_{Na}$ + Na − C$_{32}$H$_{47}$O$_6$ (Agl) − NaHSO$_4$]$^+$, 477.1 [M$_{Na}$ + Na − C$_{32}$H$_{47}$O$_6$ (Agl) − NaHSO$_4$ − C$_5$H$_8$O$_4$ (Xyl) + H]$^+$, corroborating the structure of quadrangularisoside A (1).

All these data indicate that quadrangularisoside A (1) is 3β-O-[3-O-methyl-β-D-glucopyranosyl-(1→3)-β-D-xylopyranosyl-(1→4)-β-D-quinovopyranosyl-(1→2)-4-O-sodium sulfate-β-D-xylopyranosyl]-25-peroxy-16β-acetoxyholosta-7,23E-diene.

The molecular formula of quadrangularisoside A$_1$ (2) was determined to be the same as that of 1 (C$_{55}$H$_{85}$O$_{27}$SNa) from the [M$_{Na}$ − Na]$^-$ ion peak at m/z 1209.5006 (calc. 1209.5004) in the (−)HR-ESI-MS and [M$_{Na}$ + Na]$^+$ ion peak at m/z 1255.4772 (calc. 1255.4789) in the (+)HR-ESI-MS. The signals in the ^{13}C NMR spectrum of 2 assigning to triterpene nucleus (C(1)–C(20), C(30)–C(32)) coincided with the corresponding signals in the spectrum of 1 indicating the difference of these glycoside only in the side chains structures (Table 3). An isolated spin system formed by the protons H(22)–H(24) was deduced from the ^{1}H,^{1}H-COSY spectrum of 2. The signal of H(24) was deshielded and observed at δ_H 4.51 (brt, J = 6.2 Hz) due to the attachment of a hydroperoxyl group to C(24) in the glycoside 2, which was corroborated by the deshielding of the signal of C(24) to δ_C 89.2. The signals of olefinic carbons at δ_C 144.9 (C(25)) and 113.6 (C(26)) as well as olefinic protons at δ_H 5.14 (brs, H(26)) and 5.02 (brs, H(26′)) indicated the presence of a terminal double bond in the side chain of 2. The positions of a double bond and hydroperoxyl group were confirmed by the HMBC correlations H(24)/C(26); H(26) and H(26′)/C(24), C(27); H(27)/C(24), C(25), C(26). Hence, quadrangularisosides A (1) and A$_1$ (2) are the isomers by the position of the hydroperoxy-ene fragment in their side chains.

Table 2. ^{13}C and ^{1}H NMR chemical shifts and HMBC and ROESY correlations of the aglycone moiety of quadrangularisosides A (**1**) and D$_3$ (**11**). ^{a} Recorded at 176.03 MHz in C$_5$D$_5$N/D$_2$O (4/1). ^{b} Recorded at 700.00 MHz in C$_5$D$_5$N/D$_2$O (4/1).

Position	δ_C mult. ^{a}	δ_H mult. (J in Hz) ^{b}	HMBC	ROESY
1	35.8 CH$_2$	1.33 m	-	H-19
		1.29 m	-	H-3, H-11
2	26.8 CH$_2$	1.97 m	-	-
		1.79 m	-	H-19, H-30
3	89.1 CH	3.18 dd (4.3; 12.0)	C: 4, 30, 31, C:1 Xyl1	H-1, H-5, H-31, H-1Xyl1
4	39.3 C	-	-	-
5	47.9 CH	0.91 dd (4.3; 10.5)	C: 4, 6, 7, 9, 10, 19, 30, 31	H-3, H-31
6	23.2 CH$_2$	1.94 m	C: 5, 7, 8, 10	H-19, H-30, H-31
7	120.3 CH	5.61 m	-	H-15, H-32
8	145.5 C	-	-	-
9	47.0 CH	3.31 brd (14.3)	-	H-19
10	35.4 C	-	-	-
11	22.3 CH$_2$	1.71 m	-	H-1
		1.45 m	-	H-19
12	31.1 CH$_2$	2.06 m	-	H-21
13	59.2 C	-	-	-
14	47.3 C	-	-	-
15	43.3 CH$_2$	2.52 brdd (7.3; 12.4)	C: 13, 14, 16, 17, 32	H-7, H-32
		1.64 brd (7.3)	C: 14, 16, 32	-
16	74.8 CH	5.92 q (8.5)	C: 13, 15, 17, 20, OAc	H-32
17	54.3 CH	2.76 d (8.9)	C: 12, 13, 15, 18, 21	H-12, H-21, H-32
18	180.0 C	-	-	-
19	23.8 CH$_3$	1.10 s	C: 5, 9, 10	H-2, H-6, H-9, H-11, H-30
20	84.8 C	-	-	-
21	28.2 CH$_3$	1.53 s	C: 17, 20, 22	H-12, H-17, H-22, H-23
22	41.6 CH$_2$	3.20 td (5.4; 14.0)	C: 20, 21, 23, 24	-
		2.66 dd (7.3; 14.0)	C: 17, 20, 21, 23, 24	H-21
23	124.2 CH	5.71 dt (6.6; 15.5)	C: 20, 22, 25	H-26, H-27
24	139.5 CH	5.97 d (15.8)	C: 22, 25, 26, 27	H-22, H-26, H-27
25	81.3 C	-	-	-
26	24.8 CH$_3$	1.46 s	C: 23, 24, 25, 27	H-23, H-27
27	24.6 CH$_3$	1.48 s	C: 23, 24, 25, 26	H-23, H-26
30	17.1 CH$_3$	1.00 s	C: 3, 4, 5, 31	H-2, H-6, H-19, H-31
31	28.5 CH$_3$	1.17 s	C: 3, 4, 5, 30	H-3, H-5, H-6, H-30, H-1 Xyl1
32	32.0 CH$_3$	1.09 s	C: 8, 13, 14, 15	H-7, H-12, H-15, H-16, H-17
OCOCH$_3$	170.7 C	-	-	-
OCOCH$_3$	21.1 CH$_3$	1.97 s	C: 16, OAc	-

Table 3. ^{13}C and ^{1}H NMR chemical shifts and HMBC and ROESY correlations of the aglycone moiety of quadrangularisosides A$_1$ (**2**) and D$_4$ (**11**). ^{a} Recorded at 176.03 MHz in C$_5$D$_5$N/D$_2$O (4/1). ^{b} Recorded at 700.00 MHz in C$_5$D$_5$N/D$_2$O (4/1).

Position	δ_C mult. ^{a}	δ_H mult. (J in Hz) ^{b}	HMBC	ROESY
1	35.9 CH$_2$	1.32 m	-	H-3, H-5, H-11, H-19
2	26.8 CH$_2$	1.97 m	-	-
		1.79 m	-	H-19, H-30
3	89.1 CH	3.18 dd (3.9; 12.0)	C:1 Xyl1	H-1, H-5, H-6, H-31, H-1Xyl1
4	39.3 C	-	-	-
5	47.9 CH	0.91 dd (4.6; 10.4)	C: 4, 6, 10, 19, 30	H-3, H-31
6	23.1 CH$_2$	1.94 m	-	H-19, H-30, H-31
7	120.3 CH	5.60 m	-	H-15, H-32
8	145.7 C	-	-	-
9	47.1 CH	3.29 brd (14.5)	-	H-19
10	35.4 C	-	-	-
11	22.5 CH$_2$	1.72 m	-	H-1
		1.46 m	-	-
12	31.3 CH$_2$	2.10 m	-	-
13	59.4 C	-	-	-
14	47.1 C	-	-	-
15	43.8 CH$_2$	2.58 brdd (7.3; 12.3)	C: 13, 17	H-7
		1.60 m	C: 17	H-12, H-32
16	75.5 CH	5.75 q (8.9)	-	H-21, H-32
17	54.6 CH	2.68 d (8.9)	C: 18	H-12, H-21, H-32
18	180.3 C	-	-	-
19	23.8 CH$_3$	1.10 s	C: 5, 9, 10	H-1, H-2, H-6, H-9, H-30
20	85.3 C	-	-	-
21	27.9 CH$_3$	1.52 s	C: 17, 20, 22	H-12, H-17, H-22, H-23
22	34.7 CH$_2$	2.36 td (5.0; 13.3)	-	-
		2.19 td (4.2; 13.3)	-	H-21
23	26.8 CH$_2$	1.85 m	-	H-21
		1.63 m	-	-
24	89.2 CH	4.51 t (6.2)	C: 26	H-22, H-26, H-27
25	144.9 C	-	-	-
26	113.6 CH$_2$	5.14 brs	C: 24, 27	H-24
		5.02 brs	C: 24, 27	H-27
27	17.5 CH$_3$	1.82 s	C: 24, 25, 26	H-26
30	17.2 CH$_3$	1.00 s	C: 3, 4, 5, 31	H-2, H-6, H-19, H-31, H-6 Qui2
31	28.6 CH$_3$	1.17 s	C: 3, 4, 5, 30	H-3, H-5, H-6, H-30, H-1 Xyl1
32	32.3 CH$_3$	1.15 s	C: 8, 13, 14, 15	H-15, H-16, H-17
OCOCH$_3$	171.0 C	-	-	-
OCOCH$_3$	21.4 CH$_3$	2.05 s	C: OAc	-

The 24(S)-configuration was assigned to the 24(S)-hydroxy-25-dehydroechinoside A isolated earlier from the sea cucumber *Actinopyga flammea* [26]. The same configuration of C(24)-stereocenter was established by Mosher's method in the aglycone of cucumarioside A$_7$ from the sea cucumber *Eupentacta fraudatrix* [27], which differs from the aglycone of **2** only by a hydroxyl substituent at

C(24) instead of a hydroperoxyl group. Thus, 24(S)-configuration can be attributed to the aglycone of quadrangularisoside A$_1$ (2) based on its biogenetic background.

The (+) ESI-MS/MS of **2** demonstrated the fragmentation of the [M$_{Na}$ + Na − OOH]$^+$ ion at m/z 1237.5 corresponding to a dehydrated molecule, whose formation was caused by the presence of a hydroperoxyl group in the aglycone. The peaks of fragment ions were observed at m/z 1177.4 [M$_{Na}$ + Na − OOH − CH$_3$COOH]$^+$, 1117.5 [M$_{Na}$ + Na − OOH − NaHSO$_4$]$^+$. The fragmentation of the [M$_{Na}$ + Na]$^+$ ion at m/z 1237.5 resulted in the formation of fragment ions at the same m/z as in **1**: 729.2 [M$_{Na}$ + Na− C$_{32}$H$_{47}$O$_6$ (Agl) + H]$^+$, 609.2 [M$_{Na}$ + Na − C$_{32}$H$_{47}$O$_6$ (Agl) − NaHSO$_4$]$^+$, 477.1 [M$_{Na}$ + Na − C$_{32}$H$_{47}$O$_6$ (Agl) − NaHSO$_4$ − C$_5$H$_8$O$_4$ (Xyl) + H]$^+$, corroborating their isomerism.

All these data indicate that quadrangularisosides A$_1$ (**2**) is 3β-O-[3-O-methyl-β-D-glucopyranosyl-(1→3)-β-D-xylopyranosyl-(1→4)-β-D-quinovopyranosyl-(1→2)-4-O-sodium sulfate-β-D-xylopyranosyl]-24S-peroxy-16β-acetoxyholosta-7,25-diene.

The ^{1}H and ^{13}C NMR spectra corresponding to the carbohydrate chains of quadrangularisosides B (**3**), B$_1$ (**4**), and B$_2$ (**5**) (Table 4) were identical to each other and coincided with the spectra of the carbohydrate part of pseudostichoposide B isolated earlier from the sea cucumber *Pseudostichopus trachus* (=*P. mollis*) (family Pseudostichopodidae, order Persiculida) [28] and violaceusoside E from *Pseudocolochirus violaceus* [29]. This linear disulfated tetrasaccharide chain was characterized by the attachment of the second sulfate group to C(3) of the quinovose residue. The structure of the carbohydrate chain of glycosides **3–5** was established by the thorough analysis of the ^{1}H,^{1}H-COSY, HSQC, and 1D TOCSY spectra for each monosaccharide unit, and the positions of interglycosidic linkages were elucidated based on the ROESY and HMBC correlations (Table 4). The finding of sugar moieties of the glycosides with the sulfate group at C(3) of the quinovose is very rare. Only three glycosides having such structural features are found so far [28,29] among more than 150 known triterpene glycosides from the sea cucumbers.

It is necessary to note that pentactasides B and C were reported earlier to have the disulfated tetrasaccharide chains with the same monosacccharide composition as in **3–5** but differing by the position of a second sulfate group that was positioned at C(2) of the quinovose residue [14]. The analysis of the NMR data provided in the paper [14] allowed supposing the erroneous interpretation of these data by the authors. When the sulfate group is bonded to C(2) of the monosaccharide residue in the pyranose form, it resulted in the up-field shifting of the signal of anomeric carbon to δ$_C$ approximately 100 [30]. Whenever the signals of C(1) of a quinovose unit in pentactasides B and C were observed, δ$_C$ 102.5 and 102.9, correspondingly, indicating the absence of a sulfate group at C(2) of this residue. So, the signals of C(2) at δ$_C$ 81.1 and 81.4 and C(3) at δ$_C$ 74.5 and 75.0 of the quinovose units in pentactasides B and C, correspondingly, probably were displaced with each other, and the second sulfate group is located at C(3)Qui2 in these glycosides. Therefore, the structures of pentactasides B and C most likely are identical to those of quadrangularisosides B (**3**) and B$_1$ (**4**), correspondingly.

The molecular formula of quadrangularisoside B (**3**) was determined to be C$_{55}$H$_{84}$O$_{28}$S$_2$Na$_2$ from the [M$_{2Na}$ − Na]$^−$ ion peak at m/z 1279.4489 (calc. 1279.4494) and [M$_{2Na}$ − 2Na]$^{2−}$ ion peak at m/z 628.2311 (calc. 628.2301) in the (−)HR-ESI-MS as well as from the [M$_{2Na}$ + Na]$^+$ ion peak at m/z 1325.4272 (calc. 1325.4278) in the (+)HR-ESI-MS. The signals in the ^{13}C NMR spectrum of the aglycone part of **3** were very close to those in the spectrum of cucumarioside A$_1$ from *E. fraudatrix* [28] and pentactaside B [14], indicating the identity of their aglycones (Table 5). This holostane-type aglycone with 7(8)- and 24(25)-double bonds and a 16β-acetoxy-group is quite common for the glycosides of sea cucumbers of the order Dendrochirotida [2,4,5].

The (−)ESI-MS/MS of **3** showed the fragmentation of the [M$_{2Na}$ − Na]$^−$ ion at m/z 1279.5. The peaks of fragment ions were observed at m/z 1219.4 [M$_{2Na}$ − Na − CH$_3$COOH]$^−$, 1177.5 [M$_{2Na}$ − Na − NaSO$_3$ + H]$^−$. The (+)ESI-MS/MS of **3** showed that the fragmentation of the [M$_{2Na}$ + Na]$^+$ ion at m/z 1325.4 resulted in the formation of fragment ions whose peaks were observed at m/z 1223.5 [M$_{2Na}$ + Na − NaSO$_3$ + H]$^+$, 915.4 [M$_{2Na}$ + Na − NaSO$_3$ − C$_7$H$_{12}$O$_5$ (MeGlc) − C$_5$H$_8$O$_4$ (Xyl) + H]$^+$, 813.4 [M$_{2Na}$ + Na − C$_{32}$H$_{47}$O$_5$ (Agl) − H]$^+$, 711.1 [M$_{2Na}$ + Na − C$_{32}$H$_{47}$O$_5$ (Agl) − SO$_3$Na]$^+$, 579.1 [M$_{2Na}$ + Na −

$C_{32}H_{47}O_5$ (Agl) − $C_5H_7O_7SNa$ (XylSO$_3$Na) − H]$^+$, 535.3 [M$_{2Na}$ + Na − $C_{32}H_{47}O_5$ (Agl) − SO$_3$Na − $C_7H_{12}O_5$ (MeGlc)]$^+$, 403.0 [M$_{2Na}$ + Na − $C_{32}H_{47}O_5$ (Agl) − SO$_3$Na − $C_7H_{12}O_5$ (MeGlc) − $C_5H_8O_4$ (Xyl)]$^+$, and 331.1 [M$_{2Na}$ + Na − $C_{32}H_{47}O_5$ (Agl) − $C_5H_7O_7SNa$ (XylSO$_3$Na) − $C_6H_9O_7SNa$ (QuiSO$_3$Na) − H]$^+$, which corroborate the monosaccharide sequence in the carbohydrate chain of **3**.

All these data indicate that quadrangularisoside B (**3**) is 3β-O-[3-O-methyl-β-D-glucopyranosyl-(1→3)-β-D-xylopyranosyl-(1→4)-3-O-sodium sulfate-β-D-quinovopyranosyl-(1→2)-4-O-sodium sulfate-β-D-xylopyranosyl]-16β-acetoxyholosta-7,24-diene.

Table 4. ^{13}C and ^{1}H NMR chemical shifts and HMBC and ROESY correlations of carbohydrate moiety of quadrangularisosides B (**3**), B$_1$ (**4**), and B$_2$ (**5**). ^{a} Recorded at 176.03 MHz in C$_5$D$_5$N/D$_2$O (4/1). ^{b} Bold = interglycosidic positions. ^{c} Italic = sulfate position. ^{d} Recorded at 700.00 MHz in C$_5$D$_5$N/D$_2$O (4/1). Multiplicity by 1D TOCSY.

Atom	δ_C mult. ^{a,b,c}	δ_H mult. ^{d} (J in Hz)	HMBC	ROESY
		Xyl1 (1→C-3)		
1	104.6 CH	4.63 d (7.7)	C-3; C: 5 Xyl1	H-3; H-3, 5 Xyl1
2	**81.9** CH	3.96 dd (7.3; 8.9)	C: 1 Qui2; 1, 3 Xyl1	H-1 Qui2
3	75.3 CH	4.22 t (8.9)	C: 2, 4 Xyl1	H-1, 5 Xyl1
4	76.0 CH	4.96 m	C: 3 Xyl1	-
5	64.1 CH$_2$	4.79 dd (5.4; 11.6)	C: 1, 3, 4 Xyl1	-
		3.73 dd (9.3; 11.6)	C: 1, 4 Xyl1	H-1 Xyl1
		Qui2 (1→2Xyl1)		
1	103.5 CH	5.10 d (7.1)	C: 2 Xyl1	H-2 Xyl1; H-3, 5 Qui2
2	75.7 CH	4.00 t (8.7)	C: 1, 3 Qui2	-
3	*81.5* CH	4.98 t (8.7)	C: 2, 4 Qui2	H-1, 5 Qui2
4	**79.2** CH	3.82 t (8.7)	C: 1 Xyl3	H-1 Xyl3
5	71.7 CH	3.65 dd (6.3; 8.7)	C: 1 Qui2	H-1 Qui2
6	18.3 CH$_3$	1.53 d (5.7)	C: 4, 5 Qui2	H-4, 5 Qui2
		Xyl3 (1→4Qui2)		
1	102.8 CH	5.09 d (6.8)	C: 4 Qui2; 5 Xyl3	H-4 Qui2; H-3,5 Xyl3
2	73.2 CH	4.10 t (9.1)	C: 1, 3 Xyl3	-
3	**86.0** CH	4.13 t (9.1)	C: 1 MeGlc4; 2, 4 Xyl3	H-1 MeGlc4
4	69.4 CH	4.03 m	C: 3 Xyl3	-
5	65.9 CH$_2$	4.46 dd (5.3; 12.1)	C: 1, 3, 4 Xyl3	-
		3.77 dd (8.3; 12.1)	C: 1, 4 Xyl3	H-1 Xyl3
		MeGlc4 (1→3Xyl3)		
1	104.3 CH	5.12 d (8.3)	C: 3 Xyl3	H-3 Xyl3; H-3, 5 MeGlc4
2	74.5 CH	3.85 t (8.3)	C: 1, 3 MeGlc4	-
3	86.8 CH	3.65 t (8.3)	C: 2, 4 MeGlc4, OMe	-
4	70.3 CH	3.86 t (8.3)	C: 5 MeGlc4	-
5	77.4 CH	3.86 m	C: 4 MeGlc4	H-1, 3 MeGlc4
6	61.8 CH$_2$	4.33 d (12.8)	C: 4 MeGlc4	-
		4.00 dd (6.1; 12.1)	C: 5 MeGlc4	-
OMe	60.5 CH$_3$	3.78 s	C: 3 MeGlc4	-

Table 5. ^{13}C and ^{1}H NMR chemical shifts and HMBC and ROESY correlations of the aglycone moiety of quadrangularisosides B (3) and D (8).[a] Recorded at 176.03 MHz in C_5D_5N/D_2O (4/1). [b] Recorded at 700.00 MHz in C_5D_5N/D_2O (4/1).

Atom	δ_C mult. [a]	δ_H mult. [b] (J in Hz)	HMBC	ROESY
1	35.8 CH$_2$	1.32 m	-	-
		1.28 m	-	-
2	26.7 CH$_2$	1.94 m	-	-
		1.76 m	-	H-19, H-30
3	89.2 CH	3.14 dd (4.2; 11.8)	C: 4, 30, 31, C:1 Xyl1	H-5, H-1Xyl1
4	39.3 C	-	-	-
5	47.8 CH	0.90 dd (4.5; 11.2)	C: 4, 6, 10, 30	H-1, H-3, H-31
6	23.1 CH$_2$	1.93 m	-	H-31
7	120.3 CH	5.60 m	C: 9	H-15, H-32
8	145.6 C	-	-	-
9	47.0 CH	3.30 brd (16.5)	-	H-19
10	35.3 C	-	-	-
11	22.4 CH$_2$	1.71 m	-	H-1
		1.47 m	-	-
12	31.2 CH$_2$	2.09 m	C: 13, 14, 18	-
13	59.3 C	-	-	-
14	47.3 C	-	-	-
15	43.5 CH$_2$	2.56 brdd (7.3; 12.2)	C: 13, 14, 17, 32	H-7, H-32
		1.60 brd (6.0)	-	-
16	75.2 CH	5.85 q (8.5)	C: 13, 15, 17, 20, OAc	H-32
17	54.3 CH	2.69 d (8.9)	C: 12, 13, 15, 18, 21	H-12, H-21, H-32
18	180.3 C	-	-	-
19	23.8 CH$_3$	1.09 s	C: 1, 5, 9, 10	H-2, H-9, H-30
20	85.5 C	-	-	-
21	28.1 CH$_3$	1.55 s	C: 17, 20, 22	H-12, H-17, H-23
22	38.5 CH$_2$	2.42 dt (4.3; 12.3)	C: 20, 21	-
		1.82 dt (5.2; 12.3)	C: 17, 20, 21	-
23	23.5 CH	2.01 m	-	-
		1.92 m	-	-
24	123.9 CH	4.99 m	C: 26, 27	H-22, H-26
25	132.3 C	-	-	-
26	25.4 CH$_3$	1.60 s	C: 24, 25, 27	H-24
27	17.6 CH$_3$	1.54 s	C: 24, 25, 26	H-24
30	17.2 CH$_3$	1.00 s	C: 3, 4, 5, 31	H-2, H-6, H-19, H-31
31	28.6 CH$_3$	1.13 s	C: 3, 4, 5, 30	H-3, H-5, H-6, H-30, H-1 Xyl1
32	32.1 CH$_3$	1.15 s	C: 8, 13, 14, 15	H-7, H-12, H-15, H-16, H-17
OCOCH$_3$	170.9 C	-	-	-
OCOCH$_3$	21.0 CH$_3$	1.96 s	C: 16, OAc	-

The molecular formula of quadrangularisoside B$_1$ (4) was determined to be $C_{55}H_{84}O_{28}S_2Na_2$ from the [M$_{2Na}$ − Na]$^-$ ion peak at m/z 1279.4502 (calc. 1279.4494) and [M$_{2Na}$ − 2Na]$^{2-}$ ion peak at m/z 628.2320 (calc. 628.2301) in the (−)HR-ESI-MS as well as from the [M$_{2Na}$ + Na]$^+$ ion peak at m/z 1325.4272 (calc. 1325.4278) in the (+)HR-ESI-MS, which was coincident with the formula of quadrangularisoside B (3) and indicated their isomerism. In the ^{1}H and ^{13}C NMR spectra of the aglycone part of **4**, the signals of holostane-type aglycone having 7(8)- and 25(26)-double bonds as well as a 16β-acetoxy-group were observed (Table 6). This aglycone is identical to that of pentactasides C [14] and II [15] isolated earlier from the same species and is frequently occurred in the glycosides of the sea cucumbers of the order Dendrochirotida [2,4,5,21,30].

Table 6. ^{13}C and ^{1}H NMR chemical shifts and HMBC and ROESY correlations of the aglycone moiety of quadrangularisosides B$_1$ (**4**) and D$_1$ (**9**). ^{a} Recorded at 176.03 MHz in C$_5$D$_5$N/D$_2$O (4/1). ^{b} Recorded at 700.00 MHz in C$_5$D$_5$N/D$_2$O (4/1).

Atom	δ_C mult. ^{a}	δ_H mult. ^{b} (J in Hz)	HMBC	ROESY
1	35.9 CH$_2$	1.40 m	-	H-5, H-11, H-19
2	26.7 CH$_2$	2.03 m	-	-
		1.95 m	-	-
3	89.2 CH	3.31 dd (4.2; 11.6)	-	H-5, H-31, H-1Xyl1
4	39.4 C	-	-	-
5	47.8 CH	1.00 dd (5.0; 10.0)	C: 4, 10, 19, 30	H-1, H-3
6	23.1 CH$_2$	2.00 m	-	H-30, H-31
7	120.2 CH	5.69 m	-	H-15, H-32
8	145.6 C	-	-	-
9	47.0 CH	3.40 brd (14.0)	-	H-19
10	35.3 C	-	-	-
11	22.4 CH$_2$	1.81 m	-	H-1
		1.59 m	-	H-1
12	31.2 CH$_2$	2.21 m	-	H-17, H-21
13	59.3 C	-	-	-
14	47.3 C	-	-	-
15	43.5 CH$_2$	2.66 dd (7.4; 12.2)	-	H-7
		1.71 m	-	-
16	75.3 CH	5.93 brq (8.7)	-	H-32
17	54.5 CH	2.78 d (9.0)	C: 12, 13, 18, 21	H-12, H-21, H-32
18	180.3 C	-	-	-
19	23.8 CH$_3$	1.16 s	C: 1, 5, 9, 10	H-2, H-9
20	85.6 C	-	-	-
21	28.1 CH$_3$	1.62 s	C: 17, 20, 22	H-17, H-22
22	38.3 CH$_2$	2.35 m	-	-
		1.91 m	-	-
23	22.9 CH$_2$	1.56 m	-	-
		1.44 m	-	-
24	38.2 CH$_2$	2.01 m	-	-
25	145.4 C	-	-	-
26	110.9 CH$_2$	4.83 brs	C: 24, 25, 27	
		4.84 brs	C: 24, 25, 27	
27	22.1 CH$_3$	1.75 s	C: 24, 25, 26	
30	17.3 CH$_3$	1.15 s	C: 3, 4, 5, 31	H-6
31	28.6 CH$_3$	1.28 s	C: 3, 4, 5, 30	H-3, H-6
32	32.2 CH$_3$	1.27 s	C: 8, 13, 14, 15	H-7, H-16, H-17
OCOCH$_3$	170.8 C	-	-	-
OCOCH$_3$	21.3 CH$_3$	2.12 s	-	-

The (+)ESI-MS/MS of **4** showed the fragmentation of the [M$_{2Na}$ + Na]$^+$ ion at *m/z* 1325.4. The peaks of fragment ions were observed at *m/z* 1223.5 [M$_{2Na}$ + Na − NaSO$_3$ + H]$^+$, 1205.5 [M$_{2Na}$ + Na − NaHSO$_4$]$^+$, 1085.5 [M$_{2Na}$ + Na − 2NaHSO$_4$]$^+$, 897.4 [M$_{2Na}$ + Na − NaHSO$_4$ − C$_7$H$_{12}$O$_5$ (MeGlc) − C$_5$H$_8$O$_4$ (Xyl)]$^+$, 711.1 [M$_{2Na}$ + Na − C$_{32}$H$_{47}$O$_5$ (Agl) − SO$_3$Na]$^+$, 579.1 [M$_{2Na}$ + Na − C$_{32}$H$_{47}$O$_5$ (Agl) − C$_5$H$_7$O$_7$SNa (XylSO$_3$Na) − H]$^+$, 403.0 [M$_{2Na}$ + Na − C$_{32}$H$_{47}$O$_5$ (Agl) − SO$_3$Na − C$_7$H$_{12}$O$_5$ (MeGlc) − C$_5$H$_8$O$_4$ (Xyl)]$^+$, and 331.1 [M$_{2Na}$ + Na − C$_{32}$H$_{47}$O$_5$ (Agl) − C$_5$H$_7$O$_7$SNa (XylSO$_3$Na) − C$_6$H$_9$O$_7$SNa (QuiSO$_3$Na) − H]$^+$, corroborating the structure of quadrangularisoside B$_1$ (**4**).

All these data indicate that quadrangularisoside B$_1$ (**4**) is 3β-*O*-[3-*O*-methyl-β-D-glucopyranosyl-(1→3)-β-D-xylopyranosyl-(1→4)-3-*O*-sodium sulfate-β-D-quinovopyranosyl-(1→2)-4-*O*-sodium sulfate-β-D-xylopyranosyl]-16β-acetoxyholosta-7,25-diene.

The molecular formula of quadrangularisoside B$_2$ (**5**) was determined to be C$_{53}$H$_{80}$O$_{27}$S$_2$Na$_2$ from the [M$_{2Na}$ − Na]$^-$ ion peak at *m/z* 1235.4243 (calc. 1235.4232) and [M$_{2Na}$ − 2Na]$^{2-}$ ion peak at *m/z* 606.2189 (calc. 606.2170) in the (−)HR-ESI-MS as well as the [M$_{2Na}$ + Na]$^+$ ion peak at *m/z* 1281.4004 (calc. 1281.4016) in the (+)HR-ESI-MS. The signals in the ^{1}H and ^{13}C NMR spectra of the aglycone part of **5** were characteristic of holostane-type aglycone having 9(11)- and 25(26)-double bonds and a 16-keto-group (Table 7). This aglycone is known as holotoxinogenin, and it was found first in the glycosides named as holotoxins A$_1$ and B$_1$, which were isolated from the sea cucumber *Apostichopus japonicus* (Stichopodidae, Synallactida) [31] and are rather common for the glycosides of the sea cucumbers of different orders [2,4,5].

The (+)ESI-MS/MS of **5** demonstrated the fragmentation of the [M$_{2Na}$ + Na]$^+$ ion at *m/z* 1281.4. The peaks of fragment ions were observed at *m/z* 1179.4 [M$_{2Na}$ + Na − NaSO$_3$ + H]$^+$, 1059.5 [M$_{2Na}$ + Na − NaSO$_3$ − NaHSO$_4$ + H]$^+$, confirming the presence of two sulfate groups. The peaks of fragment ions at *m/z* 711.1, 579.1, 403.0, and 331.1 were the same as in the mass spectra of the glycosides **3** and **4** due to the identity of their carbohydrate chains.

All these data indicate that quadrangularisoside B$_2$ (**5**) is 3β-*O*-[3-*O*-methyl-β-D-glucopyranosyl-(1→3)-β-D-xylopyranosyl-(1→4)-3-*O*-sodium sulfate-β-D-quinovopyranosyl-(1→2)-4-*O*-sodium sulfate-β-D-xylopyranosyl]-16-ketoholosta-7,25-diene.

The ^{13}C NMR spectra of the carbohydrate moieties of quadrangularisosides C (**6**) and C$_1$ (**7**) were identical to each other (Table 8) and to those of hemoiedemoside A isolated first from the sea cucumber *Hemoiedema spectabilis* [23] and identified by us in the glycosidic sum of *C. quadrangularis*. The glycosides **6** and **7** have a tetrasaccharide linear carbohydrate chain differing from that of **1** and **2** by the sulfated by C(6) glucose residue as the third unit in the chain instead of a xylose residue. The carbohydrate chain structure of quadrangularisosides C (**6**) and C$_1$ (**7**) was elucidated based on a thorough analysis of 1D and 2D NMR spectra (Table 8). Besides compounds **6**, **7**, and hemoiedemoside A, such a sugar moiety is a part of another six glycosides [32–37] isolated from the sea cucumbers of the order Dendrochirotida.

The molecular formula of quadrangularisoside C (**6**) was determined to be C$_{56}$H$_{86}$O$_{29}$S$_2$Na$_2$ from the [M$_{2Na}$ − Na]$^-$ ion peak at *m/z* 1309.4608 (calc. 1309.4599) and [M$_{2Na}$ − 2Na]$^{2-}$ ion peak at *m/z* 643.2369 (calc. 643.2354) in the (−)HR-ESI-MS. In the (+)HR-ESI-MS, the [M$_{2Na}$ + Na]$^+$ ion peak observed at *m/z* 1355.4373 (calc. 1355.4384) corresponded to the same molecular formula. The signals of C(1)–C(4) and C(15)–C(32) in the ^{13}C NMR spectrum of **6** (Table 9) were close to those in the spectrum of quadrangularisoside B$_1$ (**4**), but the signals characteristic for the 9(11)-double bond in the triterpene nucleus [at δ_C 150.6 (C(9)) and 110.9 (C(11)) as well as δ_H 5.16 (m, H(11))] were observed instead of the signals assigned to the 7(8)-double bond in **4**. So, these compounds were the isomers by the double bond position in the aglycone nuclei. The aglycone identical to that of quadrangularisoside C (**6**) was earlier found only in cladoloside A$_3$ from the sea cucumber *Cladolabes schmeltzii* [36].

Table 7. ^{13}C and ^{1}H NMR chemical shifts and HMBC and ROESY correlations of the aglycone moiety of quadrangularisosides B$_2$ (**5**), D$_2$ (**10**) and E (**13**). [a] Recorded at 176.03 MHz in C$_5$D$_5$N/D$_2$O (4/1). [b] Recorded at 700.00 MHz in C$_5$D$_5$N/D$_2$O (4/1).

Atom	δ$_C$ mult. [a]	δ$_H$ mult. [b] (J in Hz)	HMBC	ROESY
1	36.0 CH$_2$	1.69 m	C: 3	H-11, H-19
		1.28 m	C: 2	H-3
2	26.6 CH$_2$	2.00 m	-	-
		1.80 brd (12.4)	-	H-19, H-30
3	88.8 CH	3.09 dd (4.2; 12.4)	C: 4, 30, 31, C:1 Xyl1	H-5, H-31, H-1 Xyl1
4	39.7 C	-	-	-
5	52.7 CH	0.78 brd (11.9)	C: 6, 10, 19, 30	H-3, H-7, H-31
6	20.9 CH$_2$	1.60 m	-	H-31
		1.40 m	-	H-19, H-30
7	28.3 CH$_2$	1.58 m	-	-
		1.17 m	-	H-5, H-32
8	38.6 CH	3.12 brd (14.5)	-	H-15, H-19
9	150.9 C	-	-	-
10	39.4 C	-	-	-
11	111.1 CH	5.26 brd (4.7)	C: 8, 10, 12, 13	H-1
12	31.9 CH$_2$	2.62 brd (18.1)	C: 9, 11, 13, 18	H-17, H-32
		2.46 dd (6.2; 18.1)	C: 9, 11, 13, 14, 18	H-21
13	55.8 C	-	-	-
14	41.9 C	-	-	-
15	51.9 CH$_2$	2.38 d (15.6)	C: 13, 16, 17, 32	H-7, H-32
		2.09 d (15.6)	C: 8, 14, 16, 18, 32	H-8
16	214.4 C	-	-	-
17	61.2 CH	2.84 s	C: 12, 13, 16, 18, 20, 21	H-12, H-21, H-32
18	176.7 C	-	-	-
19	21.8 CH$_3$	1.24 s	C: 1, 5, 9, 10	H-1, H-2, H-6, H-8, H-30
20	83.5 C	-	-	-
21	26.7 CH$_3$	1.42 s	C: 17, 20, 22	H-12, H-17, H-23
22	38.1 CH$_2$	1.71 m	C: 20, 21, 23, 24	H-21
		1.55 m	C: 21, 23	-
23	22.0 CH$_2$	1.70 m	-	-
		1.43 m	-	-
24	37.7 CH$_2$	1.88 dd (7.8; 15.0)	C: 22, 23, 25, 26	H-21, H-26
25	145.5 C	-	-	-
26	110.4 CH$_2$	4.70 brs	C: 24, 27	H-27
		4.68 brs	C: 24, 27	H-24, H-27
27	22.1 CH$_3$	1.62 s	C: 24, 25, 26	-
30	16.5 CH$_3$	0.96 s	C: 3, 4, 5, 31	H-2, H-6, H-19, H-31, H-6 Qui2
31	27.9 CH$_3$	1.10 s	C: 3, 4, 5, 30	H-3, H-5, H-6, H-30, H-1 Xyl1
32	20.5 CH$_3$	0.88 s	C: 8, 13, 14, 15	H-7, H-12, H-15, H-17

Table 8. ^{13}C and ^{1}H NMR chemical shifts and HMBC and ROESY correlations of carbohydrate moiety of quadrangularisosides C (6) and C$_1$ (7). ^{a} Recorded at 176.03 MHz in C$_5$D$_5$N/D$_2$O (4/1). ^{b} Bold = interglycosidic positions. ^{c} Italic = sulfate position. ^{d} Recorded at 700.00 MHz in C$_5$D$_5$N/D$_2$O (4/1). Multiplicity by 1D TOCSY.

Atom	δ_C mult. ^{a,b,c}	δ_H mult. ^{d} (J in Hz)	HMBC	ROESY
		Xyl1 (1→C-3)		
1	104.7 CH	4.67 d (7.3)	C-3	H-3; H-3, 5 Xyl1
2	82.1 CH	3.95 t (7.3)	C: 1 Qui2; 1, 3 Xyl1	H-1 Qui2
3	74.6 CH	4.24 t (8.6)	C: 2, 4 Xyl1	H-1, 5 Xyl1
4	76.1 CH	4.97 m	-	-
5	63.7 CH$_2$	4.75 dd (4.9; 11.6)	C: 3, 4 Xyl1	-
		3.73 dd (9.8; 11.6)	-	H-1, 3 Xyl1
		Qui2 (1→2Xyl1)		
1	104.5 CH	4.93 d (7.3)	C: 2 Xyl1	H-2 Xyl1; H-3, 5 Qui2
2	75.4 CH	3.87 t (9.2)	C: 1, 3 Qui2	H-4 Qui2
3	75.0 CH	3.92 t (9.2)	C: 2 Qui2	H-1, 5 Qui2
4	86.9 CH	3.41 t (9.2)	C: 1 Glc3; 3, 5 Qui2	H-1 Glc3; H-2 Qui2
5	71.3 CH	3.60 dd (6.1; 9.2)	-	H-1, 3 Qui2
6	17.7 CH$_3$	1.59 d (6.1)	C: 4, 5 Qui2	H-4, 5 Qui2
		Glc3 (1→4Qui2)		
1	104.2 CH	4.75 d (7.6)	C: 4 Qui2	H-4 Qui2; H-3,5 Glc3
2	73.4 CH	3.85 t (8.6)	C: 1, 3 Glc3	-
3	86.0 CH	4.18 t (8.6)	C: 1 MeGlc4; 2, 4 Glc3	H-1 MeGlc4, H-1 Glc3
4	69.2 CH	3.80 t (9.5)	C: 3, 5, 6 Glc3	H-6 Glc3
5	74.9 CH	4.10 m	-	H-1, 3 Glc3
6	67.3 CH$_2$	4.99 d (8.6)	C: 5 Glc3	-
		4.60 dd (6.7; 10.5)	-	H-4 Glc3
		MeGlc4 (1→3Glc3)		
1	104.4 CH	5.21 d (7.9)	-	H-3 Glc3; H-3, 5 MeGlc4
2	74.5 CH	3.86 t (7.9)	C: 1, 3 MeGlc4	-
3	86.9 CH	3.67 t (8.8)	C: 2, 4 MeGlc4, OMe	H-1 MeGlc4
4	70.3 CH	3.90 m	C: 3, 5 MeGlc4	H-6 MeGlc4
5	77.5 CH	3.90 m	C: 6 MeGlc4	H-1, 3 MeGlc4
6	61.7 CH$_2$	4.35 d (12.4)	-	-
		4.06 dd (7.1; 12.4)	C: 5 MeGlc4	-
OMe	60.6 CH$_3$	3.80 s	C: 3 MeGlc4	-

The (−)ESI-MS/MS of **6** demonstrated the fragmentation of the [M$_{2Na}$ − Na]$^−$ ion at *m/z* 1309.5. The peaks of fragment ions were observed at *m/z* 1249.4 [M$_{2Na}$ − Na − CH$_3$COOH]$^−$, 1189.5 [M$_{2Na}$ − Na − NaHSO$_4$]$^−$, 1129.5 [M$_{2Na}$ − Na − CH$_3$COOH − NaHSO$_4$]$^−$, 677.2 [M$_{2Na}$ − Na − NaHSO$_4$ − C$_{32}$H$_{47}$O$_5$ (Agl) − H]$^−$, 563.1 [M$_{2Na}$ − Na − NaHSO$_4$ − C$_{32}$H$_{47}$O$_5$ (Agl) − C$_5$H$_7$O$_3$ (Xyl)]$^−$, 417.1 [M$_{2Na}$ − Na − NaHSO$_4$ − C$_{32}$H$_{47}$O$_5$ (Agl) − C$_5$H$_7$O$_3$ (Xyl) − C$_6$H$_{10}$O$_4$ (Qui)]$^−$, and 241.0 [M$_{2Na}$ − Na − NaHSO$_4$ − C$_{32}$H$_{47}$O$_5$ (Agl) − C$_5$H$_7$O$_3$ (Xyl) − C$_6$H$_{10}$O$_4$ (Qui) − C$_7$H$_{12}$O$_5$ (MeGlc)]$^−$.

All these data indicate that quadrangularisoside C (**6**) is 3β-O-[3-O-methyl-β-D-glucopyranosyl-(1→3)-6-O-sodium sulfate-β-D-glucopyranosyl-(1→4)-β-D-quinovopyranosyl-(1→2)-4-O-sodium sulfate-β-D-xylopyranosyl]-16β-acetoxyholosta-9(11),25-diene.

Table 9. ^{13}C and ^{1}H NMR chemical shifts and HMBC and ROESY correlations of the aglycone moiety of quadrangularisoside C (6) [a] Recorded at 176.03 MHz in C_5D_5N/D_2O (4/1). [b] Recorded at 700.00 MHz in C_5D_5N/D_2O (4/1).

Position	δ_C mult. [a]	δ_H mult. (J in Hz) [b]	HMBC	ROESY
1	36.1 CH$_2$	1.69 m	-	H-11
		1.28 m	-	H-3, H-11
2	26.7 CH$_2$	2.02 m	-	
		1.81 m	-	H-19, H-30
3	88.7 CH	3.11 dd (3.8; 11.5)	C: 30, 1 Xyl1	H-1, H-5, H-31, H-1Xyl1
4	39.6 C			
5	52.6 CH	0.78 brd (12.0)	C: 10, 19, 30	H-1, H-3, H-7, H-31
6	20.9 CH$_2$	1.61 m	-	
		1.41 m	-	H-30
7	27.7 CH$_2$	1.60 m	-	H-15
		1.17 m	-	H-32
8	39.4 CH	3.15 brd (12.5)	-	H-15, H-19
9	150.6 C	-	-	-
10	39.2 C	-	-	-
11	110.9 CH	5.16 m	C: 10, 13	H-1
12	33.8 CH$_2$	2.52 brd (16.8)	C: 18	H-17, H-32
		2.41 brdd (5.8; 17.0)	C: 11, 14, 18	H-21
13	59.0 C	-	-	-
14	42.9 C	-	-	-
15	43.7 CH$_2$	2.21 dd (6.7; 11.5)	C: 13, 16, 17, 32	H-7, H-32
		1.35 brt (11.5)	C: 14, 16, 32	H-8
16	75.3 CH	5.72 q (9.6)	C: 20, OAc	H-32
17	52.5 CH	2.69 d (9.6)	C: 12, 13, 15, 18, 21	H-12, H-21, H-32
18	177.5 C	-	-	-
19	22.0 CH$_3$	1.25 s	C: 1, 5, 9, 10	H-1, H-2, H-8, H-9, H-30
20	85.5 C	-	-	-
21	28.3 CH$_3$	1.45 s	C: 17, 20, 22	H-12, H-17, H-22
22	37.9 CH$_2$	2.08 m	-	-
		1.91 m	C: 20	-
23	22.8 CH$_2$	1.47 m	-	-
		1.39 m	-	-
24	38.1 CH$_2$	1.91 m	C: 22, 23, 25, 26, 27	H-26
25	145.4 C	-	-	-
26	110.7 CH$_2$	4.73 brs	C: 24, 27	H-27
		4.72 brs	C: 24, 27	H-24
27	22.0 CH$_3$	1.65 s	C: 24, 25, 26	H-26
30	16.4 CH$_3$	0.95 s	C: 3, 4, 5, 31	H-2, H-6, H-19, H-31
31	27.9 CH$_3$	1.14 s	C: 3, 4, 5, 30	H-3, H-5, H-30, H-1 Xyl1
32	21.0 CH$_3$	0.88 s	C: 8, 13, 14, 15	H-7, H-12, H-15, H-16, H-17
OCOCH$_3$	171.1 C	-	-	-
OCOCH$_3$	21.3 CH$_3$	2.10 s	C: OAc	-

The molecular formula of quadrangularisoside C_1 (7) was determined to be $C_{56}H_{88}O_{29}S_2Na_2$ from the $[M_{2Na} - Na]^-$ ion peak at m/z 1311.4763 (calc. 1311.4756), $[M_{2Na} - 2Na]^{2-}$ ion peak at m/z

644.2447 (calc. 644.2432), and [M$_{2Na}$ + Na]$^+$ ion peak at m/z 1357.4520 (calc. 1357.4540) in the (−) and (+)HR-ESI-MS, correspondingly. The signals of carbons corresponding to the holostane-type nucleus in the ^{13}C NMR spectrum of **7** (Table 10) were coincident with those in the spectra of quadrangularisosides A (**1**), A$_1$ (**2**), B (**3**), and B$_1$ (**4**), indicating the presence of the aglycone having a 7(8)-double bond and 16β-acetoxy-group. The signals of H(22)–H(27) form the isolated spin system in the ^{1}H,^{1}H-COSY spectrum of **7**. So, the presence of an unsubstituted saturated side chain was supposed for this compound. Actually, the ^{13}C NMR spectrum of the aglycone part of **7** was coincident with that of lefevreoside A$_2$, isolated first from *A. lefevrei* [21] and identified in the glycosidic sum of *C. quadrangularis*. The aglycone identical to that of quadrangularisoside C$_1$ (**7**) is frequently occurred in the glycosides of representatives of the order Dendrochirotida [2,4,5].

The (−)ESI-MS/MS of **7** demonstrated the fragmentation of the [M$_{2Na}$ − Na]$^-$ ion at m/z 1311.5. The peaks of fragment ions were observed at m/z 797.1 [M$_{2Na}$ − Na − C$_{32}$H$_{49}$O$_5$ (Agl) − H]$^-$, 677.2 [M$_{2Na}$ − Na − NaHSO$_4$ − C$_{32}$H$_{49}$O$_5$ (Agl) − H]$^-$, 563.1 [M$_{2Na}$ − Na − NaHSO$_4$ − C$_{32}$H$_{49}$O$_5$ (Agl) − C$_5$H$_7$O$_3$ (Xyl)]$^-$, 417.1 [M$_{2Na}$ − Na − NaHSO$_4$ − C$_{32}$H$_{49}$O$_5$ (Agl) − C$_5$H$_7$O$_3$ (Xyl) − C$_6$H$_{10}$O$_4$ (Qui)]$^-$, and 241.0 [M$_{2Na}$ − Na − NaHSO$_4$ − C$_{32}$H$_{49}$O$_5$ (Agl) − C$_5$H$_7$O$_3$ (Xyl) − C$_6$H$_{10}$O$_4$ (Qui) − C$_7$H$_{12}$O$_5$ (MeGlc)]$^-$, which were coincident with those in the MS/MS spectrum of **6**, confirming the identity of their carbohydrate chains.

All these data indicate that quadrangularisoside C$_1$ (**7**) is 3β-O-[3-O-methyl-β-D-glucopyranosyl-(1→3)-6-O-sodium sulfate-β-D-glucopyranosyl-(1→4)-β-D-quinovopyranosyl-(1→2)-4-O-sodium sulfate-β-D-xylopyranosyl]-16β-acetoxyholost-7-ene.

The ^{13}C NMR spectra of the carbohydrate moieties of quadrangularisosides D–D$_4$ (**8–12**) were coincident to each other (Table 11), indicating the presence and identity of sugar moieties in these glycosides. In the ^{1}H and ^{13}C NMR spectra of the carbohydrate part of **8–12**, four characteristic doublets at δ$_H$ 4.63–5.12 (J = 7.1–8.0 Hz), and corresponding to them, four signals of anomeric carbons at δ$_C$ 102.8–104.6 were indicative of a tetrasaccharide chain and β-configurations of glycosidic bonds. The ^{1}H,^{1}H-COSY, HSQC, and 1D TOCSY spectra of **8–12** showed the signals of the isolated spin systems assigned to two xylose residues, one quinovose residue, and one 3-O-methylglucose residue. These data indicated the same monosaccharide composition of the sugar chain of **8–12** as in quadrangularisosides of the groups A (**1, 2**) and B (**3–5**). The comparison of the ^{13}C NMR spectra of **8–12** and **3–5** showed the coincidence of the signals corresponding to the monosaccharide residues from the first to the third. The signals, assigning to the terminal 3-O-methylglucose residue in **8–12**, were deduced by the analysis of ^{1}H,^{1}H-COSY and 1D TOCSY spectra. The signal of C(4) MeGlc4 was observed at δ$_C$ 76.2, the signal of C(3) was observed at δ$_C$ 85.2, and the signal of C(5) was observed at δ$_C$ 76.3 in the spectra of **8–12**. Hence, the α- and β-shifting effects due to the attachment of a sulfate group to C(4) MeGlc4 of quadrangularisosides of the group D (**8–12**) were observed in comparison with the δ$_C$ values of the corresponding signals in the spectra of quadrangularisosides of the group B (**3–5**) (δ$_C$ 70.3 for C(4) MeGlc4, δ$_C$ 86.8 for C(3) MeGlc4, and δ$_C$ 77.4 for C(5) MeGlc4) having non-sulfated 3-O-methylglucose residue in the same position of the carbohydrate chain.

Hence, three sulfate groups are present in the carbohydrate chain of quadrangularisosides of the group D (**8–12**): at C(4) Xyl1—the common position of this functionality for the sea cucumber glycosides, at C(3) Qui2—the rare position of the group, and finally, at C(4) MeGlc4—the unique for the glycosides position of a sulfate group. The similar structural feature was found earlier in the carbohydrate chains of some glycosides from *Psolus fabricii*, but the sulfate group was attached to C(4) of the terminal disulfated glucose residue having an additional sulfate group at the C(2) or C(6) position [37] and in the carbohydrate chain of stichorrenoside B isolated from *Stichopus horrens* [38], where the sulfate group was attached to C(4) of the glucose residue terminal in its disaccharide chain. The majority of known sulfated glycosides contain terminal 3-O-methylglucose residue with the sulfate group attached to C(6); in contrast, the sulfation of C(4) of the 3-O-methylglucose residue in the linear tetrasaccharidechain as in compounds **8–12** has never been discovered earlier in the sea cucumbers glycosides.

Table 10. ^{13}C and ^1H NMR chemical shifts and HMBC and ROESY correlations of the aglycone moiety of quadrangularisoside C_1 (7). [a] Recorded at 176.03 MHz in C_5D_5N/D_2O (4/1). [b] Recorded at 700.00 MHz in C_5D_5N/D_2O (4/1).

Position	δ_C mult. [a]	δ_H mult. (J in Hz) [b]	HMBC	ROESY
1	35.7 CH$_2$	1.34 m	-	H-11
		1.30 m	-	H-11
2	26.7 CH$_2$	1.98 m	-	-
		1.80 brdd (2.7; 11.9)	-	H-19, H-30
3	88.8 CH	3.19 dd (3.6; 11.9)	C: 4, 30, 1 Xyl1	H-1, H-5, H-31, H-1Xyl1
4	39.3 C	-	-	-
5	47.7 CH	0.93 dd (4.6; 11.0)	C: 4, 10, 19, 30, 31	H-1, H-3, H-31
6	22.9 CH$_2$	1.94 m	-	H-19, H-30, H-31
7	120.0 CH	5.61 m	-	H-15, H-32
8	145.5 C	-	-	-
9	46.9 CH	3.33 brd (14.6)	-	H-12, H-19
10	35.2 C	-	-	-
11	22.3 CH$_2$	1.73 m	-	H-1
		1.48 m	-	H-32
12	31.1 CH$_2$	2.10 m	C: 13, 14	H-17, H-32
13	59.1 C	-	-	-
14	47.1 C	-	-	-
15	43.3 CH$_2$	2.55 dd (7.3; 11.9)	C: 13, 14, 17, 32	H-7, H-32
		1.62 m	C: 14, 16, 32	-
16	74.7 CH	5.85 q (9.1)	C: 13, OAc	H-32
17	54.3 CH	2.66 d (9.1)	C: 12, 13, 18, 21	H-12, H-21, H-32
18	179.8 C	-	-	-
19	23.6 CH$_3$	1.11 s	C: 1, 5, 9, 10	H-1, H-2, H-6, H-9, H-30
20	85.5 C	-	-	-
21	27.8 CH$_3$	1.53 s	C: 17, 20, 22	H-12, H-17, H-23, H-24
22	39.2 CH$_2$	1.10 m	-	-
		0.99 m	-	-
23	22.4 CH$_2$	1.27 m	-	-
		1.17 m	-	-
24	38.8 CH$_2$	2.27 td (4.6; 13.7)	C: 25	-
		1.75 m	C: 20	-
25	28.0 CH	1.55 m	-	-
26	22.5 CH$_3$	0.80 s	C: 24, 25, 27	-
27	22.0 CH$_3$	0.79 s	C: 24, 25, 26	-
30	17.0 CH$_3$	1.01 s	C: 3, 4, 5, 31	H-2, H-6, H-19, H-31
31	28.4 CH$_3$	1.18 s	C: 3, 4, 5, 30	H-3, H-5, H-6, H-30, H-1 Xyl1
32	31.9 CH$_3$	1.15 s	C: 8, 13, 14, 15	H-7, H-11, H-12, H-15, H-17
O<u>C</u>OCH$_3$	170.1 C	-	-	-
OCO<u>C</u>H$_3$	21.0 CH$_3$	2.01 s	C: OAc	-

Table 11. ^{13}C and ^{1}H NMR chemical shifts and HMBC and ROESY correlations of carbohydrate moiety of quadrangularisosides D (8), D$_1$ (9), D$_2$ (10), D$_3$ (11), and D$_4$ (12). ^{a} Recorded at 176.03 MHz in C$_5$D$_5$N/D$_2$O (4/1). ^{b} Bold = interglycosidic positions. ^{c} Italic = sulfate position. ^{d} Recorded at 700.00 MHz in C$_5$D$_5$N/D$_2$O (4/1). Multiplicity by 1D TOCSY.

Atom	δ_C mult. ^{a,b,c}	δ_H mult. ^{d} (J in Hz)	HMBC	ROESY
		Xyl1 (1→C-3)		
1	104.6 CH	4.63 d (7.1)	C-3	H-3; H-3, 5 Xyl1
2	81.9 CH	3.96 t (8.6)	C: 1 Qui2; 1, 3 Xyl1	H-1 Qui2; H-4 Xyl1
3	75.3 CH	4.23 t (8.6)	C: 2, 4 Xyl1	H-1, 5 Xyl1
4	76.0 CH	4.97 m	-	H-2 Xyl1
5	64.1 CH$_2$	4.79 dd (5.7; 12.1)	C: 1, 3, 4 Xyl1	-
		3.74 brt (10.7)	C: 1 Xyl1	H-1, 3 Xyl1
		Qui2 (1→2Xyl1)		
1	103.5 CH	5.11 d (7.8)	C: 2 Xyl1	H-2 Xyl1; H-3, 5 Qui2
2	75.7 CH	4.00 t (8.7)	C: 1, 3 Qui2	H-4 Qui2
3	81.5 CH	4.99 t (8.7)	C: 2, 4 Qui2	H-5 Qui2
4	79.3 CH	3.82 t (8.7)	C: 1 Xyl3; 3, 5, 6 Qui2	H-1 Xyl3; H-2 Qui2
5	71.8 CH	3.65 dd (6.1; 9.6)	C: 1 Qui2	H-1, 3 Qui2
6	18.3 CH$_3$	1.54 d (6.1)	C: 4, 5 Qui2	H-4, 5 Qui2
		Xyl3 (1→4Qui2)		
1	102.8 CH	5.09 d (7.1)	C: 4 Qui2; 5 Xyl3	H-4 Qui2; H-3,5 Xyl3
2	73.3 CH	4.08 t (8.9)	C: 1, 3 Xyl3	-
3	86.1 CH	4.13 t (8.9)	C: 1 MeGlc4; 2 Xyl3	H-1, 5 Xyl3
4	69.4 CH	4.01 m	C: 3 Xyl3	-
5	65.9 CH$_2$	4.46 dd (5.3; 12.5)	C: 1, 3, 4 Xyl3	-
		3.78 dd (8.0; 12.5)	C: 1, 3, 4 Xyl3	H-1 Xyl3
		MeGlc4 (1→3Xyl3)		
1	104.2 CH	5.12 d (8.0)	C: 3 Xyl3	H-3 Xyl3; H-3, 5 MeGlc4
2	74.0 CH	3.87 dd (7.1; 9.8)	C: 1, 3 MeGlc4	H-4 MeGlc4
3	85.2 CH	3.71 t (8.9)	C: 2, 4 MeGlc4, OMe	H-1 MeGlc4; OMe
4	76.2 CH	4.85 t (8.9)	C: 3, 5, 6 MeGlc4	H-2, 6 MeGlc4
5	76.3 CH	3.83 m	-	-
6	61.7 CH$_2$	4.48 dd (2.7; 13.3)	C: 5 MeGlc4	-
		4.29 dd (6.2; 11.8)	C: 5 MeGlc4	-
OMe	60.6 CH$_3$	3.92 s	C: 3 MeGlc4	-

The positions of interglycosidic linkages were established by the ROESY and HMBC spectra of 8–12 (Table 11) where the cross-peaks between H(1) of the xylose and H(3) (C(3)) of an aglycone, H(1) of the second residue (quinovose) and H(2) (C(2)) of the xylose, H(1) of the third residue (xylose) and H(4) (C(4)) of the second residue (quinovose), H(1) of the fourth residue (3-O-methylglucose) and H-3 (C(3)) of the third residue (xylose) were observed.

The molecular formula of quadrangularisoside D (8) was determined to be C$_{55}$H$_{83}$O$_{31}$S$_3$Na$_3$ from the [M$_{3Na}$ − Na]$^-$ ion peak at m/z 1381.3888 (calc. 1381.1881), [M$_{3Na}$ − 2Na]$^{2-}$ ion peak at m/z 679.2012 (calc. 679.1995), [M$_{3Na}$ − 3Na]$^{3-}$ ion peak at m/z 445.1387 (calc. 445.1366), and [M$_{3Na}$ + Na]$^+$ ion peak at m/z 1427.3663 (calc. 1427.3666) in the (−) and (+) HR-ESI-MS, respectively. The ^{13}C NMR spectrum of the aglycone part of 8 (Table 5) coincided with that of quadrangularisoside B (3), indicating the identity of their aglycones.

The (−)ESI-MS/MS of quadrangularisoside D (**8**) demonstrated the fragmentation of the [M$_{3Na}$ − Na]$^-$ ion at m/z 1381.4. The peaks of fragment ions were observed at m/z 1261.4 [M$_{3Na}$ − Na − NaHSO$_4$]$^-$, 1103.4 [M$_{3Na}$ − Na − C$_7$H$_{11}$O$_8$SNa (MeGlcSO$_3$Na)]$^-$, 751.3 [M$_{3Na}$ − Na − NaHSO$_4$ − C$_{32}$H$_{47}$O$_5$ (Agl) + H]$^-$, 533.1 [M$_{3Na}$ − Na − 2NaSO$_3$ − C$_{33}$H$_{47}$O$_5$ (Agl) − C$_5$H$_8$O$_4$ (Xyl) + H]$^-$, 387.1 [M$_{3Na}$ − Na − 2NaSO$_3$ − C$_{33}$H$_{47}$O$_5$ (Agl) − C$_5$H$_8$O$_4$ (Xyl) − C$_6$H$_{10}$O$_4$ (Qui) + H]$^-$, and 255.0 [M$_{3Na}$ − Na − 2NaSO$_3$ − C$_{33}$H$_{47}$O$_5$ (Agl) − C$_5$H$_8$O$_4$ (Xyl) − C$_6$H$_{10}$O$_4$ (Qui) − C$_5$H$_8$O$_4$ (Xyl) + 2H]$^-$.

All these data indicate that quadrangularisoside D (**8**) is 3β-O-[4-O-sodium sulfate-3-O-methyl-β-D-glucopyranosyl-(1→3)-β-D-xylopyranosyl-(1→4)-3-O-sodium sulfate-β-D-quinovopyranosyl-(1→2)-4-O-sodium sulfate-β-D-xylopyranosyl]-16β-acetoxyholosta-7,24-diene.

The molecular formula of quadrangularisoside D$_1$ (**9**) was determined to be the same as for quadrangularisoside D (**8**) (C$_{55}$H$_{83}$O$_{31}$S$_3$Na$_3$) from the [M$_{3Na}$ − Na]$^-$ ion peak at m/z 1381.3891 (calc. 1381.3881), [M$_{3Na}$ − 2Na]$^{2-}$ ion peak at m/z 679.2015 (calc. 679.1995), and [M$_{3Na}$ − 3Na]$^{3-}$ ion peak at m/z 445.1390 (calc. 445.1366) in the (−)HR-ESI-MS as well as from the [M$_{3Na}$ + Na]$^+$ ion peak at m/z 1427.3653 (calc. 1427.3666) in the (+)HR-ESI-MS. The aglycone of quadrangularisoside D$_1$ (**9**) was identical to that of quadrangularisoside B$_1$ (**4**), which was deduced from the coincidence of their ^{13}C NMR spectra (Table 6).

The (−)ESI-MS/MS of **9** demonstrated the fragmentation of the [M$_{3Na}$ − Na]$^-$ ion at m/z 1381.4. The peaks of fragment ions were observed at m/z 1279.5 [M$_{3Na}$ − Na − NaSO$_3$ + H]$^-$, 1177.5 [M$_{3Na}$ − Na − 2NaSO$_3$ + 2H]$^-$, 1001.4 [M$_{3Na}$ − Na − 2NaSO$_3$−C$_7$H$_{12}$O$_5$ (MeGlc) + 2H]$^-$, 941.4 [M$_{3Na}$ − Na − 2NaSO$_3$−C$_7$H$_{12}$O$_5$ (MeGlc) − CH$_3$COO + H]$^-$, 751.3 [M$_{3Na}$ − Na − NaHSO$_4$ − C$_{32}$H$_{47}$O$_5$ (Agl) + H]$^-$, and 255.0 [M$_{3Na}$ − Na − 2NaSO$_3$ − C$_{33}$H$_{47}$O$_5$ (Agl) − C$_5$H$_8$O$_4$ (Xyl) − C$_6$H$_{10}$O$_4$ (Qui) − C$_5$H$_8$O$_4$ (Xyl) + 2H]$^-$. The (+)ESI-MS/MS of **9** demonstrated the sequential loss by the [M$_{3Na}$ + Na]$^+$ ion at m/z 1427.4 of three sulfate groups (ion peaks at m/z 1325.4 [M$_{3Na}$ + Na − NaSO$_3$ + H]$^+$, 1223.5 [M$_{3Na}$ + Na − 2NaSO$_3$ + 2H]$^+$, and 1121.5 [M$_{3Na}$ + Na − 3NaSO$_3$ + 3H]$^+$).

All these data indicate that quadrangularisoside D$_1$ (**9**) is 3β-O-[4-O-sodium sulfate-3-O-methyl-β-D-glucopyranosyl-(1→3)-β-D-xylopyranosyl-(1→4)-3-O-sodium sulfate-β-D-quinovopyranosyl-(1→2)-4-O-sodium sulfate-β-D-xylopyranosyl]-16β-acetoxyholosta-7,25-diene.

The molecular formula of quadrangularisoside D$_2$ (**10**) was determined to be C$_{53}$H$_{79}$O$_{30}$S$_3$Na$_3$ from the [M$_{3Na}$ − Na]$^-$ ion peak at m/z 1337.3625 (calc. 1337.3619), [M$_{3Na}$ − 2Na]$^{2-}$ ion peak at m/z 657.1881 (calc. 657.1863), and [M$_{3Na}$ − 3Na]$^{3-}$ ion peak at m/z 430.4633 (calc. 430.4612) in the (−)HR-ESI-MS as well as from the [M$_{3Na}$ + Na]$^+$ ion peak at m/z 1383.3390 (calc. 1383.3404) in the (+)HR-ESI-MS. The aglycone of quadrangularisoside D$_2$ (**10**) was identical to that of quadrangularisoside B$_2$ (**5**) (Table 7), having holotoxinogenin as a triterpenoid nucleus [31].

The (−)ESI-MS/MS of **10** demonstrated the fragmentation of the [M$_{3Na}$ − Na]$^-$ ion at m/z 1381.4. The peaks of fragment ions were observed at m/z 1217.4 [M$_{3Na}$ − Na − NaHSO$_4$]$^-$, 1059.4 [M$_{3Na}$ − Na − C$_7$H$_{11}$O$_8$SNa (MeGlcSO$_3$Na)]$^-$, 939.4 [M$_{3Na}$ − Na − NaHSO$_4$ − C$_7$H$_{11}$O$_8$SNa (MeGlcSO$_3$Na)]$^-$, 533.1 [M$_{3Na}$ − Na − 2NaSO$_3$ − C$_{30}$H$_{43}$O$_4$ (Agl) − C$_5$H$_8$O$_4$ (Xyl) + H]$^-$, 387.1 [M$_{3Na}$ − Na − 2NaSO$_3$ − C$_{30}$H$_{43}$O$_4$ (Agl) − C$_5$H$_8$O$_4$ (Xyl) − C$_6$H$_{10}$O$_4$ (Qui) + H]$^-$, and 255.0 [M$_{3Na}$ − Na − 2NaSO$_3$ − C$_{30}$H$_{43}$O$_4$ (Agl) − C$_5$H$_8$O$_4$ (Xyl) − C$_6$H$_{10}$O$_4$ (Qui) − C$_5$H$_8$O$_4$ (Xyl) + 2H]$^-$, corroborating the identity of the carbohydrate chains of compounds **8**–**10**. The (+)ESI-MS/MS of **10** demonstrated the loss of two sulfate groups: ion peaks at m/z 1264.4 [M$_{3Na}$ + Na − NaSO$_4$]$^+$ and 1143.4 [M$_{3Na}$ + Na − 2NaSO$_4$]$^+$.

All these data indicate that quadrangularisoside D$_2$ (**10**) is 3β-O-[4-O-sodium sulfate-3-O-methyl-β-D-glucopyranosyl-(1→3)-β-D-xylopyranosyl-(1→4)-3-O-sodium sulfate-β-D-quinovopyranosyl-(1→2)-4-O-sodium sulfate-β-D-xylopyranosyl]-16-ketoholosta-9(11),25-diene.

The molecular formula of quadrangularisoside D$_3$ (**11**) was determined to be C$_{55}$H$_{83}$O$_{33}$S$_3$Na$_3$ from the [M$_{3Na}$ − Na]$^-$ ion peak at m/z 1413.3785 (calc. 1413.3780), [M$_{3Na}$ − 2Na]$^{2-}$ ion peak at m/z 695.1963 (calc. 695.1944), and [M$_{3Na}$ − 3Na]$^{3-}$ ion peak at m/z 455.8006 (calc. 455.7998) in the (−)HR-ESI-MS as well as from the [M$_{3Na}$ + Na]$^+$ ion peak at m/z 1459.3534 (calc. 1459.3564) in the (+)HR-ESI-MS. The aglycone of quadrangularisoside D$_3$ (**11**) was established to be 25-peroxy-16β-acetoxyholosta-7,23E-diene-3β-ol and was identical to the aglycone of quadrangularisoside A (1) (Table 2), which was deduced from the comparison of their ^{13}C NMR spectra.

The (−)ESI-MS/MS of **11** demonstrated the fragmentation of the [M$_{3Na}$ − Na]$^-$ ion at *m/z* 1413.4. The peaks of fragment ions were observed at *m/z* 1261.4 [M$_{Na}$ − Na − OOH − NaSO$_4$]$^-$, 1103.3 [M$_{Na}$ − Na − OOH − C$_7$H$_{11}$O$_8$SNa (MeGlcSO$_3$Na) + H]$^-$, 723.3 [M$_{3Na}$ − Na − OOH −C$_7$H$_{11}$O$_8$SNa (MeGlcSO$_3$Na) − C$_5$H$_8$O$_4$ (Xyl) − C$_6$H$_9$O$_7$SNa (QuiSO$_3$Na) + H]$^-$, as well as the ion peaks at the same *m/z* as in the mass spectra of the other quadrangularisosides of the group D (**8–10**): 751.3 [M$_{3Na}$ − Na − NaHSO$_4$ − C$_{32}$H$_{47}$O$_6$ (Agl)+ H]$^-$, 387.1 [M$_{3Na}$ − Na − 2NaSO$_3$ − C$_{32}$H$_{47}$O$_6$ (Agl) − C$_5$H$_8$O$_4$ (Xyl) − C$_6$H$_{10}$O$_4$ (Qui) + H]$^-$, and 255.0 [M$_{3Na}$ − Na − 2NaSO$_3$ − C$_{32}$H$_{47}$O$_6$ (Agl) − C$_5$H$_8$O$_4$ (Xyl) − C$_6$H$_{10}$O$_4$ (Qui) − C$_5$H$_8$O$_4$ (Xyl) + H]$^-$.

All these data indicate that quadrangularisoside D$_3$ (**11**) is 3β-*O*-[4-*O*-sodium sulfate-3-*O*-methyl-β-D-glucopyranosyl-(1→3)-β-D-xylopyranosyl-(1→4)-3-*O*-sodium sulfate-β-D-quinovopyranosyl-(1→2)-4-*O*-sodium sulfate-β-D-xylopyranosyl]-25-peroxy-16β-acetoxyholosta-7,23*E*-diene.

The molecular formula of quadrangularisoside D$_4$ (**12**) was determined to be the same as that for **11** (C$_{55}$H$_{83}$O$_{33}$S$_3$Na$_3$) from the [M$_{3Na}$ − Na]$^-$ ion peak at *m/z* 1413.3762 (calc. 1413.3780), [M$_{3Na}$ − 2Na]$^{2-}$ ion peak at *m/z* 695.1954 (calc. 695.1944), and [M$_{3Na}$ − 3Na]$^{3-}$ ion peak at *m/z* 455.8011 (calc. 455.7998) in the (−)HR-ESI-MS as well as from the [M$_{3Na}$ + Na]$^+$ ion peak at *m/z* 1459.3512 (calc. 1459.3564) in the (+)HR-ESI-MS, indicating the isomerism of these glycosides. The comparison of the ^{13}C NMR spectra of the aglycone parts of quadrangularisosides D$_4$ (**12**) and A$_1$ (**2**) showed their identity (Table 3). Thus, the aglycone of quadrangularisoside D$_4$ (**12**) was established to be 24*S*-peroxy-16β-acetoxyholosta-7,25-diene-3β-ol.

The (−)ESI-MS/MS of **12** demonstrated the fragmentation of the [M$_{3Na}$ − Na]$^-$ ion at *m/z* 1413.4. The peaks of fragment ions were observed at *m/z* 999.4 [M$_{Na}$ − Na − OOH−NaSO$_3$ − C$_7$H$_{11}$O$_8$SNa (MeGlcSO$_3$Na)]$^-$, 867.4 [M$_{Na}$ − Na − OOH − NaSO$_3$ − C$_7$H$_{11}$O$_8$SNa (MeGlcSO$_3$Na) − C$_5$H$_8$O$_4$ (Xyl)]$^-$, and 255.0 [M$_{3Na}$ − Na − 2NaSO$_3$ − C$_{32}$H$_{47}$O$_6$ (Agl) − C$_5$H$_8$O$_4$ (Xyl) − C$_6$H$_{10}$O$_4$ (Qui) − C$_5$H$_8$O$_4$ (Xyl) + H]$^-$.

All these data indicate that quadrangularisoside D$_4$ (**12**) is 3β-*O*-[4-*O*-sodium sulfate-3-*O*-methyl-β-D-glucopyranosyl-(1→3)-β-D-xylopyranosyl-(1→4)-3-*O*-sodium sulfate-β-D-quinovopyranosyl-(1→2)-4-*O*-sodium sulfate-β-D-xylopyranosyl]-24*S*-peroxy-16β-acetoxyholosta-7,25-diene.

In the ^{1}H and ^{13}C NMR spectra of the carbohydrate moiety of quadrangularisoside E (**13**), four characteristic doublets at δ$_H$ 4.67–5.19 (*J* = 7.3–7.7 Hz) and corresponding to them four signals of anomeric carbons at δ$_C$ 104.2–104.7 were indicative of a tetrasaccharide chain and β-configurations of glycosidic bonds (Table 12). The ^{1}H,^{1}H-COSY and 1D TOCSY spectra of **13** showed the signals of the isolated spin systems assigned to the xylose, quinovose, glucose, and 3-*O*-methylglucose residues. So, the monosaccharide composition of **13** was identical to that in the quadrangularisosides of group C (**6, 7**). The comparison of their ^{13}C NMR spectra showed the coincidence of the signals corresponding to the monosaccharide residues from the first to the third. The signals of terminal 3-*O*-methylglucose residue in the ^{13}C NMR spectrum of **13** differed from the corresponding signals in the spectrum of **6, 7** due to the attachment of the third sulfate group to C(4) MeGlc4, causing α- and β-shifting effects (δ$_C$ 76.1 (C(4) MeGlc4); δ$_C$ 85.2 (C(3) MeGlc4); δ$_C$ 76.4 (C(5) MeGlc4)) in quadrangularisoside E (**13**). Actually, the signals of terminal sugar moieties in the spectra of quadrangularisosides E (**13**) and D (**8**) were coincident, corroborating the sulfation of C(4) MeGlc4 in glycoside **13**. Hence, compound **13** has a novel carbohydrate chain with an unusual position of the third sulfate group in the terminal sugar unit.

The molecular formula of quadrangularisoside E (**13**) was determined to be C$_{54}$H$_{81}$O$_{31}$S$_3$Na$_3$ from the [M$_{3Na}$ − Na]$^-$ ion peak at *m/z* 1367.3739 (calc. 1367.3725), [M$_{3Na}$ − 2Na]$^{2-}$ ion peak at *m/z* 672.1941 (calc. 672.1916), and [M$_{3Na}$ − 3Na]$^{3-}$ ion peak at *m/z* 440.4674 (calc. 440.4647) in the (−)HR-ESI-MS as well as from the [M$_{3Na}$ + Na]$^+$ ion peak at *m/z* 1413.3488 (calc. 1413.3509) in the (+)HR-ESI-MS. The aglycone of quadrangularisoside E (**13**) was identical to the aglycone of quadrangularisosides B$_2$ (**5**) and D$_2$ (**10**)—holotoxinogenin (Table 7).

Table 12. ^{13}C and ^{1}H NMR chemical shifts and HMBC and ROESY correlations of carbohydrate moiety of quadrangularisoside E (**13**). ^{a} Recorded at 176.03 MHz in C$_5$D$_5$N/D$_2$O (4/1). ^{b} Bold = interglycosidic positions. ^{c} Italic = sulfate position. ^{d} Recorded at 700.00 MHz in C$_5$D$_5$N/D$_2$O (4/1). Multiplicity by 1D TOCSY.

Atom	δ_C mult. ^{a,b,c}	δ_H mult. ^{d} (J in Hz)	HMBC	ROESY
		Xyl1 (1→C-3)		
1	104.7 CH	4.67 d (7.3)	C: 3; C: 5 Xyl1	H-3; H-3, 5 Xyl1
2	**82.2** CH	3.94 t (8.2)	C: 1 Qui2; 3 Xyl1	H-1 Qui2
3	74.6 CH	4.23 t (9.1)	C: 2, 4 Xyl1	H-1, 5 Xyl1
4	75.6 CH	4.96 m	C: 3 Xyl1	H-2 Xyl1
5	63.7 CH$_2$	4.75 dd (5.5; 11.0)	C: 1, 3, 4 Xyl1	-
		3.73 t (10.1)	-	H-1 Xyl1
		Qui2 (1→2Xyl1)		
1	104.5 CH	4.92 d (7.6)	C: 2 Xyl1; 5 Qui2	H-2 Xyl1; H-3, 5 Qui2
2	75.3 CH	3.83 t (9.1)	C: 1, 3 Qui2	-
3	74.9 CH	3.89 t (9.1)	C: 2, 4 Qui2	H-1, 5 Qui2
4	**87.1** CH	3.41 t (9.1)	C: 1 Glc3; 3, 5 Qui2	H-1 Glc3; H-6 Qui2
5	71.3 CH	3.60 m	C: 1, 3, 4 Qui2	H-1 Qui2
6	17.7 CH$_3$	1.59 d (6.0)	C: 4, 5 Qui2	H-4, 5 Qui2
		Glc3 (1→4Qui2)		
1	104.2 CH	4.76 d (7.3)	C: 4 Qui2	H-4 Qui2; H-3,5 Glc3
2	73.5 CH	3.84 t (8.9)	C: 1, 3 Glc3	H-4 Glc3
3	**86.0** CH	4.17 t (8.9)	C: 1 MeGlc4; 2, 4 Glc3	H-1 MeGlc4, H-1, 5 Glc3
4	69.2 CH	3.76 t (8.9)	C: 3, 5, 6 Glc3	H-6 Glc3
5	74.8 CH	4.11 t (8.9)	-	H-1, 3 Glc3
6	67.5 CH$_2$	4.99 d (9.7)	C: 4 Glc3	-
		4.56 dd (6.3; 11.3)	C: 5 Glc3	-
		MeGlc4 (1→3Glc3)		
1	104.4 CH	5.19 d (7.7)	C: 3 Glc3, 5 MeGlc4	H-3 Glc3; H-3, 5 MeGlc4
2	74.0 CH	3.87 t (7.7)	C: 1, 3 MeGlc4	H-4 MeGlc4
3	85.2 CH	3.72 t (9.6)	C: 2, 4 MeGlc4, OMe	H-1 MeGlc4; OMe
4	76.1 CH	4.87 t (9.6)	C: 3, 5, 6 MeGlc4	H-2 MeGlc4
5	76.4 CH	3.85 t (9.6)	-	H-1 MeGlc4
6	61.6 CH$_2$	4.48 d (11.5)	C: 5 MeGlc4	-
		4.31 dd (5.8; 11.5)		
OMe	60.6 CH$_3$	3.92 s	C: 3 MeGlc4	

The (−)ESI-MS/MS of **13** demonstrated the fragmentation of the [M$_{3Na}$ − Na]$^−$ ion at m/z 1367.4. The peaks of fragment ions were observed at m/z 1247.4 [M$_{Na}$ − Na − NaHSO$_4$]$^−$, 1089.4 [M$_{Na}$ − Na − C$_7$H$_{11}$O$_8$SNa (MeGlcSO$_3$Na)]$^−$, 969.4 [M$_{3Na}$ − Na − NaHSO$_4$−C$_7$H$_{11}$O$_8$SNa (MeGlcSO$_3$Na)]$^−$, 825.4 [M$_{3Na}$ − Na − C$_7$H$_{11}$O$_8$SNa(MeGlcSO$_3$Na) − C$_6$H$_{10}$O$_8$SNa(GlcSO$_3$Na) + H]$^−$, and 255.0 [M$_{3Na}$ − Na − C$_{30}$H$_{43}$O$_4$ (Agl) − C$_5$H$_7$O$_7$SNa(XylSO$_3$Na) − C$_6$H$_{10}$O$_4$ (Qui) − C$_6$H$_9$O$_8$SNa(GlcSO$_3$Na) − H]$^−$. As result of the fragmentation of the [M$_{3Na}$ + Na]$^+$ ion at m/z 1413.4 in the (+)ESI-MS/MS of **13**, the peaks of fragment ions were observed at m/z 963.5 [M$_{3Na}$ + Na − C$_{30}$H$_{43}$O$_3$ (Agl) + H]$^+$ and 685.4 [M$_{3Na}$ + Na − C$_{30}$H$_{43}$O$_3$ (Agl) − C$_7$H$_{11}$O$_8$SNa (MeGlcSO$_3$Na) + H]$^+$.

All these data indicate that quadrangularisoside E (**13**) is 3β-O-[4-O-sodium sulfate-3-O-methyl-β-D-glucopyranosyl-(1→3)-6-O-sodium sulfate-β-D-glucopyranosyl-(1→4)-β-D-quinovopyranosyl-(1→2)-4-O-sodium sulfate-β-D-xylopyranosyl]-16-ketoholosta-9(11),25-diene.

Thus, 13 unknown earlier triterpene glycosides were isolated from the Vietnamese sea cucumber *Colochirus quadrangularis*. The glycosides include five different carbohydrate chains (quadrangularisosides of the groups A–E) and seven holostane aglycones. The trisulfated carbohydrate chains of quadrangularisosides of the groups D and E are novel and characterized by the position of one of the sulfate groups at C(4) of the terminal 3-O-methylglucose residue, which is unusual for the glycosides from sea cucumbers. Two novel aglycones having hydroperoxyl groups in the side chains were discovered in quadrangularisosides A (**1**) and D_3 (**11**) (hydroperoxyl group at C(25)) as well as in quadrangularisosides A_1 (**2**) and D_4 (**12**) (hydroperoxyl group at C(24)). The finding of such functionalities in the aglycones of triterpene glycosides from the sea cucumbers is rare, and two other cases were reported only last year [24,25].

As to the structures of the glycosides isolated earlier by the Chinese researchers from the same species [12–15], only two compounds—philinopsides A and F—were identified by us in the glycosidic fraction of *C. quadrangularis*. Other two compounds, isolated earlier—pentactasides B and C—are presumably the glycosides identical to quadrangularisosides B (**4**) and B_1 (**5**), because their carbohydrate chain structures were established incorrectly due to inaccuracies made by the authors in the NMR data interpretation. The glycosides with di- (pentactaside III) and trisaccharide chains (pentactasides I and II) as well as pentactaside E, having 16-ketoholosta-7,25-diene-3β-ol as the aglycone, have not been found in the glycosidic sum obtained by us from *C. quadrangularis*.

2.3. Bioactivity of the Glycosides

The cytotoxic activities of compounds **1–13** as well as known earlier cladoloside C (used as positive control) against mouse erythrocytes (hemolytic activity), neuroblastoma Neuro 2a cells, and normal epithelial JB-6 cells are presented in Table 13. The erythrocytes were more sensitive (all of the compounds were rather strong hemolytics) to the action of the glycosides than Neuro 2a or JB-6 cells, but the structure–activity relationships (SARs) observed for the glycosides **1–13** were similar for three cell lines investigated. For instance, the quadrangularisosides of the groups B (**3, 4**) and C (**6, 7**), as well as quadrangularisosides D (**8**) and D_1 (**9**) demonstrated high hemolytic action and slightly decreased cytotoxicity against Neuro 2a and JB-6 cells. These compounds contain holostane aglycones without hydroperoxyl groups and di- or trisulfated tetrasaccharide chains. Such a combination of structural features provides high membranolytic activity even if three sulfate groups are present.

The membranolytic activity of monosulfated quadrangularisosides of the group A (**1, 2**) were decreased in comparison with that for the most active glycosides **3, 4, 6–9** due to the presence of the hydroperoxyl group. However, the combination of the aglycones with the hydroperoxy-group in the side chains and trisulfated carbohydrate chains, as in quadrangularisosides D_3 (**11**) and D_4 (**12**), significantly decreased the activity.

The unusual position of the third sulfate group at C-4 MeGlc4 in the carbohydrate chain of quadrangularisoside E (**13**) does not significantly influence the membranolytic activity, and the glycoside is rather strong hemolytic and cytotoxin.

The glycosides in this series having aglycones with a 7(8)-double bond and 16β-O-acetic group were more active in comparison with those having aglycones characterized by a 9(11)-double bond.

To detect the influence of compounds **1–13** on the cell viability, formation, and growth of colonies of human colorectal adenocarcinoma HT-29 cells, the cells were treated with various concentrations of the compounds (0–20 µM) for 24 h, and then cell viability was assessed by MTS (3-(4,5-dimethylthiazol-2-yl)-5-(3-carboxymethoxyphenyl)-2-(4-sulfophenyl)-2H-tetrazolium) assay. The concentrations of glycosides **1–13** that cause 50% of the inhibition of HT-29 cells viability are given in Table 13. It was shown that quadrangularisosides A (**1**), A_1 (**2**), D_2 (**10**), D_3 (**11**), and D_4 (**12**) are non-cytotoxic against HT-29 cells at the dose up to 20 µM. Compounds **6, 7**, and **13** possess moderate cytotoxic activity, while the rest (**3–5, 8, 9**) effectively suppressed the cell viability of HT-29 cells (Table 13).

Table 13. The cytotoxic activities of glycosides 1–13 and cladoloside C (positive control) against mouse erythrocytes, neuroblastoma Neuro 2a cells, and normal epithelial JB-6 cells. The inhibiting concentration of the glycosides 1–13 on cell viability (IC_{50}) and colony formation ($ICCF_{50}$) of HT-29 cells.

Glycoside	ED_{50}, µM	Cytotoxicity EC_{50}, µM		IC_{50}, µM	$ICCF_{50}$, µM
	Erythrocytes	Neuro-2a	JB-6	HT-29	HT-29
quadrangularisoside A (1)	1.57 ± 0.16	27.43 ± 2.23	>50.00	>20	18.3 ± 0.8
quadrangularisoside A_1 (2)	1.11 ± 0.08	21.34 ± 1.32	27.91 ± 2.19	>20	7.2 ± 0.3
quadrangularisoside B (3)	0.51 ± 0.05	9.79 ± 0.76	18.62 ± 0.80	0.49 ± 0.03	0.28 ± 0.04
quadrangularisoside B_1 (4)	0.23 ± 0.02	11.52 ± 0.26	17.01 ± 0.81	0.48 ± 0.01	0.25 ± 0.07
quadrangularisoside B_2 (5)	0.51 ± 0.01	16.27 ± 1.70	19.43 ± 0.88	4.8 ± 0.1	0.46 ± 0.05
quadrangularisoside C (6)	0.56 ± 0.02	22.34 ± 0.82	11.35 ± 0.85	12.6 ± 1.5	0.65 ± 0.08
quadrangularisoside C_1 (7)	0.11 ± 0.01	14.68 ± 0.33	9.13 ± 0.37	19.0 ± 2.0	1.38 ± 0.4
quadrangularisoside D (8)	0.24 ± 0.01	10.98 ± 0.78	12.71 ± 1.76	3.0 ± 0.2	0.84 ± 0.07
quadrangularisoside D_1 (9)	0.41 ± 0.02	10.68 ± 0.94	16.50 ± 2.32	4.1 ± 0.2	1.31 ± 0.08
quadrangularisoside D_2 (10)	3.31 ± 0.09	24.49 ± 1.09	37.87 ± 1.51	>20	6.75 ± 1.25
quadrangularisoside D_3 (11)	6.03 ± 0.42	>50.00	>50.00	>20	>20
quadrangularisoside D_4 (12)	5.45 ± 0.15	>50.00	>50.00	>20	>20
quadrangularisoside E (13)	2.04 ± 0.05	19.48 ± 1.47	19.01 ± 0.47	16.8 ± 0.4	1.87 ± 0.94
cladoloside C	0.20 ± 0.02	16.24 ± 2.41	11.20 ± 0.27	—	—

To investigate the effect of glycosides 1–13 on the colony formation of HT-29 cells, the concentrations lower than IC_{50} were chosen. The data concerning the inhibitory activity of the compounds on colony formation are presented as a concentration that causes 50% of the inhibition of colonies number ($ICCF_{50}$) (Table 13). The glycosides having hydroperoxyl groups in the aglycones (11, 12, as well as 1) were shown to not inhibit the colony formation and growth of HT-29 cells for 50% under concentration even at 20 µM or demonstrated only a slight effect, correspondingly. Meanwhile, quadrangularisoside A_1 (2) having this functionality was surprisingly active. Interestingly, quadrangularisosides C (6), C_1 (7), and E (13) possessed strong inhibitory activity on colony formation in HT-29 cells at concentrations much lower that their IC_{50} values. This can indicate that their mechanism of action is related with the regulation of specific signaling pathways rather than a direct toxic effect. The structure–activity relationships (SARs) observed for HT-29 cells were largely similar with the SARs of the glycosides in relation to the other cell lines investigated. The main contributors influencing the SARs were the hydroperoxyl and sulfate groups presented in the glycosides. Generally, the quadrangularisosides of group B (disulfated compounds with the second sulfate group attached to C-3 Qui2 and without hydroperoxyls in the aglycones) were the most active in all tests.

Initially, the effects of X-ray irradiation of 1 Gy or the individual compounds at a concentration of 0.02 µM on the colony formation of HT-29 cells were checked. None of the glycosides 1–13 influenced the process of colony formation and proliferation at a dose of 0.02 µM (data not shown). The number of colonies of HT-29 cells was found to be decreased by 32% after radiation exposure at a dose of 1 Gy. Noticeably, the synergic effects of the glycosides (0.02 µM) and radioactive irradiation (1 Gy) decreasing the number of colonies was observed. Quadrangularisosides A (1), B_1 (4), and D_1 (9) enhanced the effect of radiation by about 30%, while compounds 3, 5, 6, and 8 enhanced the radiation effect by about 20%, and glycosides 2 and 10 enhanced the radiation effect by less than 10% (Figure 2).

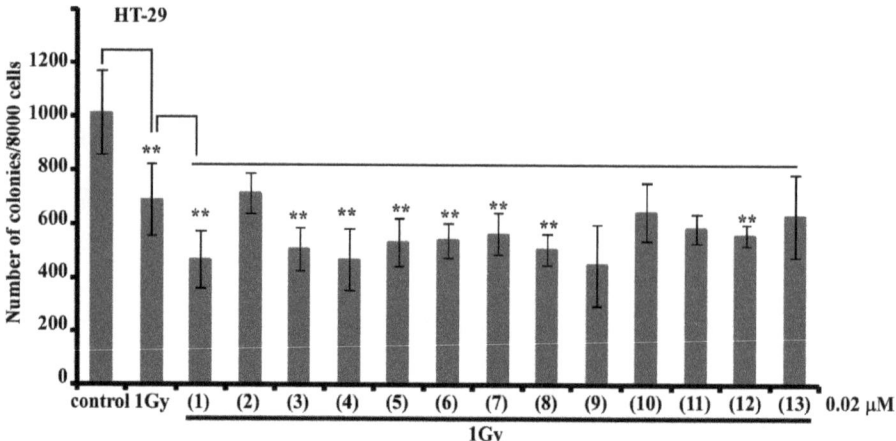

Figure 2. The effect of radioactive irradiation and a combination of radioactive irradiation and glycosides **1–13** on HT-29 cancer cells colony formation. HT-29 cells (8.0×10^3) were cultured in the presence or absence of 0.02 µM compounds for an additional 24 h before irradiation at the dose of 1 Gy. Immediately after irradiation, cells were returned to the incubator for recovery. Three hours later, the cells were harvested and used for soft agar assay. Data are represented as the mean ± SD as determined from triplicate experiments. A Student's t-test was used to evaluate the data with the following significance levels: ** $p < 0.01$.

3. Materials and Methods

3.1. General Experimental Procedures

Specific rotation, Perkin-Elmer 343 Polarimeter; NMR, Bruker Avance III 500 (Bruker BioSpin GmbH, Rheinstetten, Germany) (500.13/125.77 MHz) or Avance III 700 Bruker FT-NMR (Bruker BioSpin GmbH, Rheinstetten, Germany) (700.00/176.03 MHz) (^{1}H/^{13}C) spectrometers; ESI MS (positive and negative ion modes), Agilent 6510 Q-TOF apparatus, sample concentration 0.01 mg/mL; HPLC, Agilent 1100 apparatus with a differential refractometer; columns Supelcosil LC-Si (4.6 × 150 mm, 5 µm), Supelco Discovery HS F5-5 (10 × 250 mm, 5 µm).

3.2. Animals and Cells

Specimens of the sea cucumber *Colochirus quadrangularis* (family Cucumariidae; order Dendrochirotida) were collected on the coral reefs near the seashore of Vietnam in the South China Sea. Sampling was performed by scuba diving in July 2016 (collector T.N. Dautova) at a depth of 7–9 m. Sea cucumbers were identified by S. Sh. Dautov; voucher specimens are preserved in A.V. Zhirmunsky National Scientific Center of Marine Biology, Vladivostok, Russia.

CD-1 mice weighing 18–20 g were purchased from RAMS 'Stolbovaya' nursery (Russia) and kept at the animal facility in standard conditions. All experiments were conducted in compliance with all of the rules and international recommendations of the European Convention for the Protection of Vertebrate Animals Used for Experimental Studies.

Mouse epithelial JB-6 cells Cl 41-5a and mouse neuroblastoma cell line Neuro 2a (ATCC® CCL-131) were purchased from ATCC (Manassas, VA, USA).

HT-29 cell line (ATCC# HTB-28) was cultured in McCoy's 5A medium supplemented with 10% fetal bovine serum (FBS) and penicillin–streptomycin solution. Cells were maintained in a sterile environment and kept in an incubator at 5% CO_2 and 37 °C to promote growth. HT-29 cells were sub-cultured every 3–4 days by their rinsing with phosphate-buffered saline (PBS), adding trypsin to detach the cells from the tissue culture flask, and transferring 10–20% of the harvested cells to a new flask containing fresh growth media.

3.3. Extraction and Isolation

The sea cucumbers were extracted twice with refluxing 60% EtOH. The extract was evaporated to dryness and dissolved in water followed by chromatography on a Polychrom-1 column (powdered Teflon, Biolar, Latvia). The glycosides were eluted with 50% EtOH and evaporated (2500 mg of crude glycoside sum were obtained). Its subsequent chromatography on an Si gel column with the gradient of solvent systems $CHCl_3/EtOH/H_2O$ (100:100:17) followed by (100:125:25) as the mobile phase gave three fractions (I–III) containing different groups of glycosides. Fraction I (525 mg) was submitted to HPLC on a Supelco Discovery HS F5-5 column with $MeOH/H_2O/NH_4OAc$ (1 M water solution) (70/28/2) as the mobile phase, which resulted in the isolation of six known earlier compounds (lefevreoside A_2 (2.3 mg), philinopside A (29.8 mg), lefevreoside C (39.8 mg), neothyonidioside (25 mg), philinopside F (or violaceoside B) (8 mg), and colochiroside B_3 (6.6 mg)) and two other subfractions (1.1 and 1.2). The HPLC of subfraction 1.2 on the same column but with $CH_3CN/H_2O/NH_4OAc$ (1 M water solution) (28/71/1) as the mobile phase gave 4.1 mg of known earlier colochiroside B_2 and 16 mg of quadrangularisoside A (**1**). The rechromatography of the subfraction 1.1 under the same conditions gave 2.8 mg of quadrangularisoside A_1 (**2**) and 1.8 mg of known colochiroside B_1. The fraction II (709 mg) was submitted to HPLC on a Supelco Discovery HS F5-5 column with $CH_3CN/H_2O/NH_4OAc$ (1 M water solution) (35/63.5/1.5) as the mobile phase, which lead to the isolation of individual quadrangularisoside C_1 (**7**) (3.8 mg) as well as two other subfractions (2.1 and 2.2). The subsequent HPLC of subfraction 2.2 on the same column but with $MeOH/H_2O/NH_4OAc$ (67/31/2) as the mobile phase was followed by different ratios of the same solvents: (1) (75/22/3) gave 20.4 mg of quadrangularisoside B_1 (**4**); (2) (66/32/2) gave 4.5 mg of quadrangularisoside C (**6**); (3) (63/35/2) gave 12.3 mg of quadrangularisoside B (**3**). The rechromatography of subfraction 2.1 on the silica-based column Supelcosil LC-Si with $CHCl_3/MeOH/H_2O$ (65/25/2) as the mobile phase resulted in the isolation of 53 mg of known earlier hemioedemoside A and 30 mg of quadrangularisoside B_2 (**5**). The most polar fraction III (195 mg) was submitted to HPLC on a Supelco Discovery HS F5-5 column with $MeOH/H_2O/NH_4OAc$ (60/38.5/1.5) as the mobile phase to give four subfractions, 3.1–3.4. The subsequent HPLC of 3.4 on the same column with an $MeOH/H_2O/NH_4OAc$ (58/40/2) solvent system resulted in the isolation of individual quadrangularisosides D (**8**) (6.2 mg) and D_1 (**9**) (3.2 mg). Quadrangularisosides D_2 (**10**) (3.4 mg) and E (**13**) (5.2 mg) were isolated by HPLC of subfraction 3.3 on a silica-based column Supelcosil LC-Si with $CHCl_3/MeOH/H_2O$ (50/28/3) as the mobile phase followed by the rechromatography of two fractions obtained on a Supelco Discovery HS F5-5 column with $MeOH/H_2O/NH_4OAc$ (60/38/2) as the mobile phase. The HPLC of subfraction 3.2 on a Supelco Discovery HS F5-5 column with $MeOH/H_2O/NH_4OAc$ (60/37/3) gave 2.2 mg of quadrangularisoside D_3 (**11**). The HPLC of subfraction 3.1 on the same column with $MeOH/H_2O/NH_4OAc$ (62/35/3) gave 2.3 mg of quadrangularisoside D_4 (**12**).

3.3.1. Quadrangularisoside A (**1**)

Colorless powder; $[\alpha]_D^{20}$ − 16 (c 0.1, 50% MeOH). NMR: See Tables 1 and 2. (−)-HR-ESI-MS m/z: 1209.5004 (calc. 1209.5004) $[M_{Na} - Na]^-$; (+)HR-ESI-MS m/z: 1255.4779 (calc. 1255.4789) $[M_{Na} + Na]^+$; (+)ESI-MS/MS m/z: 1223.5 $[M_{Na} + Na - OOH + H]^+$, 1103.5 $[M_{Na} + Na - OOH - NaSO_4 + H]^+$, 927.5 $[M_{Na} + Na - OOH - NaSO_4 - C_7H_{12}O_5 (MeGlc) + H]^+$, 795.4 $[M_{Na} + Na - OOH - NaSO_4 - C_7H_{12}O_5 (MeGlc) - C_5H_8O_4 (Xyl) + H]^+$, 729.2 $[M_{Na} + Na - C_{32}H_{47}O_6 (Agl) + H]^+$, 649.3 $[M_{Na} + Na - OOH - NaSO_4 - C_7H_{12}O_5 (MeGlc) - C_5H_8O_4 (Xyl) - C_6H_{10}O_4 (Qui) + H]^+$, 609.2 $[M_{Na} + Na - C_{32}H_{47}O_6 (Agl) - NaHSO_4]^+$, 477.1 $[M_{Na} + Na - C_{32}H_{47}O_6 (Agl) - NaHSO_4 - C_5H_8O_4 (Xyl) + H]^+$.

3.3.2. Quadrangularisoside A$_1$ (2)

Colorless powder; $[\alpha]_D^{20}$ − 25 (c 0.1, 50% MeOH). NMR: See Tables 1 and 3. (−)HR-ESI-MS m/z: 1209.5006 (calc. 1209.5004) [M$_{Na}$ − Na]$^-$; (+)HR-ESI-MS m/z: 1255.4772 (calc. 1255.4789) [M$_{Na}$ + Na]$^+$; (+)ESI-MS/MS m/z: 1237.5 [M$_{Na}$ + Na − H$_2$O]$^+$, 1177.4 [M$_{Na}$ + Na − H$_2$O − CH$_3$COOH]$^+$, 1117.5 [M$_{Na}$ + Na − H$_2$O − NaHSO$_4$]$^+$, 729.2 [M$_{Na}$ + Na− C$_{32}$H$_{47}$O$_6$ (Agl) + H]$^+$, 609.2 [M$_{Na}$ + Na− C$_{32}$H$_{47}$O$_6$ (Agl) − NaHSO$_4$]$^+$, 477.1 [M$_{Na}$ + Na − C$_{32}$H$_{47}$O$_6$ (Agl) − NaHSO$_4$ − C$_5$H$_8$O$_4$ (Xyl) + H]$^+$.

3.3.3. Quadrangularisoside B (3)

Colorless powder; $[\alpha]_D^{20}$ − 22 (c 0.1, 50% MeOH). NMR: See Tables 4 and 5. (−)HR-ESI-MS m/z: 1279.4489 (calc. 1279.4494) [M$_{2Na}$ − Na]$^-$, 628.2311 (calc. 628.2301) [M$_{2Na}$ − 2Na]$^{2-}$; (+)HR-ESI-MS m/z: 1325.4272 (calc. 1325.4278) [M$_{2Na}$ + Na]$^+$; (−)ESI-MS/MS m/z: 1219.4 [M$_{2Na}$ − Na − CH$_3$COOH]$^-$, 1177.5 [M$_{2Na}$ − Na − NaSO$_3$ + H]$^-$; (+)ESI-MS/MS m/z:1223.5 [M$_{2Na}$ + Na − NaSO$_3$ + H]$^+$, 915.4 [M$_{2Na}$ + Na − NaSO$_3$ − C$_7$H$_{12}$O$_5$ (MeGlc) − C$_5$H$_8$O$_4$ (Xyl) + H]$^+$, 813.4 [M$_{2Na}$ + Na − C$_{32}$H$_{47}$O$_5$ (Agl) − H]$^+$, 711.1 [M$_{2Na}$ + Na − C$_{32}$H$_{47}$O$_5$ (Agl) − SO$_3$Na]$^+$, 579.1 [M$_{2Na}$ + Na − C$_{32}$H$_{47}$O$_5$ (Agl) − C$_5$H$_7$O$_7$SNa (XylSO$_3$Na) − H]$^+$, 535.3 [M$_{2Na}$ + Na − C$_{32}$H$_{47}$O$_5$ (Agl) − SO$_3$Na − C$_7$H$_{12}$O$_5$ (MeGlc)]$^+$, 403.0 [M$_{2Na}$ + Na − C$_{32}$H$_{47}$O$_5$ (Agl) − SO$_3$Na − C$_7$H$_{12}$O$_5$ (MeGlc) − C$_5$H$_8$O$_4$ (Xyl)]$^+$, 331.1 [M$_{2Na}$ + Na − C$_{32}$H$_{47}$O$_5$ (Agl) − C$_5$H$_7$O$_7$SNa (XylSO$_3$Na) − C$_6$H$_9$O$_7$SNa (QuiSO$_3$Na) − H]$^+$.

3.3.4. Quadrangularisoside B$_1$ (4)

Colorless powder; $[\alpha]_D^{20}$ − 23 (c 0.1, 50% MeOH). NMR: See Tables 4 and 6. (−)HR-ESI-MS m/z: 1279.4502 (calc. 1279.4494) [M$_{2Na}$ − Na]$^-$, 628.2320 (calc. 628.2301) [M$_{2Na}$ − 2Na]$^{2-}$; (+)HR-ESI-MS m/z: 1325.4272 (calc. 1325.4278) [M$_{2Na}$ + Na]$^+$; (+)ESI-MS/MS m/z: 1223.5 [M$_{2Na}$ + Na − NaSO$_3$ + H]$^+$, 1205.5 [M$_{2Na}$ + Na − NaHSO$_4$]$^+$, 1085.5 [M$_{2Na}$ + Na − 2NaHSO$_4$]$^+$, 897.4 [M$_{2Na}$ + Na − NaHSO$_4$ − C$_7$H$_{12}$O$_5$ (MeGlc) − C$_5$H$_8$O$_4$ (Xyl)]$^+$, 711.1 [M$_{2Na}$ + Na − C$_{32}$H$_{47}$O$_5$ (Agl) − SO$_3$Na]$^+$, 579.1 [M$_{2Na}$ + Na − C$_{32}$H$_{47}$O$_5$ (Agl) − C$_5$H$_7$O$_7$SNa (XylSO$_3$Na) − H]$^+$, 403.0 [M$_{2Na}$ + Na − C$_{32}$H$_{47}$O$_5$ (Agl) − SO$_3$Na − C$_7$H$_{12}$O$_5$ (MeGlc) − C$_5$H$_8$O$_4$ (Xyl)]$^+$, 331.1 [M$_{2Na}$ + Na − C$_{32}$H$_{47}$O$_5$ (Agl) − C$_5$H$_7$O$_7$SNa (XylSO$_3$Na) − C$_6$H$_9$O$_7$SNa (QuiSO$_3$Na) − H]$^+$.

3.3.5. Quadrangularisoside B$_2$ (5)

Colorless powder; $[\alpha]_D^{20}$ − 55 (c 0.1, 50% MeOH). NMR: See Tables 4 and 7. (−)HR-ESI-MS m/z: 1235.4243 (calc. 1235.4232) [M$_{2Na}$ − Na]$^-$, 606.2189 (calc. 606.2170) [M$_{2Na}$ − 2Na]$^{2-}$; (+)HR-ESI-MS m/z: 1281.4004 (calc. 1281.4016) [M$_{2Na}$ + Na]$^+$; (+)ESI-MS/MS m/z: 1179.4 [M$_{2Na}$ + Na − NaSO$_3$ + H]$^+$, 1059.5 [M$_{2Na}$ + Na − NaSO$_3$ − NaHSO$_4$ + H]$^+$, 711.1 [M$_{2Na}$ + Na − C$_{30}$H$_{43}$O$_4$ (Agl) − SO$_3$Na]$^+$, 579.1 [M$_{2Na}$ + Na − C$_{30}$H$_{43}$O$_4$ (Agl) − C$_5$H$_7$O$_7$SNa (XylSO$_3$Na) − H]$^+$, 403.0 [M$_{2Na}$ + Na − C$_{30}$H$_{43}$O$_4$ (Agl) − SO$_3$Na − C$_7$H$_{12}$O$_5$ (MeGlc) − C$_5$H$_8$O$_4$ (Xyl)]$^+$, 331.1 [M$_{2Na}$ + Na − C$_{30}$H$_{43}$O$_4$ (Agl) − C$_5$H$_7$O$_7$SNa (XylSO$_3$Na) − C$_6$H$_9$O$_7$SNa (QuiSO$_3$Na) − H]$^+$.

3.3.6. Quadrangularisoside C (6)

Colorless powder; $[\alpha]_D^{20}$ − 8 (c 0.1, 50% MeOH). NMR: See Tables 8 and 9. (−)HR-ESI-MS m/z: 1309.4608 (calc. 1309.4599) [M$_{2Na}$ − Na]$^-$, 643.2369 (calc. 643.2354) [M$_{2Na}$ − 2Na]$^{2-}$; (+)HR-ESI-MS m/z: 1355.4373 (calc. 1355.4384) [M$_{2Na}$ + Na]$^+$; (−)ESI-MS/MS m/z: 1249.4 [M$_{2Na}$ − Na − CH$_3$COOH]$^-$, 1189.5 [M$_{2Na}$ − Na − NaHSO$_4$]$^-$, 1129.5 [M$_{2Na}$ − Na − CH$_3$COOH − NaHSO$_4$]$^-$, 677.2 [M$_{2Na}$ − Na − NaHSO$_4$ − C$_{32}$H$_{47}$O$_5$ (Agl) − H]$^-$, 563.1 [M$_{2Na}$ − Na − NaHSO$_4$ − C$_{32}$H$_{47}$O$_5$ (Agl) − C$_5$H$_7$O$_3$ (Xyl)]$^-$, 417.1 [M$_{2Na}$ − Na − NaHSO$_4$ − C$_{32}$H$_{47}$O$_5$ (Agl) − C$_5$H$_7$O$_3$ (Xyl) − C$_6$H$_{10}$O$_4$ (Qui)]$^-$, 241.0 [M$_{2Na}$ − Na − NaHSO$_4$ − C$_{32}$H$_{47}$O$_5$ (Agl) − C$_5$H$_7$O$_3$ (Xyl) − C$_6$H$_{10}$O$_4$ (Qui) − C$_7$H$_{12}$O$_5$ (MeGlc)]$^-$.

3.3.7. Quadrangularisoside C$_1$ (7)

Colorless powder; $[\alpha]_D^{20}$ − 10 (c 0.1, 50% MeOH). NMR: See Tables 8 and 10. (−)HR-ESI-MS m/z: 1311.4763 (calc. 1311.4756) [M$_{2Na}$ − Na]$^-$, 644.2447 (calc. 644.2432) [M$_{2Na}$ − 2Na]$^{2-}$; (+)HR-ESI-MS m/z:

1357.4520 (calc. 1357.4540) [M$_{2Na}$ + Na]$^+$; (−)ESI-MS/MS m/z:797.1 [M$_{2Na}$ − Na − − C$_{32}$H$_{49}$O$_5$ (Agl) − H]$^-$, 677.2 [M$_{2Na}$ − Na − NaHSO$_4$ − C$_{32}$H$_{49}$O$_5$ (Agl) − H]$^-$, 563.1 [M$_{2Na}$ − Na − NaHSO$_4$ − C$_{32}$H$_{49}$O$_5$ (Agl) − C$_5$H$_7$O$_3$ (Xyl)]$^-$, 417.1 [M$_{2Na}$ − Na − NaHSO$_4$ − C$_{32}$H$_{49}$O$_5$ (Agl) − C$_5$H$_7$O$_3$ (Xyl) − C$_6$H$_{10}$O$_4$ (Qui)]$^-$, 241.0 [M$_{2Na}$ − Na − NaHSO$_4$ − C$_{32}$H$_{49}$O$_5$ (Agl) − C$_5$H$_7$O$_3$ (Xyl) − C$_6$H$_{10}$O$_4$ (Qui) − C$_7$H$_{12}$O$_5$ (MeGlc)]$^-$.

3.3.8. Quadrangularisoside D (8)

Colorless powder; [α]$_D^{20}$ − 23 (c 0.1, 50% MeOH). NMR: See Tables 5 and 11. (−)HR-ESI-MS m/z: 1381.3888 (calc. 1381.1881) [M$_{3Na}$ − Na]$^-$, 679.2012 (calc. 679.1995) [M$_{3Na}$ − 2Na]$^{2-}$, 445.1387 (calc. 445.1366) [M$_{3Na}$ − 3Na]$^{3-}$; (+)HR-ESI-MS m/z: 1427.3663 (calc. 1427.3666) [M$_{3Na}$ + Na]$^+$; (−)ESI-MS/MS m/z: 1261.4 [M$_{3Na}$ − Na − NaHSO$_4$]$^-$, 1103.4 [M$_{3Na}$ − Na − C$_7$H$_{11}$O$_8$SNa (MeGlcSO$_3$Na)]$^-$, 751.3 [M$_{3Na}$ − Na − NaHSO$_4$ − C$_{32}$H$_{47}$O$_5$ (Agl)+ H]$^-$, 533.1 [M$_{3Na}$ − Na − 2NaSO$_3$ − C$_{33}$H$_{47}$O$_5$ (Agl) − C$_5$H$_8$O$_4$ (Xyl) + H]$^-$, 387.1 [M$_{3Na}$ − Na − 2NaSO$_3$ − C$_{33}$H$_{47}$O$_5$ (Agl) − C$_5$H$_8$O$_4$ (Xyl) − C$_6$H$_{10}$O$_4$ (Qui) + H]$^-$, 255.0 [M$_{3Na}$ − Na − 2NaSO$_3$ − C$_{33}$H$_{47}$O$_5$ (Agl) − C$_5$H$_8$O$_4$ (Xyl) − C$_6$H$_{10}$O$_4$ (Qui) − C$_5$H$_8$O$_4$ (Xyl) + 2H]$^-$.

3.3.9. Quadrangularisoside D$_1$ (9)

Colorless powder; [α]$_D^{20}$ − 26 (c 0.1, 50% MeOH). NMR: See Tables 6 and 11. (−)HR-ESI-MS m/z: 1381.3891 (calc. 1381.3881) [M$_{3Na}$ − Na]$^-$, 679.2015 (calc. 679.1995) [M$_{3Na}$ − 2Na]$^{2-}$, 445.1390 (calc. 445.1366) [M$_{3Na}$ − 3Na]$^{3-}$; (+)HR-ESI-MS m/z: 1427.3653 (calc. 1427.3666) [M$_{3Na}$ + Na]$^+$; (−)ESI-MS/MS m/z: 1279.5 [M$_{3Na}$ − Na − NaSO$_3$ + H]$^-$, 1177.5 [M$_{3Na}$ − Na − 2NaSO$_3$ + 2H]$^-$, 1001.4 [M$_{3Na}$ − Na − 2NaSO$_3$ − C$_7$H$_{12}$O$_5$ (MeGlc) + 2H]$^-$, 941.4 [M$_{3Na}$ − Na − 2NaSO$_3$ − C$_7$H$_{12}$O$_5$ (MeGlc) − CH$_3$COO + H]$^-$, 751.3 [M$_{3Na}$ − Na − NaHSO$_4$ − C$_{32}$H$_{47}$O$_5$ (Agl)+ H]$^-$, 255.0 [M$_{3Na}$ − Na − 2NaSO$_3$ − C$_{33}$H$_{47}$O$_5$ (Agl) − C$_5$H$_8$O$_4$ (Xyl) − C$_6$H$_{10}$O$_4$ (Qui) − C$_5$H$_8$O$_4$ (Xyl) + 2H]$^-$; (+)ESI-MS/MS m/z: 1325.4 [M$_{3Na}$ + Na − NaSO$_3$ + H]$^+$, 1223.5 [M$_{3Na}$ + Na − 2NaSO$_3$ + 2H]$^+$ and 1121.5 [M$_{3Na}$ + Na − 3NaSO$_3$ + 3H]$^+$.

3.3.10. Quadrangularisoside D$_2$ (10)

Colorless powder; [α]$_D^{20}$ − 33 (c 0.1, 50% MeOH). NMR: See Tables 7 and 11. (−)HR-ESI-MS m/z: 1337.3625 (calc. 1337.3619) [M$_{3Na}$ −Na]$^-$, 657.1881 (calc. 657.1863) [M$_{3Na}$ − 2Na]$^{2-}$, 430.4633 (calc. 430.4612) [M$_{3Na}$ − 3Na]$^{3-}$; (+)HR-ESI-MS m/z: 1383.3390 (calc. 1383.3404) [M$_{3Na}$ + Na]$^+$; (−)ESI-MS/MS m/z: 1217.4 [M$_{3Na}$ − Na − NaHSO$_4$]$^-$, 1059.4 [M$_{3Na}$ − Na − C$_7$H$_{11}$O$_8$SNa (MeGlcSO$_3$Na)]$^-$, 939.4 [M$_{3Na}$ − Na − NaHSO$_4$ − C$_7$H$_{11}$O$_8$SNa (MeGlcSO$_3$Na)]$^-$, 533.1 [M$_{3Na}$ − Na − 2NaSO$_3$ − C$_{30}$H$_{43}$O$_4$ (Agl) − C$_5$H$_8$O$_4$ (Xyl) + H]$^-$, 387.1 [M$_{3Na}$ − Na − 2NaSO$_3$ − C$_{30}$H$_{43}$O$_4$ (Agl) − C$_5$H$_8$O$_4$ (Xyl) − C$_6$H$_{10}$O$_4$ (Qui) + H]$^-$, 255.0 [M$_{3Na}$ − Na − 2NaSO$_3$ − C$_{30}$H$_{43}$O$_4$ (Agl) − C$_5$H$_8$O$_4$ (Xyl) − C$_6$H$_{10}$O$_4$ (Qui) − C$_5$H$_8$O$_4$ (Xyl) + 2H]$^-$; (+)ESI-MS/MS m/z: 1264.4 [M$_{3Na}$ + Na − NaSO$_4$]$^+$, 1143.4 [M$_{3Na}$ + Na − 2NaSO$_4$]$^+$.

3.3.11. Quadrangularisoside D$_3$ (11)

Colorless powder; [α]$_D^{20}$ − 19 (c 0.1, 50% MeOH). NMR: See Tables 2 and 11. (−)HR-ESI-MS m/z: 1413.3785 (calc. 1413.3780) [M$_{3Na}$ − Na]$^-$, 695.1963 (calc. 695.1944) [M$_{3Na}$ − 2Na]$^{2-}$, 455.8006 (calc. 455.7998) [M$_{3Na}$ − 3Na]$^{3-}$; (+)HR-ESI-MS m/z: 1459.3534 (calc. 1459.3564) [M$_{3Na}$ + Na]$^+$; (−)ESI-MS/MS m/z: 1261.4 [M$_{Na}$ − Na − OOH − NaSO$_4$]$^-$, 1103.3 [M$_{Na}$ − Na − OOH − C$_7$H$_{11}$O$_8$SNa (MeGlcSO$_3$Na) + H]$^-$, 723.3 [M$_{3Na}$ − Na − OOH − C$_7$H$_{11}$O$_8$SNa (MeGlcSO$_3$Na) − C$_5$H$_8$O$_4$ (Xyl) − C$_6$H$_9$O$_7$SNa (QuiSO$_3$Na) + H]$^-$, 751.3 [M$_{3Na}$ − Na − NaHSO$_4$ − C$_{32}$H$_{47}$O$_6$ (Agl)+ H]$^-$, 387.1 [M$_{3Na}$ − Na − 2NaSO$_3$ − C$_{32}$H$_{47}$O$_6$ (Agl) − C$_5$H$_8$O$_4$ (Xyl) − C$_6$H$_{10}$O$_4$ (Qui) + H]$^-$, 255.0 [M$_{3Na}$ − Na − 2NaSO$_3$ − C$_{32}$H$_{47}$O$_6$ (Agl) − C$_5$H$_8$O$_4$ (Xyl) − C$_6$H$_{10}$O$_4$ (Qui) − C$_5$H$_8$O$_4$ (Xyl) + H]$^-$.

3.3.12. Quadrangularisoside D$_4$ (12)

Colorless powder; $[\alpha]_D^{20}$ − 25 (c 0.1, 50% MeOH). NMR: See Tables 3 and 11. (−)-HR-ESI-MS m/z: 1413.3762 (calc. 1413.3780) [M$_{3Na}$ − Na]$^-$, 695.1954 (calc. 695.1944) [M$_{3Na}$ − 2Na]$^{2-}$, 455.8011 (calc. 455.7998) [M$_{3Na}$ − 3Na]$^{3-}$; (+)-HR-ESI-MS m/z: 1459.3512 (calc. 1459.3564)[M$_{3Na}$ + Na]$^+$; (−)-ESI-MS/MS m/z: 999.4 [M$_{Na}$ − Na − OOH − NaSO$_3$ − C$_7$H$_{11}$O$_8$SNa (MeGlcSO$_3$Na)]$^-$, 867.4 [M$_{Na}$ − Na − OOH − NaSO$_3$ − C$_7$H$_{11}$O$_8$SNa (MeGlcSO$_3$Na) − C$_5$H$_8$O$_4$ (Xyl)]$^-$, 255.0 [M$_{3Na}$ − Na − 2NaSO$_3$ − C$_{32}$H$_{47}$O$_6$ (Agl) − C$_5$H$_8$O$_4$ (Xyl) − C$_6$H$_{10}$O$_4$ (Qui) − C$_5$H$_8$O$_4$ (Xyl) + H]$^-$.

3.3.13. Quadrangularisoside E (13)

Colorless powder; $[\alpha]_D^{20}$ − 38 (c 0.1, 50% MeOH). NMR: See Tables 7 and 12. (−)-HR-ESI-MS m/z: 1367.3739 (calc. 1367.3725) [M$_{3Na}$ − Na]$^-$, 672.1941 (calc. 672.1916) [M$_{3Na}$ − 2Na]$^{2-}$, 440.4674 (calc. 440.4647) [M$_{3Na}$ − 3Na]$^{3-}$; (+)-HR-ESI-MS m/z: 1413.3488 (calc. 1413.3509) [M$_{3Na}$ + Na]$^+$; (−)-ESI-MS/MS m/z: 1247.4 [M$_{Na}$ − Na − NaHSO$_4$]$^-$, 1089.4 [M$_{Na}$ − Na − C$_7$H$_{11}$O$_8$SNa (MeGlcSO$_3$Na)]$^-$, 969.4 [M$_{3Na}$ − Na − NaHSO$_4$ − C$_7$H$_{11}$O$_8$SNa (MeGlcSO$_3$Na)]$^-$, 825.4 [M$_{3Na}$ − Na − C$_7$H$_{11}$O$_8$SNa (MeGlcSO$_3$Na) − C$_6$H$_{10}$O$_8$SNa (GlcSO$_3$Na) + H]$^-$, 255.0 [M$_{3Na}$ − Na − C$_{30}$H$_{43}$O$_4$ (Agl) − C$_5$H$_7$O$_7$SNa (XylSO$_3$Na) − C$_6$H$_{10}$O$_4$ (Qui) − C$_6$H$_9$O$_8$SNa (GlcSO$_3$Na) − H]$^-$; (+)-ESI-MS/MS m/z: 963.5 [M$_{3Na}$ + Na − C$_{30}$H$_{43}$O$_3$ (Agl) + H]$^+$, 685.4 [M$_{3Na}$ + Na − C$_{30}$H$_{43}$O$_3$ (Agl) − C$_7$H$_{11}$O$_8$SNa (MeGlcSO$_3$Na) + H]$^+$.

3.4. Cytotoxic Activity (MTT Assay)

All compounds were tested in concentrations from 1.5 µM to 100 µM using two-fold dilution in dH$_2$O. The solutions (20 µL) of tested substances in different concentrations and cell suspension (180 µL) were added in wells of 96-well plates (1 × 10^4 cells/well) and incubated 24 h at 37 °C and 5% CO$_2$. After incubation, the medium with tested substances was replaced by 100 µL of fresh medium. Then, 10 µL of MTT (thiazoyl blue tertrazolium bromide) stock solution (5 mg/mL) was added to each well, and the microplate was incubated for 4 h. After that, 100 µL of SDS-HCl solution (1 g SDS/10 mL dH$_2$O/17 µL 6 N HCl) was added to each well followed by incubation for 4–18 h. The absorbance of the converted dye formazan was measured using a Multiskan FC microplate photometer (Thermo Scientific, Waltham, MA, USA) at a wavelength of 570 nm. The cytotoxic activity of the substances was calculated as the concentration that caused 50% metabolic cell activity inhibition (IC$_{50}$). All the experiments were made in triplicate, $p < 0.05$.

3.5. Cytotoxic Activity (MTS Assay)

HT-29 cells (1.0 × 10^4/200 µL) were seeded in 96-well plates for 24 h at 37 °C in a 5% CO$_2$ incubator. The cells were treated with compounds **1–13** at concentrations ranging from 0 to 20 µM for an additional 24 h. Subsequently, cells were incubated with 15 µL MTS reagent for 3 h, and the absorbance in each well was measured at 490/630 nm using a microplate reader "Power Wave XS" (Bio Tek, Winooski, VT, USA). All the experiments were repeated three times, and the mean absorbance values were calculated. The results are expressed as the percentage of inhibition that produced a reduction in absorbance by the compound's treatment compared to the non-treated cells (control). All the experiments were made in triplicate, $p < 0.01$.

3.6. Hemolytic Activity

Blood was taken from CD-1 mice (18–20 g). Erythrocytes were isolated from the blood of albino CD-1 mice by centrifugation with phosphate-buffered saline (pH 7.4) during 5 minutes at 4 °C by 450 g on a centrifuge LABOFUGE 400R (Heraeus, Germany) for three times. Then, the residue of erythrocytes was resuspended in ice cold phosphate saline buffer (pH 7.4) to a final optical density of 1.5 at 700 nm and kept on ice [39]. For the hemolytic assay, 180 µL of erythrocyte suspension was mixed with 20 µL of test compound solution in V-bottom 96-well plates. After 1 h of incubation at 37 °C, plates were exposed to centrifugation 10 min at 900 g on a laboratory centrifuge LMC-3000 (Biosan,

Riga, Latvia) [40]. Then, we carefully separated 100 µL of supernatant and transferred it onto new flat plates, respectively. The lysis of erythrocytes was determined by measuring of the concentration of hemoglobin in the supernatant with a microplate photometer Multiskan FC (Themo Scientific, USA), $\lambda = 570$ nm [41]. The effective dose causing 50% hemolysis of erythrocytes (ED_{50}) was calculated using the computer program SigmaPlot 10.0. All the experiments were made in triplicate, $p < 0.05$.

3.7. Soft Agar Assay

HT-29 cells (2.4×10^4/mL) were seeded into 6-well plates and treated with compounds **1–13** at a concentrations range 0–20 µM in 1 mL of 0.3% Basal Medium Eagle (BME) agar containing 10% FBS, 2 mM L-glutamine, and 25 µg/mL gentamicin. The cultures were maintained at 37 °C in a 5% CO_2 incubator for 14 days, and the cell's colonies were scored using a microscope "Motic AE 20" (Scientific Instrument Company, Campbell, CA, USA) and the Motic Image Plus (Scientific Instrument Company, Campbell, CA, USA) computer program.

3.8. Radiation Exposure

Irradiation was delivered at room temperature using 1 Gy of the X-ray system XPERT 80 (KUB Technologies, Inc., Milford, CT, USA). The absorber dose was measured using an X-ray radiation clinical dosimeter DRK-1 (Akselbant, Moscow, Russia).

3.9. Cell Irradiation

HT-29 cells (5.0×10^5/5 mL) were plated at 60 mm dishes and incubated for 24 h. After the incubation, the cells were cultured in the presence or absence of 0.02 µM of compounds **1–13** for an additional 24 h before irradiation at the dose of 1 Gy. Immediately after irradiation, the cells were returned to the incubator for recovery. Three hours later, cells were harvested and used for soft agar assay to establish the synergism between irradiation and the investigated compounds.

4. Conclusions

It is interesting to note that the aglycones having both 7(8)- and 9(11)-double bonds are present in the glycosidic sum of *C. quadrangularis* whenever the majority of sea cucumber species usually biosynthesize the aglycones with the certain position of double bond in the triterpene nucleus. Only six species of the holothurians besides *C. quadrangularis* are known so far to produce simultaneously the aglycones with different positions of double bonds in the nuclei: *Cucumaria frondosa* [42], *Australostichopus mollis* [43], and *Colochirus robustus* [20]—the aglycones with 7(8)- and 9(11)-double bonds; *Synapta maculata*—the aglycones with 7(8)- and 8(9)-double bonds [44]; and *Psolus fabricii* and *Cucumaria fallax*—the aglycones with 7(8)-, 8(9)-, and 9(11)-double bonds [37,45].

This peculiarity is interesting from the viewpoint of the biosynthesis of triterpene precursors of these aglycones. The species of sea cucumbers selectively biosynthesizing the aglycones with a certain position of the intra-nucleus double bond and the other species that can produce the aglycones having different positions of the double bond probably have diversely functioning oxydosqualene cyclases—the enzymes cyclizing 2,3-oxidosqualene to different triterpene alcohols—precursors of the aglycones. The reasons for such differences between the organisms and the producers of the glycosides are still unclear and have to be studied.

Triterpene glycosides of the sea cucumbers are metabolites that are formed by the mosaic type of biosynthesis [30,37], i.e., the aglycones and carbohydrate moieties are biosynthesized simultaneously and independently from each other. One of the results of such biosynthesis is the appearance of the glycosides having sugar chains identical to each other but structurally diverse aglycones. Such glycosides are usually attributed to one group. The glycosidic composition of *C. quadrangularis* is not an exception, since the glycosides of five groups have been isolated: the quadrangularisosides of group A (with a tetrasaccharide monosulfated chain), group B (with tetrasaccharide disulfated chain having the second sulfate group at C(3)Qui2), group C (with a tetrasaccharide disulfated chain having the sulfated by C(6) glucose residue as the third unit), group D (with a tetrasaccharide trisulfated chain having the sulfate groups at C(4)Xyl1, C(3)Qui2, and C(4)MeGlc4) and finally group E (with a tetrasaccharide trisulfated chain having the sulfate groups at C(4)Xyl1, C(6)Glc3, and C(4)MeGlc4). The majority of known compounds found in C. quadrangularis have carbohydrate chains identical to that of the quadrangularisoside of group A. Among them are colochirosides B_1–B_3 [20], lefevreosides A_2 and C [21], neothyonidioside [22], and philinopside A [12]. The biogenetic relationships between the groups of these glycosides are obvious (Figure 3): the carbohydrate chain of quadrangularisosides of group A is a biosynthetic precursor of the di- and trisulfated carbohydrate chains of groups B and D. The carbohydrate chain of the quadrangularisosides of group C is a biosynthetic precursor of the sugar chain of quadrangularisoside E.

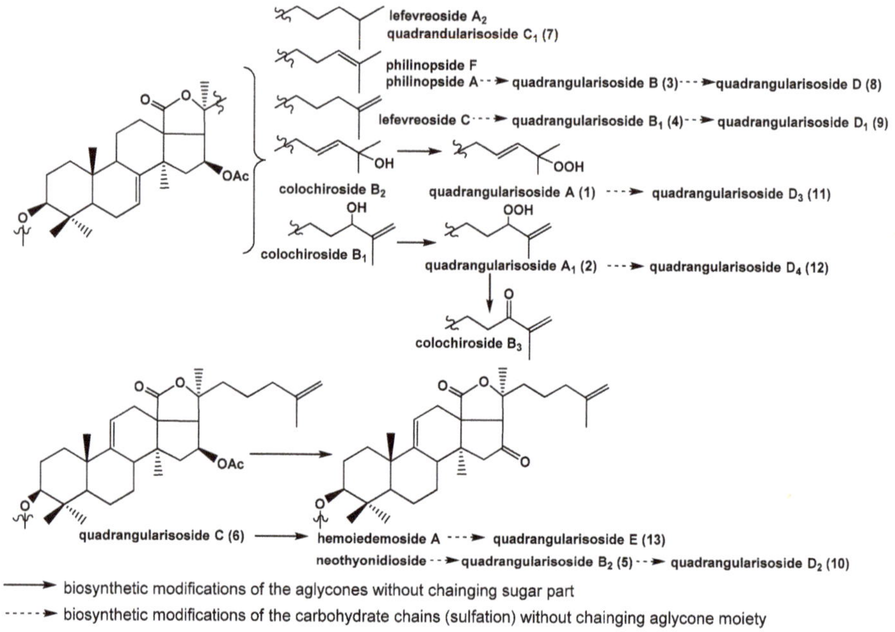

Figure 3. The biosynthetic network of triterpene glycosides from C. quadrangularis.

The mosaicism of the biosynthetic network of the glycosides is also illustrated by the biogenetic relationships of the aglycone parts of their molecules (Figure 3). Thus, the same aglycones can be glycosylated by different carbohydrate moieties as in quadrangularisosides A (**1**) and D_3 (**11**); A_1 (**2**) and D_4 (**12**); philinopside A [12], quadrangularisosides B (**3**) and D (**8**); lefevreoside C [21], quadrangularisosides B_1 (**4**) and D_1 (**9**); neothyonidioside [22], quadrangularisosides B_2 (**5**), D_2 (**10**), and E (**14**). It is peculiar that only quadrangularisoside C (**6**) has the aglycone that is not represented in the other groups of quadrangularisosides.

It is known that sea cucumber triterpene glycosides are taxonomically specific and can be used as chemotaxonomic markers for different systematic groups of holothuroids [7–10]. Since the systematic position of the species under investigation was revised more than once and it was classified earlier as representative of the genus Pentacta, it seems to be important to analyze the glycosides isolated from C. quadrangularis from the viewpoint of chemotaxonomy. Chemically studied species of the sea cucumbers systematically related to C. quadrangularis are Colochirus robustus (=Pentacta robustus) and Pseudocolochirus violaceus (=Colochirus violaceus). It is also interesting to compare the glycosides of C. quadrangularis with those isolated from Plesiocolochirus australis (=Pentacta australis, =Colochirus australis).

Colochirosides B$_1$–B$_3$ isolated initially from *Colochirus robustus* [20] were identified in the glycosidic fraction of *C. quadrangularis*. Another four glycosides common to these species of sea cucumbers are hemoiedemoside A [20,23], philinopside F (=violaceuside B) [13,20,46], lefevreoside F [20,21], and neothyonidioside [20,22]. All these data indicate the systematic closeness of *Colochirus robustus* and *Colochirus quadrangularis*, which share seven identical compounds having holostane aglycones and tetrasaccharide chains and the reasonableness of their assignment to one genus.

Philinopside F found earlier in *C. quadrangularis* [13] was also identified in *Pseudocolochirus violaceus* but was discussed as a new glycoside named violaceuside B [46]. This compound was also identified by us in the glycosidic sum of *C. quadrangularis*. These species of sea cucumbers also have glycosides that are common for both of them such as philinopsides A, E, and F [12,13,46] and lefevreoside C [21,30]. This indicates that *Pseudocolochirus violaceus* and *C. quadrangularis* are systematically close species.

On the other hand, the glycosides from *Plesiocolochirus australis* (=*Pentacta australis*) [47] were significantly different from those from *C. quadrangularis* both by the aglycones structures (non-holostane aglycones of ds-penaustrosides A and B) and by the carbohydrate chains structures (pentasaccharide branched chains in ds-penaustrosides A–D [47]). So, the exclusion of *C. quadrangularis* from the genus *Pentacta* seems accurate.

Supplementary Materials: The following are available online at http://www.mdpi.com/1660-3397/18/8/394/s1, Figure S1:The 13C NMR (176.03 MHz) spectrum of quadrangularisoside A (1) in C5D5N/D2O (4/1), Figure S2: The 1H NMR (700.00 MHz) spectrum of quadrangularisoside A (1) in C5D5N/D2O (4/1), Figure S3: The COSY (700.00 MHz) spectrum of quadrangularisoside A (1) in C5D5N/D2O (4/1), Figure S4: The HSQC (700.00 MHz) spectrum of quadrangularisoside A (1) in C5D5N/D2O (4/1), Figure S5: The HMBC (700.00 MHz) spectrum of quadrangularisoside A (1) in C5D5N/D2O (4/1), Figure S6: The ROESY (700.00 MHz) spectrum of quadrangularisoside A (1) in C5D5N/D2O (4/1), Figure S7: 1 D TOCSY (700.00 MHz) spectra of quadrangularisoside A (1) in C5D5N/D2O (4/1), Figure S8: 1 D TOCSY (700.00 MHz) spectra of quadrangularisoside A (1) in C5D5N/D2O (4/1), Figure S9: The 13C NMR (176.03 MHz) spectrum of quadrangularisoside A1 (2) in C5D5N/D2O (4/1), Figure S10: The 1H NMR (700.00 MHz) spectrum of quadrangularisoside A1 (2) in C5D5N/D2O (4/1), Figure S11: The COSY (700.00 MHz) spectrum of quadrangularisoside A1 (2) in C5D5N/D2O (4/1), Figure S12: The HSQC (700.00 MHz) spectrum of quadrangularisoside A1 (2) in C5D5N/D2O (4/1), Figure S13: The ROESY (700.00 MHz) spectrum of quadrangularisoside A1 (2) in C5D5N/D2O (4/1), Figure S14. The HMBC (700.00 MHz) spectrum of quadrangularisoside A1 (2) in C5D5N/D2O (4/1), Figure S15: The 13C NMR (176.03 MHz) spectrum of quadrangularisoside B (3) in C5D5N/D2O (4/1), Figure S16: The 1H NMR (700.00 MHz) spectrum of quadrangularisoside B (3) in C5D5N/D2O (4/1), Figure S17: The COSY (700.00 MHz) spectrum of quadrangularisoside B (3) in C5D5N/D2O (4/1), Figure S18: The HSQC (700.00 MHz) spectrum of quadrangularisoside B (3) in C5D5N/D2O (4/1), Figure S19: The HMBC (700.00 MHz) spectrum of quadrangularisoside B (3) in C5D5N/D2O (4/1), Figure S20: The ROESY (700.00 MHz) spectrum of quadrangularisoside B (3) in C5D5N/D2O (4/1), Figure S21: 1D TOCSY (700.00 MHz) spectra of quadrangularisoside B (3) in C5D5N/D2O (4/1), Figure S22: 1D TOCSY (700.00 MHz) spectra of quadrangularisoside B (3) in C5D5N/D2O (4/1), Figure S23: The 13C NMR (176.03 MHz) spectrum of quadrangularisoside B1 (4) in C5D5N/D2O (4/1), Figure S24: The 1H NMR (700.00 MHz) spectrum of quadrangularisoside B1 (4) in C5D5N/D2O (4/1), Figure S25: HR-ESI-MS and ESI-MS/MS spectra of quadrangularisoside B1 (4), Figure S26: The 13C NMR (176.03 MHz) spectrum of quadrangularisoside B2 (5) in C5D5N/D2O (4/1), Figure S27: The 1H NMR (700.00 MHz) spectrum of quadrangularisoside B2 (5) in C5D5N/D2O (4/1), Figure S28: The COSY (700.00 MHz) spectrum of quadrangularisoside B2 (5) in C5D5N/D2O (4/1), Figure S29: The HSQC (700.00 MHz) spectrum of quadrangularisoside B2 (5) in C5D5N/D2O (4/1), Figure S30: The ROESY (700.00 MHz) spectrum of quadrangularisoside B2 (5) in C5D5N/D2O (4/1), Figure S31: The HMBC (700.00 MHz) spectrum of quadrangularisoside B2 (5) in C5D5N/D2O (4/1), Figure S32: The 13C NMR (176.03 MHz) spectrum of quadrangularisoside C (6) in C5D5N/D2O (4/1), Figure S33: The 1H NMR (700.00 MHz) spectrum of quadrangularisoside C (6) in C5D5N/D2O (4/1), Figure S34: The COSY (700.00 MHz) spectrum of quadrangularisoside C (6) in C5D5N/D2O (4/1), Figure S35: The HSQC (700.00 MHz) spectrum of quadrangularisoside C (6) in C5D5N/D2O (4/1), Figure S36: The HMBC (700.00 MHz) spectrum of quadrangularisoside C (6) in C5D5N/D2O (4/1), Figure S37: The ROESY (700.00 MHz) spectrum of quadrangularisoside C (6) in C5D5N/D2O (4/1), Figure S38: 1D TOCSY (700.00 MHz) spectra of quadrangularisoside C (6) in C5D5N/D2O (4/1), Figure S39: 1D TOCSY (700.00 MHz) spectra of quadrangularisoside C (6) in C5D5N/D2O (4/1), Figure S40: HR-ESI-MS and ESI-MS/MS spectra of quadrangularisoside C (6), Figure S41: The 13C NMR (176.03 MHz) spectrum of quadrangularisoside C1 (7) in C5D5N/D2O (4/1), Figure S42: The 1H NMR (700.00 MHz) spectrum of quadrangularisoside C1 (7) in C5D5N/D2O (4/1), Figure S43: The COSY (700.00 MHz) spectrum of the aglycone part of quadrangularisoside C1 (7) in C5D5N/D2O (4/1), Figure S44: The HSQC (700.00 MHz) spectrum of the aglycone part of quadrangularisoside C1 (7) in C5D5N/D2O (4/1), Figure S45: The ROESY (700.00 MHz) spectrum of the aglycone part of quadrangularisoside C1 (7) in C5D5N/D2O (4/1), Figure S46: HR-ESI-MS and ESI-MS/MS spectra of quadrangularisoside C1 (7), Figure S47: The 13C NMR (176.03 MHz) spectrum of quadrangularisoside D (8) in C5D5N/D2O (4/1), Figure S48: The 1H

NMR (700.00 MHz) spectrum of quadrangularisoside D (8) in C5D5N/D2O (4/1), Figure S49: The COSY (700.00 MHz) spectrum of quadrangularisoside D (8) in C5D5N/D2O (4/1), Figure S50: The HSQC (700.00 MHz) spectrum of quadrangularisoside D (8) in C5D5N/D2O (4/1), Figure S51: The HMBC (700.00 MHz) spectrum of quadrangularisoside D (8) in C5D5N/D2O (4/1), Figure S52: The ROESY (700.00 MHz) spectrum of quadrangularisoside D (8) in C5D5N/D2O (4/1), Figure S53: 1D TOCSY (700.00 MHz) spectra of quadrangularisoside D (8) in C5D5N/D2O (4/1), Figure S54: 1D TOCSY (700.00 MHz) spectra of quadrangularisoside D (8) in C5D5N/D2O (4/1), Figure S55: The 13C NMR (176.03 MHz) spectrum of quadrangularisoside D1 (9) in C5D5N/D2O (4/1), Figure S56: The 1H NMR (700.00 MHz) spectrum of quadrangularisoside D1 (9) in C5D5N/D2O (4/1), Figure S57: HR-ESI-MS and ESI-MS/MS spectra of quadrangularisoside D1 (9), Figure S58: The 13C NMR (176.03 MHz) spectrum of quadrangularisoside D2 (10) in C5D5N/D2O (4/1), Figure S59: The 1H NMR (700.00 MHz) spectrum of quadrangularisoside D2 (10) in C5D5N/D2O (4/1), Figure S60: HR-ESI-MS and ESI-MS/MS spectra of quadrangularisoside D2 (10), Figure S61: The 13C NMR (176.03 MHz) spectrum of quadrangularisoside D3 (11) in C5D5N/D2O (4/1), Figure S62: The 1H NMR (700.00 MHz) spectrum of quadrangularisoside D3 (11) in C5D5N/D2O (4/1), Figure S63. HR-ESI-MS and ESI-MS/MS spectra of quadrangularisoside D3 (11), Figure S64: The 13C NMR (176.03 MHz) spectrum of quadrangularisoside D4 (12) in C5D5N/D2O (4/1), Figure S65: The 1H NMR (700.00 MHz) spectrum of quadrangularisoside D4 (12) in C5D5N/D2O (4/1), Figure S66: HR-ESI-MS and ESI-MS/MS spectra of quadrangularisoside D4 (12), Figure S67: The 13C NMR (176.03 MHz) spectrum of quadrangularisoside E (13) in C5D5N/D2O (4/1), Figure S68: The 1H NMR (700.00 MHz) spectrum of quadrangularisoside E (13) in C5D5N/D2O (4/1), Figure S69: The COSY (700.00 MHz) spectrum of quadrangularisoside E (13) in C5D5N/D2O (4/1), Figure S70. The HSQC (700.00 MHz) spectrum of quadrangularisoside E (13) in C5D5N/D2O (4/1), Figure S71. The HMBC (700.00 MHz) spectrum of uadrangularisoside E (13) in C5D5N/D2O (4/1), Figure S72: The ROESY (700.00 MHz) spectrum of quadrangularisoside E (13) in C5D5N/D2O (4/1), Figure S73: 1D TOCSY (700.00 MHz) spectra of quadrangularisoside E (13) in C5D5N/D2O (4/1), Figure S74: 1D TOCSY (700.00 MHz) spectra of quadrangularisoside E (14) in C5D5N/D2O (4/1).

Author Contributions: Conceptualization, A.S.S., V.I.K.; methodology, A.S.S., S.A.A., S.P.E., P.S.D.; investigation, A.S.S., A.I.K., S.A.A., R.S.P., E.A.C., P.V.A., S.P.E., O.S.M., S.S.D.; writing—original draft preparation, A.S.S., V.I.K.; writing—review and editing, A.S.S., V.I.K. All authors have read and agreed to the published version of the manuscript.

Funding: This research was partially funded by the Grant of the Russian Foundation for Basic Research No. 19-04-000-14 and by the Grant of the Russian Science Foundation No. 16-14-10131. The APC was funded by the MDPI as full discount for invited articles for the SI "Echinoderms Metabolites: Structure, Function and Biomedical Perspectives".

Acknowledgments: The chemical structure and part of the bioassay were carried out with the partial financial support of the Grant of the Russian Foundation for Basic Research No. 19-04-000-14 for partial financial support. The studies of cytotoxic activities on a series of human cancer cell lines and its synergy with radioactive irradiation were supported by the Grant of the Russian Science Foundation No. 16-14-10131. The study was carried out on the equipment of the Collective Facilities Center "The Far Eastern Center for Structural Molecular Research (NMR/MS) PIBOC FEB RAS". The authors are very appreciative to Professor Valentin A. Stonik (G.B. Elyakov Pacific Institute of Bioorganic Chemistry) for reading and discussion of the manuscript.

Conflicts of Interest: The authors declare no conflict of interest.

References

1. Stonik, V.A.; Kalinin, V.I.; Avilov, S.A. Toxins from sea cucumbers (holothuroids): Chemical structures, properties, taxonomic distribution, biosynthesis and evolution. *J. Nat. Toxins* **1999**, *8*, 235–248.
2. Mondol, M.A.M.; Shin, H.J.; Rahman, M.A. Sea cucumber glycosides: Chemical structures, producing species and important biological properties. *Mar. Drugs* **2017**, *15*, 317. [CrossRef]
3. Kalinin, V.I.; Silchenko, A.S.; Avilov, S.A.; Stonik, V.A. Non-holostane aglycones of sea cucumber triterpene glycosides. Structure, biosynthesis, evolution. *Steroids* **2019**, *147*, 42–51. [CrossRef] [PubMed]
4. Claereboudt, E.J.S.; Gualier, G.; Decroo, C.; Colson, E.; Gerbaux, P.; Claereboudt, M.R.; Schaller, H.; Flammang, P.; Deleu, M.; Eeckhaut, I. Triterpenoids in echinoderms: Fundamental differences in diversity and biosynthetic pathways. *Mar. Drugs* **2019**, *17*, 352. [CrossRef] [PubMed]
5. Kalinin, V.I.; Aminin, D.L.; Avilov, S.A.; Silchenko, A.S.; Stonik, V.A. Triterpene glycosides from sea cucumbers (Holothurioidea, Echinodermata). Biological activities and functions. In *Studies in Natural Product Chemistry (Bioactive Natural Products)*; Atta-ur-Rahman, Ed.; Elsevier Science Publisher: Amsterdam, The Netherlands, 2008; Volume 35, pp. 135–196.
6. Aminin, D.L.; Menchinskaya, E.S.; Pisliagin, E.A.; Silchenko, A.S.; Avilov, S.A.; Kalinin, V.I. Sea cucumber triterpene glycosides as anticancer agents. In *Studies in Natural Product Chemistry*; Atta-ur-Rahman, Ed.; Elsevier B.V.: Amsterdam, The Netherlands, 2016; Volume 49, pp. 55–105.

7. Avilov, S.A.; Kalinin, V.I.; Smirnov, A.V. Use of triterpene glycosides for resolving taxonomic problems in the sea cucumber genus *Cucumaria* (Holothorioidea, Echinodermata). *Biochem. Syst. Ecol.* **2004**, *32*, 715–733. [CrossRef]
8. Honey-Escandon, M.; Arreguin-Espinosa, R.; Solis-Martin, F.A.; Samyn, Y. Biological and taxonomic perspective of triterpenoid glycosides of sea cucumbers of the family Holothuriidae (Echinodermata, Holothuroidea). *Comp. Biochem. Physiol.* **2015**, *180B*, 16–39. [CrossRef] [PubMed]
9. Kalinin, V.I.; Avilov, S.A.; Silchenko, A.S.; Stonik, V.A. Triterpene glycosides of sea cucumbers (Holothuroidea, Echinodermata) as taxonomic markers. *Nat. Prod. Commun.* **2015**, *10*, 21–26. [CrossRef] [PubMed]
10. Kalinin, V.I.; Silchenko, A.S.; Avilov, S.A. Taxonomic significance and ecological role of triterpene glycosides from holothurians. *Biol. Bull.* **2016**, *43*, 532–540. [CrossRef]
11. Zhang, S.-L.; Li, L.; Yi, Y.-H.; Zou, Z.R.; Sun, P. Philinopgenin A, B and C, three new triterpenoid aglycones from the sea cucumber *Pentacta quadrangulasis*. *Mar. Drugs* **2004**, *2*, 185–191. [CrossRef]
12. Yi, Y.-H.; Xu, Q.-Z.; Li, L.; Zhang, S.-L.; Wu, H.-M.; Ding, J.; Tong, Y.G.; Tan, W.-F.; Li, M.-H.; Tian, F.; et al. Philinopsides A and B, two new sulfated triterpene glycosides from the sea cucumber *Pentacta quadrangularis*. *Helv. Chim. Acta* **2006**, *89*, 54–63. [CrossRef]
13. Zhang, S.-L.; Li, L.; Yi, Y.-H.; Sun, P. Philinopsides E and F, two new sulfated triterpene glycosides from the sea cucumber *Pentacta quadrangularis*. *Nat. Prod. Res.* **2006**, *20*, 399–407. [CrossRef]
14. Han, H.; Xa, Q.-Z.; Yi, Y.-H.; Gong, W.; Jiao, B.-H. Two new cytotoxic disulfated holostane glycosides from the sea cucumber *Pentacta quadrangularis*. *Chem. Biodivers.* **2010**, *7*, 158–167. [CrossRef] [PubMed]
15. Han, H.; Xu, Q.-Z.; Tang, H.-F.; Yi, Y.-H.; Gong, W. Cytotoxic holostane type glycosides from the sea cucumber *Pentacta quadrangularis*. *Planta Med.* **2010**, *76*, 1900–1904. [CrossRef] [PubMed]
16. Kalinin, V.I.; Kalinovskii, A.I.; Stonik, V.A. Onekotanogenin—A new triterpene genin from the sea cucumber *Psolus fabricii*. *Chem. Nat. Compd.* **1987**, *23*, 560–563. [CrossRef]
17. Kalinovsky, A.I.; Silchenko, A.S.; Avilov, S.A.; Kalinin, V.I. The assignment of the absolute configuration of C-22 chiral center in the aglycones of triterpene glycosides from the sea cucumber *Cladolabes schmeltzii* and chemical transformations of cladoloside C. *Nat. Prod. Commun.* **2015**, *10*, 1167–1170. [CrossRef] [PubMed]
18. Silchenko, A.S.; Kalinovsky, A.I.; Avilov, S.A.; Kalinin, V.I.; Andrijaschenko, P.V.; Dmitrenok, P.S.; Chingizova, E.A.; Ermakova, S.P.; Malyarenko, O.S.; Dautova, T.N. Nine new triterpene glycosides, magnumosides A_1–A_4, B_2, C_1, C_2 and C_4, from the Vietnamese sea cucumber *Neothyonidium* (=*Massinum*) *magnum*: Structures and avtivities against tumor cells independently and in synergy with radioactive irradiation. *Mar. Drugs* **2017**, *15*, 256. [CrossRef] [PubMed]
19. Kitagawa, I.; Nishino, T.; Matsuno, T.; Akutsu, H.; Kyogoku, Y. Structure of holothurin B a pharmacologically active triterpene-oligoglycoside from the sea cucumber *Holothuria leucospilota* Brandt. *Tetrahedron Lett.* **1978**, *11*, 985–988. [CrossRef]
20. Silchenko, A.S.; Kalinovsky, A.I.; Avilov, S.A.; Andryjaschenko, P.V.; Dmitrenok, P.S.; Kalinin, V.I.; Yurchenko, E.V.; Dolmatov, I.Y. Colochirosides B_1, B_2, B_3 and C, novel sulfated triterpene glycosides from the sea cucumber *Colochirus robustus* (Cucumariidae, Dendrochirotida). *Nat. Prod. Commun.* **2015**, *10*, 1687–1694. [CrossRef]
21. Rodriguez, J.; Riguera, R. Lefevreosides: Four novel triterpenoid glycosides from the sea cucumber *Cucumaria lefevrei*. *Chem. Inform.* **1989**, *21*, 2620–2636.
22. Zurita, M.B.; Ahond, A.; Poupat, C.; Potier, P. Invertebresmarins du lagon Neo-Caledonien, VII. Etude structurale d'un nouveau saponoside sulfate extrait de l'holothurie *Neothyonidium magnum*. *J. Nat. Prod.* **1986**, *49*, 809–813. [CrossRef]
23. Chludil, H.D.; Muniain, C.C.; Seldes, A.M.; Maier, M.S. Cytotoxic and antifungal triterpene glycosides from the Patagonian sea cucumber *Hemoidema spectabilis*. *J. Nat. Prod.* **2002**, *65*, 860–865. [CrossRef]
24. Silchenko, A.S.; Avilov, S.A.; Kalinovsky, A.I.; Kalinin, V.I.; Andrijaschenko, P.V.; Dmitrenok, P.S.; Popov, R.S.; Chingizova, E.A.; Kasakin, M.F. Psolusosides C_3 and D_2–D_5, five novel triterpene hexaosides from the sea cucumber *Psolusfabricii* (Psolidae, Dendrochirotida): Chemical structures and bioactivities. *Nat. Prod. Commun.* **2019**, *14*, 1–12. [CrossRef]
25. Hoanga, L.; Vien, L.T.; Hanh, T.T.H.; Thanh, N.V.; Cuonga, N.X.; Nam, N.H.; Thung, D.C.; Ivanchina, N.V.; Thao, D.T.; Dmitrenok, P.S.; et al. Triterpene glycosides from the Vietnamese sea cucumber *Holothuria edulis*. *Nat. Prod. Res.* **2020**, *34*, 1061–1067. [CrossRef]

26. Bhatnagar, S.; Dudoet, B.; Ahond, A.; Poupat, C.; Thoison, O.; Clastres, A.; Laurent, D.; Potier, P. Invertebresmarins du lagonneocaledonien IV. Saponines et sapogenines d'une holothurie, *Actinopyga flammea*. *Bull. Soc. Chim. Fr.* **1985**, *1*, 124–129.
27. Silchenko, A.S.; Kalinovsky, A.I.; Avilov, S.A.; Andryjaschenko, P.V.; Dmitrenok, P.V.; Martyyas, E.A.; Kalinin, V.I. Triterpene glycosides from the sea cucumber *Eupentacta fraudatrix*. Structure and cytotoxic action of cucumariosides A_2, A_7, A_9, A_{10}, A_{11}, A_{13} and A_{14}, seven new minor non-sulatedtetraosides and an aglycone with an uncommon 18-hydroxy group. *Nat. Prod. Commun.* **2012**, *7*, 845–852. [CrossRef]
28. Silchenko, A.S.; Avilov, S.A.; Kalinin, V.I.; Kalinovsky, A.I.; Stonik, V.A.; Smirnov, A.V. Pseudostichoposide B—New triterpene glycoside with unprecedent type of sulfatation from deep-water North-Pacific sea cucumber *Pseudostichopus trachus*. *Nat. Prod. Res.* **2004**, *18*, 565–570. [CrossRef]
29. Silchenko, A.S.; Kalinovsky, A.I.; Avilov, S.A.; Andryjaschenko, P.V.; Dmitrenok, P.S.; Kalinin, V.I.; Yurchenko, E.A.; Dautov, S.S. Structures of violaceusosides C, D, E and G, sulfated triterpene glycosides from the sea cucumber *Pseudocolochirus violaceus* (Cucumariidae, Denrochirotida). *Nat. Prod. Commun.* **2014**, *9*, 391–399.
30. Silchenko, A.S.; Kalinovsky, A.I.; Avilov, S.A.; Kalinin, V.I.; Andrijaschenko, P.V.; Dmitrenok, P.S.; Popov, R.S.; Chingizova, E.A.; Ermakova, S.P.; Malyarenko, O.S. Structures and bioactivities of six new triterpene glycosides, psolusosides E, F, G, H, H_1 and I and the corrected structure of psolusoside B from the sea cucumber *Psolus fabricii*. *Mar. Drugs* **2019**, *17*, 358. [CrossRef]
31. Maltsev, I.I.; Stonik, V.A.; Kalinovsky, A.I.; Elyakov, G.B. Triterpene glycosides from sea cucumber *Stichopus japonicus* Selenka. *Comp. Biochem. Physiol.* **1984**, *78B*, 421–426. [CrossRef]
32. Silchenko, A.S.; Kalinovsky, A.I.; Avilov, S.A.; Andryjaschenko, P.V.; Dmitrenok, P.S.; Martyyas, E.A.; Kalinin, V.I.; Jayasandhya, P.; Rajan, G.C.; Padmakumar, K.P. Structures and biological activities of typicosideds A_1, A_2, B_1, C_1 and C_2, triterpene glycosides from the sea cucumbers *Actinocucumis typica*. *Nat. Prod. Commun.* **2013**, *8*, 301–310.
33. Antonov, A.S.; Avilov, S.A.; Kalinovsky, A.I.; Anastyuk, S.D.; Dmitrenok, P.S.; Evtushenko, E.V.; Kalinin, V.I.; Smirnov, A.V.; Taboada, S.; Ballesteros, M.; et al. Triterpene glycosides from Antarctic sea cucumbers I. Structure of liouvillosides A_1, A_2, A_3, B_1 and B_2, from the sea cucumber *Staurocucumis liouvillei*, new procedure for separation of highly polar glycoside fractions and taxonomic revision. *J. Nat. Prod.* **2008**, *71*, 1677–1685. [CrossRef] [PubMed]
34. Murray, A.P.; Muniain, C.; Seldes, A.M.; Maier, M. Patagonicoside A: A novel antifungal disulfated triterpene glycoside from the sea cucumber *Psolus patagonicus*. *Tetrahedron* **2001**, *57*, 9563–9568. [CrossRef]
35. Careaga, V.P.; Bueno, C.; Muniain, C.; Alche, L.; Maier, M.S. Pseudocnoside A, a new cytotoxic and antiproliferative triterpene glycoside from the sea cucumber *Pseudocnus dubiosus leoninus*. *Nat. Prod. Res.* **2014**, *28*, 213–220. [CrossRef]
36. Silchenko, A.S.; Kalinovsky, A.I.; Avilov, S.A.; Andryjaschenko, P.V.; Dmitrenok, P.S.; Yurchenko, E.A.; Dolmatov, I.Y.; Savchenko, A.M.; Kalinin, V.I. Triterpene glycosides from the sea cucumber *Cladolabes schmeltzii* II. Structure and biological action of cladolosides A_1–A_6. *Nat. Prod. Commun.* **2014**, *9*, 1421–1428. [CrossRef]
37. Silchenko, A.S.; Kalinovsky, A.I.; Avilov, S.A.; Kalinin, V.I.; Andrijaschenko, P.V.; Dmitrenok, P.S.; Popov, R.S.; Chingizova, E.A. Structures and bioactivities of psolusosides B_1, B_2, J, K, L, M, N, O, P, and Q from the sea cucumber *Psolus fabricii*. The first finding of tetrasulfated marine low molecular weight metabolites. *Mar. Drugs* **2019**, *7*, 631. [CrossRef]
38. Cuong, N.X.; Vien, L.T.; Hoang, L.; Hanh, T.T.H.; Thao, D.T.; Thann, N.V.; Nam, N.H.; Thung, D.C.; Kiem, P.V.; Minh, C.V. Cytotoxic triterpene glycosides from the sea cucumber *Stichopus horrens*. *Bioorg. Med. Chem. Lett.* **2017**, *27*, 2939–2942. [CrossRef]
39. Prokofieva, N.G.; Likhatskaya, G.N.; Volkova., O.V.; Anisimov, M.M.; Kiseleva, M.I.; Iliyn, S.G.; Budina, T.A.; Pokhilo, N.D. Action of betulafolientetraol on the erythrocyte and model mombranes. *Biol. Membr.* **1992**, *9*, 954–960.
40. Taniyama, S.; Arakawa, O.; Terada, M.; Nishio, S.; Takatani, T.; Mahmud, Y.; Noguchi, T. *Ostreopsis* sp., a possible origin of palytoxin (PTX) in parrotfish *Scarus ovifrons*. *Toxicon* **2003**, *42*, 29–33. [CrossRef]
41. Malagoli, D. *A Full-Length Protocol to Test Hemolytic Activity of Palytoxin on Human Erythrocytes*; Technical Report; Department of Animal Biology, University of Modena and Reggio Emilia: Modena, Italy, 2007; ISJ 4; pp. 92–94.

42. Silchenko, A.S.; Avilov, S.A.; Kalinovsky, A.I.; Dmitrenok, P.S.; Kalinin, V.I.; Morre, J.; Deinzer, M.L.; Woodward, C.; Collin, P.D. Glycosides from the North Atlantic sea cucumber *Cucumaria frondosa* V—Structures of five new minor trisulfated triterpene oligoglycosides, frondosides A_7-1, A_7-3, A_7-4, and isofrondoside C. *Can. J. Chem.* **2007**, *85*, 626–636. [CrossRef]
43. Moraes, G.; Northcote, P.T.; Silchenko, A.S.; Antonov, A.S.; Kalinovsky, A.I.; Dmitrenok, P.S.; Avilov, S.A.; Kalinin, V.I.; Stonik, V.A. Mollisosides A, B_1 and B_2: Minor triterpene glycosides from the New Zealand and South Australian sea cucumber *Australostichopus mollis*. *J. Nat. Prod.* **2005**, *68*, 842–847. [CrossRef]
44. Avilov, S.A.; Silchenko, A.S.; Antonov, A.S.; Kalinin, V.I.; Kalinovsky, A.I.; Smirnov, A.V.; Dmitrenok, P.S.; Evtushenko, E.V.; Fedorov, S.N.; Savina, A.S.; et al. Synaptosides A and A_1, two triterpene glycosides from the sea cucumber *Synapta maculata* containing 3-*O*-methylglucuronic acid and their cytotoxic activity against tumor cells. *J. Nat. Prod.* **2008**, *71*, 525–531. [CrossRef] [PubMed]
45. Silchenko, A.S.; Kalinovsky, A.I.; Avilov, S.A.; Andryjaschenko, P.V.; Dmitrenok, P.S.; Kalinin, V.I.; Chingizova, E.A.; Minin, K.V.; Stonik, V.A. Structures and biogenesis of fallaxosides D_4, D_5, D_6 and D_7, trisulfated non-holostane triterpene glycosides from the sea cucumber *Cucumaria fallax*. *Molecules* **2016**, *21*, 939. [CrossRef] [PubMed]
46. Zhang, S.-Y.; Yi, Y.-H.; Tang, H.-F.; Li, L.; Sun, P.; Wu, J. Two new bioactive triterpene glycosides from the sea cucumber *Pseudocolochirus violaceus*. *J. Asian Nat. Prod. Res.* **2006**, *8*, 1–8. [CrossRef] [PubMed]
47. Miyamoto, T.; Togawa, K.; Higuchi, R.; Komori, T.; Sasaki, T. Structures of four new triterpenoid oligoglycosides: Ds-penaustrosides A, B, C and D from the sea cucumber *Pentacta australis*. *J. Nat. Prod.* **1992**, *55*, 940–946. [CrossRef]

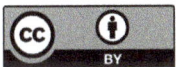

© 2020 by the authors. Licensee MDPI, Basel, Switzerland. This article is an open access article distributed under the terms and conditions of the Creative Commons Attribution (CC BY) license (http://creativecommons.org/licenses/by/4.0/).

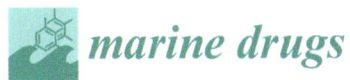

Article

Kurilosides A_1, A_2, C_1, D, E and F—Triterpene Glycosides from the Far Eastern Sea Cucumber *Thyonidium (= Duasmodactyla) kurilensis* (Levin): Structures with Unusual Non-Holostane Aglycones and Cytotoxicities

Alexandra S. Silchenko, Anatoly I. Kalinovsky, Sergey A. Avilov, Pelageya V. Andrijaschenko, Roman S. Popov, Pavel S. Dmitrenok, Ekaterina A. Chingizova and Vladimir I. Kalinin *

G.B. Elyakov Pacific Institute of Bioorganic Chemistry, Far Eastern Branch of the Russian Academy of Sciences, Pr. 100-letya Vladivostoka 159, 690022 Vladivostok, Russia; sialexandra@mail.ru (A.S.S.); kaaniv@piboc.dvo.ru (A.I.K.); avilov-1957@mail.ru (S.A.A.); pandryashchenko@mail.ru (P.V.A.); prs_90@mail.ru (R.S.P.); paveldmt@piboc.dvo.ru (P.S.D.); martyyas@mail.ru (E.A.C.)
* Correspondence: kalininv@piboc.dvo.ru; Tel./Fax: +7-(423)2-31-40-50

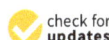

Received: 20 October 2020; Accepted: 4 November 2020; Published: 6 November 2020

Abstract: Six new monosulfated triterpene tetra-, penta- and hexaosides, namely, the kurilosides A_1 (**1**), A_2 (**2**), C_1 (**3**), D (**4**), E (**5**) and F (**6**), as well as the known earlier kuriloside A (**7**), having unusual non-holostane aglycones without lactone, have been isolated from the sea cucumber *Thyonidium (= Duasmodactyla) kurilensis* (Levin) (Cucumariidae, Dendrochirotida), collected in the Sea of Okhotsk near Onekotan Island from a depth of 100 m. Structures of the glycosides were established by 2D NMR spectroscopy and HR-ESI mass spectrometry. Kurilosides of the groups A and E contain carbohydrate moieties with a rare architecture (a pentasaccharide branched by C(4) Xyl1), differing from each other in the second monosaccharide residue (quinovose or glucose, correspondingly); kurilosides of the group C are characterized by a unique tetrasaccharide branched by a C(4) Xyl1 sugar chain; and kurilosides of the groups D and F are hexaosides differing from each other in the presence of an O-methyl group in the fourth (terminal) sugar unit. All these glycosides contain a sulfate group at C-6 of the glucose residue attached to C-4 Xyl1 and the non-holostane aglycones have a 9(11) double bond and lack γ-lactone. The cytotoxic activities of compounds **1**–**7** against mouse neuroblastoma Neuro 2a, normal epithelial JB-6 cells and erythrocytes were studied. Kuriloside A_1 (**1**) was the most active compound in the series, demonstrating strong cytotoxicity against the erythrocytes and JB-6 cells and a moderate effect against Neuro 2a cells.

Keywords: *Thyonidium kurilensis*; triterpene glycosides; kurilosides; sea cucumber; cytotoxic activity

1. Introduction

Triterpene glycosides isolated from different species of the sea cucumbers demonstrate promising biological activities [1,2] and a great structural diversity, including some recently found structural features unique for the glycosides [3–5] of terrestrial or marine origin. These glycosides usually form an extremely complicated mixture in the organism producer. So, its separation and isolation of dozens of pure individual compounds, especially minor ones, became possible only as a result of the development of chromatographic equipment and methodology. Thus, the glycoside compositions of some sea cucumber species were reinvestigated during last years, and novel minor glycosides were found, and the structures of some known substances were corrected [2,5–7].

The reinvestigation of the glycoside composition of the sea cucumber *Thyonidium* (= *Duasmodactuyla*) *kurilensis* (Levin) was undertaken for the same reason. Earlier studies of the glycosides of this species showed the complexity of its glycoside mixture. So, a part of the glycoside sum was subjected to acid hydrolysis followed by the separation of the obtained derivatives. As a result, the structures of two genins, kurilogenin [8] and nemogenin [9], were established. Later, two glycosides, kurilosides A (**7**) and C, were isolated [10]. The absolute configurations of the monosaccharide residues, composed of the carbohydrate chains of kurilosides A (**7**) and C, were assigned as D [10]. However, the remaining part of the glycoside fraction, containing more polar and minor glycosides, remained unexplored.

Herein, we report the isolation and structure elucidation of six glycosides, kurilosides A_1 (**1**), A_2 (**2**), C_1 (**3**), D (**4**), E (**5**) and F (**6**), as well as of the known kuriloside, A (**7**), obtained in native form from the glycoside mixture. The animals were collected near Onekotan Island in the Sea of Okhotsk. The structures of the novel compounds **1–6** were established and the structure of **7** was corroborated through analyses of the ^{1}H, ^{13}C NMR, 1D TOCSY and 2D NMR (^{1}H,^{1}H-COSY, HMBC, HSQC and ROESY) spectra, as well as through HR-ESI mass spectra. All the original spectra are presented in Figures S1–S58 in the supplementary data. The hemolytic activities against mouse erythrocytes and the cytotoxic activities against mouse neuroblastoma Neuro 2a and normal epithelial JB-6 cells were also studied.

2. Results and Discussion

2.1. Structural Elucidation of the Glycosides

The concentrated ethanolic extract of the sea cucumber *Thyonidium* (= *Duasmodactyla*) *kurilensis* was chromatographed on a Polychrom-1 column (powdered Teflon, Biolar, Latvia), repeated chromatography on Si gel columns, to give five fractions (I–V). Fraction I was subsequently subjected to HPLC on a reversed-phase semipreparative column to yield the compounds **1–6** (Figure 1) as well as kuriloside A (**7**), isolated earlier from this species.

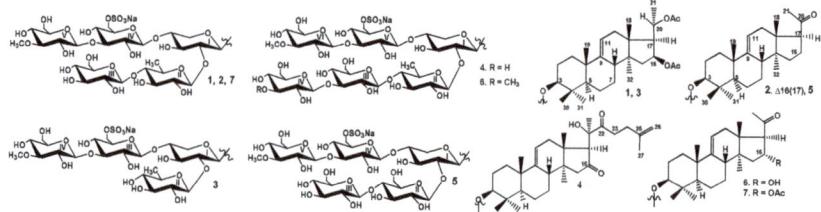

Figure 1. Chemical structures of the glycosides isolated from *Thyonidium kurilensis*: **1**—kuriloside A_1; **2**—kuriloside A_2; **3**—kuriloside C_1; **4**—kuriloside D; **5**—kuriloside E; **6**—kuriloside F; **7**—kuriloside A.

The ^{1}H and ^{13}C NMR spectra corresponding to the carbohydrate chains of kurilosides A_1 (**1**) and A_2 (**2**) (Table 1) were identical to each other and to that of the known kuriloside A (**7**), isolated from this species earlier and repeatedly this time. The structure of the sugar chain of kuriloside A (**7**) was established earlier by the ^{13}C NMR and chemical transformations (periodate oxidation, Smith degradation, Hakomori methylation followed by methanolysis, acetylation and GLC-MS analysis of the obtained products) [10]. The analysis of the 2D NMR spectra of the carbohydrate chain of the kurilosides of group A (**1, 2, 7**) was made for the first time (Table 1) and the structure established earlier was confirmed.

Table 1. ^{13}C and ^{1}H NMR chemical shifts and HMBC and ROESY correlations of the carbohydrate moiety of kurilosides A$_1$ (1), A$_2$ (2) and A (7).

Atom.	δ_C mult. ^{a,b,c}	δ_H mult. ^{d} (J in Hz)	HMBC	ROESY
Xyl1 (1→C-3)				
1	105.0 CH	4.69 d (7.2)	C-3; C: 5 Xyl1	H-3; H-3, 5 Xyl1
2	83.2 CH ^{b}	3.95 t (8.8)	C: 3 Xyl1	H-1 Qui2
3	75.7 CH	4.13 t (9.0)	C: 2, 4 Xyl1	
4	79.8 CH ^{b}	4.07 m		H-1 Glc4
5	63.8 CH$_2$	4.29 dd (5.3; 11.3)	C: 1, 3 Xyl1	
		3.58 t (11.3)	C: 1 Xyl1	H-1 Xyl1
Qui2 (1→2Xyl1)				
1	105.3 CH	5.02 d (7.6)	C: 2 Xyl1	H-2 Xyl1; H-3, 5 Qui2
2	76.1 CH	3.98 t (8.3)	C: 1, 3 Qui2	
3	75.3 CH	4.13 t (8.3)		
4	86.8 CH ^{b}	3.57 t (8.3)	C: 1 Glc3; C: 3, 5 Qui2	H-1 Glc3
5	71.7 CH	3.76 dd (6.2; 8.3)		H-1 Qui2
6	17.9 CH$_3$	1.70 d (6.2)	C: 4, 5 Qui2	
Glc3 (1→4Qui2)				
1	105.3 CH	4.92 d (8.0)	C: 4 Qui2	H-4 Qui2; H-3,5 Glc3
2	74.7 CH	4.00 t (8.5)	C: 1, 3 Glc3	
3	78.2 CH	4.21 t (9.1)	C: 2, 4 Glc3	H-1 Glc3
4	71.4 CH	4.11 t (8.5)	C: 5, 6 Glc3	
5	78.4 CH	4.05 m		H-1 Glc3
6	62.3 CH$_2$	4.55 brd (10.7)		
		4.23 dd (6.4; 11.7)		
Glc4 (1→4Xyl1)				
1	103.7 CH	4.87 d (8.0)	C: 4Xyl1	H-4 Xyl1; H-3, 5 Glc4
2	73.2 CH	3.89 t (8.9)	C: 1, 3 Glc4	
3	86.9 CH ^{b}	4.16 t (8.9)	C: 2, 4 Glc4, C: 1 MeGlc5	H-1 MeGlc5; H-1 Glc4
4	69.6 CH	3.90 t (8.9)	C: 3, 5, 6 Glc4	
5	75.7 CH	4.13 m		H-1 Glc4
6	67.3 CH$_2$ ^{c}	5.18 d (9.8)		
		4.75 dd (6,3; 11.6)	C: 5 Glc4	
MeGlc5 (1→3Glc4)				
1	105.3 CH	5.25 d (8.7)	C: 3 Glc4	H-3 Glc4; H-3, 5 MeGlc5
2	74.9 CH	3.95 t (8.7)	C: 1, 3 MeGlc5	
3	87.8 CH	3.68 t (8.7)	C: 2, 4 MeGlc5, OMe	H-1 MeGlc5
4	70.3 CH	4.13 t (8.7)	C: 3, 5, 6 MeGlc5	
5	78.1 CH	3.93 m		H-1, 3 MeGlc5
6	61.9 CH$_2$	4.44 d (12.0)	C: 4 MeGlc5	
		4.26 dd (5.5; 12.0)		
OMe	60.5 CH$_3$	3.85 s	C: 3 MeGlc5	

^{a} Recorded at 176.03 MHz in C$_5$D$_5$N/D$_2$O (4/1). ^{b} Bold = interglycosidic positions. ^{c} Italic = sulphate position. ^{d} Recorded at 700.00 MHz in C$_5$D$_5$N/D$_2$O (4/1). Multiplicity by 1D TOCSY.

In the ^{1}H and ^{13}C NMR spectra of the carbohydrate part of 1, 2 and 7, five characteristic doublets at δ_H = 4.69–5.25 (J = 7.2–8.7 Hz), and corresponding to them signals of anomeric carbons at δ_C = 103.7–105.3, were indicative of a pentasaccharide chain and β-configurations of the glycosidic bonds. The ^{1}H,^{1}H-COSY, HSQC and 1D TOCSY spectra of 1, 2 and 7 showed the signals of an isolated spin systems assigned to one xylose, one quinovose, two glucoses and one 3-O-methylglucose residue, which coincided with the monosaccharide composition of kuriloside A (7) established by chemical modifications [10]. The signal of C(6) Glc4 was observed at δ_C = 67.3, due to α-shifting effect of a sulfate group at this position.

The positions of the interglycosidic linkages were established by the ROESY and HMBC spectra of 1, 2 and 7 (Table 1) where the cross-peaks between H(1) of the xylose and H(3) (C(3)) of an aglycone, H(1) of the second residue (quinovose) and H(2) (C(2)) of the xylose, H(1) of the third residue (glucose) and H(4) (C(4)) of the second residue (quinovose), H(1) of the fourth residue (glucose) and H-4 of the first residue (xylose), and H-1 of the fifth residue (3-O-methylglucose) and H-3 (C(3)) of the fourth residue (glucose) were observed, indicating the presence of branching by the C(4) Xyl1 pentasaccharide chain. Such an architecture is very rare for the sea cucumber glycosides, as is another finding—a carbohydrate chain of cladoloside J_1 from *Cladolabes schmeltzii*, which, however, differed from kurilosides A (7), A_1 (1) and A_2 (2) in the monosaccharide composition [11].

The molecular formula of kuriloside A_1 (1) was determined to be $C_{58}H_{93}O_{31}SNa$ from the $[M_{Na} - Na]^-$ ion peak at an *m/z* of 1317.5449 (calc. 1317.5427) in the (−)HR-ESI-MS.

The analysis of the ^{13}C and ^1H NMR spectra of the aglycone part of 1 suggested the presence of an 22,23,24,25,26,27-hexa-*nor*-lanostane aglycone having a 9(11) double bond, which was deduced from the characteristic signals of the quaternary carbon C(9) at $\delta_C = 148.9$ and tertiary carbon C(11) at $\delta_C = 114.0$, with the corresponding proton signal at $\delta_H = 5.23$ (brd, $J = 5.6$ Hz; H(11)) (Table 2). The signals at $\delta_C = 169.8$ and 169.9 as well as the signals of the methyl groups at $\delta_C = 20.2$ and 21.0 corresponded to the carbons of the two acetoxy groups, whose positions at C(16) and C(20) were established by the correlations between the protons of the O-acetate methyl groups ($\delta_H = 2.12$ (s, COOC$\underline{H}_3$(16)) and H(16) ($\delta_H = 2.05$ (s, COOC$\underline{H}_3$(20)) and H(20) in the ROESY spectrum of 1. The HMBC correlations H(16) ($\delta_H = 5.64$ (ddd, $J = 5.2$; 7.7; 13.4 Hz)/$\underline{C}$OOCH$_3$(16) and H(20) ($\delta_H = 5.46$ (dd, $J = 6.1$; 10.6 Hz)/$\underline{C}$OOCH$_3$(20) corroborated these positions. Nemogenin—the aglycone with the same structure as in kuriloside A_1 (1)—was obtained earlier as result of acid hydrolysis of the glycoside sum of *T. kurilensis* [9]. Nemogenin has a β-oriented O-acetic group at C(16), which was established by the comparison of the observed ^1H NMR spectrum coupling constant $J_{16/17} = 7.7$ Hz with those calculated for the model 16α- and 16β-acetoxy-holostane derivatives as well as by the observed NOE between H(16α) and H(17α) [9]. The coupling constant ($J_{16/17} = 7.7$ Hz), observed in the ^1H NMR spectrum of 1 (Table 2), coincided with that in nemogenin. The ROE correlation H(16)/H(32) corroborated the 16β-OAc orientation. The (S)-configuration of the C(20) stereo-center in nemogenin was established by the analysis of inter-atomic distances in the models of the (20R)- and (20S)-isomers and the NOE-experiments. The correlations H(17)/H(21), H(20)/H(18) and H(18)/H(21) observed in the ROESY spectrum of 1 and the closeness of the coupling constant $J_{17/20} = 10.6$ Hz to that for nemogenin ($J_{17/20} = 10.8$ Hz) indicated the same (20S) configuration in kuriloside A_1 (1).

The (−)ESI-MS/MS of 1 demonstrated the fragmentation of the $[M_{Na}-Na]^-$ ion at an *m/z* of 1317.5. The peaks of the fragment ions were observed at an *m/z* of 1257.5 $[M_{Na}-Na-CH_3COOH]^-$, 1197.5 $[M_{Na}-Na-2CH_3COOH]^-$, 1035.4 $[M_{Na}-Na-2CH_3COOH-C_6H_{10}O_5$ (Glc)$]^-$, 889.4 $[M_{Na}-Na-2CH_3COOH-C_6H_{10}O_5$ (Glc)−$C_6H_{10}O_4$ (Qui)$]^-$ and 565.1 $[M_{Na}-Na-C_{28}H_{43}O_4$ (Agl)−$C_6H_{10}O_5$ (Glc)−$C_6H_{10}O_4$ (Qui)−H$]^-$, corroborating the structure of kuriloside A_1 (1).

All these data indicated that kuriloside A_1 (1) is 3β-O-{β-D-glucopyranosyl-(1→4)-β-D-quinovopyranosyl-(1→2)-[3-O-methyl-β-D-glucopyranosyl-(1→3)-6-O-sodium sulfate-β-D-glucopyranosyl-(1→4)]-β-D-xylopyranosyl}-22,23,24,25,26,27-hexa-*nor*-16β,(20S)-diacetoxylanost-9(11)-ene.

The molecular formula of kuriloside A_2 (2) was determined to be $C_{54}H_{85}O_{28}SNa$ from the $[M_{Na}-Na]^-$ ion peak at an *m/z* of 1213.4964 (calc. 1213.4954) in the (−)HR-ESI-MS.

Analysis of the ^{13}C NMR spectrum of 2 indicated the presence of 22,23,24,25,26,27-hexa-*nor*-lanostane aglycone with the signals from C(1) to C(11), C(30), C(31) and C(32) close to those in the spectrum of 1 (Table 3). The signals of the olefinic carbons at $\delta_C = 144.5$ (C(16)) and 152.1 (C(17)) with the corresponding olefinic proton H(16) at $\delta_H = 6.63$ (brt, $J = 2.6$ Hz) indicated the presence of an additional double bond in the polycyclic nucleus of 2. Its 16(17) position was deduced from the $^1H,^1H$-COSY spectrum where the signals of protons H(15α)–H(15β)–H(16) formed an isolated spin system and was confirmed by the HMBC correlations: H(15α)/C(16, 17), H(15β)/C(16, 17), H(18)/C(17) and H(21)/C(17). The signal of the quaternary carbon at $\delta_C = 196.3$ (C(20)) indicated the presence of a 20-oxo-group conjugated with a 16(17) double bond, which was confirmed by the correlations H(16)/C(20) and H(21)/C(20) observed in the HMBC spectrum of 2. The structure of the aglycone of kuriloside A_2 (2) was identical to that of the kurilogenin—an artificial genin—obtained from the glycoside sum of *T. kurilensis* as a result of acid hydrolysis. It was found first as a part of the native glycoside **2**.

Table 2. ^{13}C and ^{1}H NMR chemical shifts and HMBC and ROESY correlations of the aglycone moiety of kurilosides A$_1$ (**1**) and C$_1$ (**3**).

Position	δ_C mult. ^{a}	δ_H mult. (J in Hz) ^{b}	HMBC	ROESY
1	36.2 CH$_2$	1.77 m		H-11, H-19
		1.38 m		H-3, H-5, H-11
2	27.0 CH$_2$	2.19 m		H-19
		1.94 m		H-19, H-30
3	88.3 CH	3.18 dd (4.2; 11.9)	C: 1, 30, 31, C-1Xyl1	H-1, H-5, H-31, H-1Xyl1
4	39.7 C			
5	52.7 CH	0.87 brd (12.3)	C: 6, 10, 19, 30	H-1, H-3, H-7, H-31
6	21.1 CH$_2$	1.70 m		H-30, H-31
		1.50 m		H-19, H-30
7	28.0 CH$_2$	1.58 m		H-15
		1.27 m		H-5, H-32
8	41.2 CH	2.20 m		H-18
9	148.9 C			
10	39.3 C			
11	114.0 CH	5.23 brd (5.6)	C: 8, 10, 12, 14	H-1
12	35.8 CH$_2$	2.08 m		H-17, H-32
		1.78 m	C: 9, 11, 13, 15, 18	H-18, H-21
13	45.5 C			
14	43.6 C			
15	43.7 CH$_2$	2.10 dd (6.3; 13.6)	C: 32	H-32
		1.35 dd (5.0; 13.6)	C: 8, 13, 16, 32	H-18
16	73.8 CH	5.64 dd (5.2; 7.7; 13.4)	C: 15; OAc-16	H-32; OAc-16
17	53.3 CH	2.41 dd (7.7; 10.6)	C: 12, 15, 18, 20, 21	H-12, H-21, H-32
18	15.2 CH$_3$	0.82 s	C: 12, 13, 14, 17	H-8, H-12, H-19, H-20, H-21
19	22.3 CH$_3$	1.14 s	C: 1, 5, 9, 10	H-1, H-2, H-6, H-8, H-18, H-30
20	69.4 CH	5.46 dd (6.1; 10.6)	C: 16, 17, 21, OAc-20	H-21, OAc-20
21	19.6 CH$_3$	1.32 d (6.0)	C: 17, 20	H-12, H-17, H-18, H-20
30	16.4 CH$_3$	1.04 s	C: 3, 4, 5, 31	H-2, H-6, H-31
31	27.8 CH$_3$	1.24 s	C: 3, 4, 5, 30	H-3, H-5, H-6, H-30, H-1 Xyl1
32	18.9 CH$_3$	0.76 s	C: 8, 13, 14, 15	H-7, H-12, H-15, H-16, H-17
COOCH$_3$-16	169.8 C			
COOCH$_3$-16	20.2 CH$_3$	2.12 s		H-16, H-18
COOCH$_3$-20	169.9 C			
COOCH$_3$-20	21.0 CH$_3$	2.05 s		H-21

^{a} Recorded at 176.03 MHz in C$_5$D$_5$N/D$_2$O (4/1). ^{b} Recorded at 700.00 MHz in C$_5$D$_5$N/D$_2$O (4/1).

The (−)ESI-MS/MS of **2** demonstrated the fragmentation of the [M$_{Na}$−Na]$^-$ ion at an *m/z* of 1213.5. The peaks of fragment ions were observed at an *m/z* of 1037.4 [M$_{Na}$−Na−C$_7$H$_{12}$O$_5$ (MeGlc)]$^-$, 905.4 [M$_{Na}$−Na−C$_6$H$_{10}$O$_5$ (Glc)−C$_6$H$_{10}$O$_4$ (Qui)]$^-$, 565.1 [M$_{Na}$−Na−C$_{24}$H$_{35}$O (Agl)−C$_6$H$_{10}$O$_5$ (Glc)−C$_6$H$_{10}$O$_4$ (Qui)−H]$^-$, corroborating the identity of carbohydrate chains of **1** and **2**.

All these data indicated that kuriloside A$_2$ (**2**) is 3β-O-{β-D-glucopyranosyl-(1→4)-β-D-quinovopyranosyl-(1→2)-[3-O-methyl-β-D-glucopyranosyl-(1→3)-6-O-sodium sulfate-β-D-glucopyranosyl-(1→4)]-β-D-xylopyranosyl}-22,23,24,25,26,27-hexa-*nor*-20-oxo-lanosta-9(11),16-diene.

The molecular formula of kuriloside C$_1$ (**3**) was determined to be C$_{52}$H$_{83}$O$_{26}$SNa from the [M$_{Na}$−Na]$^-$ ion peak at an *m/z* of 1155.4923 (calc. 1155.4899) in the (−)HR-ESI-MS. The ^{1}H and ^{13}C NMR spectra corresponding to the carbohydrate chain of kuriloside C$_1$ (**3**) (Table 4) demonstrated four signals of anomeric doublets at δ$_H$ = 4.66–5.13 (d, *J* = 6.9–8.2 Hz) and anomeric carbons at δ$_C$ = 102.3–104.9 deduced by the HSQC spectrum. These data indicated the presence of a tetrasaccharide chain in **3**. Actually, its ^{13}C NMR spectrum was similar with that of the known kuriloside C, isolated earlier from *T. kurilensis* [10], and different from the spectra of the carbohydrate part of kurilosides A (**7**), A$_1$ (**1**) and A$_2$ (**2**) by the absence of the signals corresponding to a glucose residue attached to C(4)Qui2 in their chain. The signal of C(4)Qui2 was shielded (δ$_C$ 76.2) and the signals of C(3)Qui2 and C(5)Qui2 (δ$_C$ = 76.7 and 72.9, correspondingly) were deshielded in the spectrum of **3**, when compared with these signals in the spectra of the kurilosides of group A (Table 1) due to the lacking of the glycosylation effects. Thorough analysis of the $^1H,^1H$-COSY, the HSQC and 1D TOCSY spectra of 3 corroborated the presence of xylose, quinovose, glucose and 3-O-methylglucose residues. The positions of the interglycosidic linkages were elucidated based on the ROESY and HMBC correlations (Table 4). Hence, kurilosides C [10] and C_1 (3) have a tetrasaccharide chain branched by C(4)Xyl1 and the part of the chain attached to C(2)Xyl1 consists of one monosaccharide only (quinovose), while the part attached to C(4)Xyl1 is composed of glucose, sulfated by C(6), and 3-O-methylglucose residues. This architecture of a carbohydrate chain is unique for the sea cucumber glycosides.

Table 3. ^{13}C and ^1H NMR chemical shifts and HMBC and ROESY correlations of the aglycone moiety of kuriloside A_2 (2).

Position	δ_C mult. [a]	δ_H mult. (J in Hz) [b]	HMBC	ROESY
1	36.3 CH$_2$	1.71 m		H-11
		1.35 m		H-11
2	27.0 CH$_2$	2.15 m		
		1.89 m		H-19
3	88.5 CH	3.17 dd (4.2; 11.9)	C: 4, 30, 31, C:1 Xyl1	H-1, H-5, H-31, H-1Xyl1
4	39.7 C			
5	52.9 CH	0.90brd (1.8; 11.9)	C: 4, 6, 10, 19, 30, 31	H-1, H-3, H-31
6	21.1 CH$_2$	1.71 m	C: 8	H-31
		1.49 m		H-30
7	27.9 CH$_2$	1.65 m		
		1.31 m		H-32
8	39.4 CH	2.38 brd (9.6)		H-15, H-18, H-19
9	149.1 C			
10	39.4 C			
11	115.3 CH	5.33 brd (6.0)	C: 10, 12, 13	H-1
12	32.2 CH$_2$	2.58 dd (5.7; 16.6)	C: 9, 11, 13, 14, 18	H-18
		2.47 brdd (2.7; 16.6)	C: 9, 11, 18	H-32
13	49.7 C			
14	47.1 C			
15	41.7 CH$_2$	2.24 d (16.6)	C: 8, 14, 16, 17, 32	H-18
		2.05dd (3.0; 16.6)	C: 13, 14, 16, 17, 32	H-32
16	144.5 CH	6.63 brt (2.6)	C: 13, 14, 15, 17, 20	H-21
17	152.1 C			
18	19.4 CH$_3$	0.98 s	C: 12, 13, 14, 17	H-8, H-12, H-15
19	22.2 CH$_3$	1.10 s	C: 1, 5, 9, 10	H-1, H-2, H-6, H-8
20	196.3 C			
21	26.8 CH$_3$	2.28 s	C: 16, 17, 20	H-16
30	16.5 CH$_3$	1.06 s	C: 3, 4, 5, 31	H-2, H-6, H-31
31	27.9 CH$_3$	1.24 s	C: 3, 4, 5, 30	H-3, H-5, H-6, H-30, H-1 Xyl1
32	19.8 CH$_3$	0.86 s	C: 8, 13, 14, 15	H-7, H-12, H-15

[a] Recorded at 176.03 MHz in C_5D_5N/D_2O (4/1). [b] Recorded at 700.00 MHz in C_5D_5N/D_2O (4/1).

The NMR spectra of the aglycone part of kuriloside C_1 (3) were coincident with those of kuriloside A_1 (1), indicating the identity of their aglycones possessing two acetoxy-groups (Table 2).

The (−)ESI-MS/MS of 3 showed the fragmentation of the [M$_{Na}$−Na]$^−$ ion at an m/z of 1155.5. The peaks of the ions fragments were observed at an m/z of 1095.5 [M$_{Na}$−Na−CH$_3$COOH]$^−$, 1035.5 [M$_{Na}$−Na−2CH$_3$COOH]$^−$, 889.4 [M$_{Na}$−Na−2CH$_3$COOH−C$_6$H$_{10}$O$_4$ (Qui)]$^−$, 565.1 [M$_{Na}$−Na−C$_{28}$H$_{43}$O$_4$ (Agl)−C$_6$H$_{10}$O$_4$ (Qui)−H]$^−$, and confirmed the structure of 3.

All these data indicated that kuriloside C_1 (3) is 3β-O-{β-D-quinovopyranosyl-(1→2)-[3-O-methyl-β-D-glucopyranosyl-(1→3)-6-O-sodium sulfate-β-D-glucopyranosyl-(1→4)]-β-D-xylopyranosyl}-22,23,24,25,26,27-hexa-nor-16β,(20S)-diacetoxylanost-9(11)-ene.

The molecular formula of kuriloside D (4) was determined to be $C_{66}H_{105}O_{35}SNa$ from the [M$_{Na}$−Na]$^−$ ion peak at an m/z of 1489.6174 (calc. 1489.6163) in the (−)HR-ESI-MS.

Table 4. ^{13}C and ^{1}H NMR chemical shifts and HMBC and ROESY correlations of carbohydrate moiety of kuriloside C$_1$ (3).

Atom	δ_C mult. [a,b,c]	δ_H mult. (J in Hz) [d]	HMBC	ROESY
Xyl1 (1→C-3)				
1	104.9 CH	4.66 d (6.9)	C: 3	H-3; H-3, 5 Xyl1
2	81.8 CH [b]	3.95 t (7.5)	C: 1, 3 Xyl1	H-1 Qui2
3	74.8 CH	4.14 t (7.5)	C: 4 Xyl1	H-1, 5 Xyl1
4	78.1 CH [b]	4.14 m		H-1 Glc3
5	63.5 CH$_2$	4.37 dd (3.8; 10.7)	C: 3 Xyl1	H-3 Xyl1
		3.64 t (10.7)		H-1, 3 Xyl1
Qui2 (1→2Xyl1)				
1	104.8 CH	5.01 d (7.8)	C: 2 Xyl1	H-2 Xyl1; H-5 Qui2
2	76.2 CH	3.80 t (8.6)	C: 1 Qui2	
3	76.7 CH	3.99 t (8.6)	C: 2, 4 Qui2	H-1, 5 Qui2
4	76.2 CH	3.52 t (8.6)	C: 3, 5 Qui2	H-2, 6 Qui2
5	72.9 CH	3.67 dd (6.2; 8.6)		H-1 Qui2
6	18.3 CH$_3$	1.49 d (6.2)	C: 4, 5 Qui2	H-4 Qui2
Glc3 (1→4Xyl1)				
1	102.3 CH	4.88 d (8.2)	C: 4 Xyl1	H-4 Xyl1; H-3,5 Glc3
2	73.4 CH	3.83 t (9.0)	C: 1, 3 Glc3	
3	85.9 CH [b]	4.13 t (9.0)	C: 1 MeGlc4; C: 2, 4 Glc3	H-1 MeGlc4
4	69.1 CH	3.87 t (9.0)	C: 3, 5, 6 Glc3	H-6 Glc3
5	75.0 CH	4.01 t (9.0)		H-1 Glc3
6	67.5 CH$_2$ [c]	4.83 d (11.5)		
		4.61 dd (5.7; 11.5)		H-4 Glc3
MeGlc4 (1→3Glc3)				
1	104.3 CH	5.13 d (8.0)	C: 3 Glc3	H-3 Glc3; H-3, 5 MeGlc4
2	74.5 CH	3.78 t (8.8)	C: 1 MeGlc4	
3	86.7 CH	3.63 t (8.8)	C: 2, 4 MeGlc4, OMe	H-1 MeGlc4
4	70.3 CH	3.83 t (8.8)	C: 5 MeGlc4	
5	77.4 CH	3.83 m		H-1 MeGlc4
6	61.8 CH$_2$	4.27 d (12.0)		H-4 MeGlc4
		3.98 dd (6.4; 12.0)	C: 5 MeGlc4	
OMe	60.8 CH$_3$	3.79 s	C: 3 MeGlc4	

[a] Recorded at 176.03 MHz in C$_5$D$_5$N/D$_2$O (4/1). [b] Bold = interglycosidic positions. [c] Italic = sulphate position.
[d] Recorded at 700.00 MHz in C$_5$D$_5$N/D$_2$O (4/1). Multiplicity by 1D TOCSY.

The ^{1}H and ^{13}C NMR spectra corresponding to the carbohydrate part of kuriloside D (4) (Table 5) demonstrated six signals of anomeric doublets at δ_H = 4.70–5.28 (d, J = 7.5–8.2 Hz) as well as six signals of anomeric carbons at δ_C = 103.7–105.7 deduced from the HSQC spectrum, which indicated the presence of a hexasaccharide chain in 4. The presence of xylose, quinovose, three glucose and 3-O-methylglucose residues was deduced from the analysis of the ^{1}H,^{1}H-COSY, HSQC and 1D TOCSY spectra of 4. The positions of the interglycosidic linkages were elucidated based on the ROESY and HMBC correlations (Table 5). The comparison of the ^{13}C NMR spectra of the carbohydrate chains of kurilosides A$_1$ (1) and D (4) showed the coincidence of the signals assigned to the xylose, quinovose and glucose attached to C(4)Xyl1, sulfated by C(6), and the 3-O-methylglucose residues. The differences were observed between the signals assigned to the glucose, bonded to C(4)Qui2: the signal of C(3)Glc3 in the spectrum of 4 was deshielded (δ_C = 88.1) and the signals of C(2)Glc3 and C(4)Glc3 were shielded (δ_C = 73.6 and δ_C = 69.7, correspondingly) when compared with the spectrum of 1 (δ_C = 78.2 (C(3)Glc3), 74.7 (C(2)Glc3) and 71.4 (C(4)Glc3)). These shifting effects were observed due to the glycosylation of this glucose residue by the C(3) position with an additional glucose residue. Its signals were observed in the ^{13}C NMR spectrum of 4 and its anomeric proton correlated with H(3)Glc3 in the ROESY spectrum of 4 and with C(3)Glc3 in the HMBC spectrum, corroborating the position of its glycosidic bond (Table 5). Therefore, one of the terminal monosaccharide residues in kuriloside D (4) has no O-methyl group at C(3) in contrary with the majority of known glycosides from the sea cucumbers. Thus, kuriloside D (4) contains a sulfated hexasaccharide chain, a new finding for the glycosides of sea cucumbers. Sulfated hexaosides were earlier isolated only from one holothurian species—*Cladolabes schmeltzii* [11]—but had another monosaccharide composition and sulfate group position.

The analysis of the ^{1}H and ^{13}C NMR spectra of the aglycone part of **4** suggested the presence of a lanostane aglycone containing a non-shortened side chain (30 carbons) with a 9(11) double bond, which was deduced from the characteristic signals of the quaternary carbon C(9) at δ_C = 149.0 and tertiary carbon C(11) at δ_C = 115.0, with the corresponding proton signal at δ_H = 5.35 (brd, J = 6.2 Hz; H(11)) (Table 6). A lactone ring was absent and the signal of the methyl group C(18) was observed at δ_C = 16.9. Two strongly deshielded signals at δ_C = 216.6 and 216.5 corresponded to carbonyl groups, whose positions were deduced as C(16) and C(22), correspondingly, based on the correlations H(15)/C(16), H(17)/C(16), H(21)/C(22) and H(23)/C(22) in the HMBC spectrum of **4**. The protons of side chain H(23)-H(24)-H(26)-H(27) formed an isolated spin system and the protons H(15α) and H(15β) correlated only to each other in the ^{1}H,^{1}H-COSY spectrum of **4**, which confirmed the presence of oxo-groups at C(22) and C(16). The signals of the olefinic carbons at δ_C = 145.5 (C(25)) and 110.0 (C(26)) indicated the presence of a terminal double bond. Therefore, a new triterpene non-holostane aglycone of kuriloside D (**4**) has a normal side chain, two double bonds and two oxo-groups.

The (−)ESI-MS/MS of **4** demonstrated the fragmentation of the [M$_{Na}$−Na]$^-$ ion at an *m/z* of 1489.6. The peaks of the fragment ions were observed at an *m/z* of 1349.5 [M$_{Na}$−Na−C$_8$H$_{13}$O$_2$+H]$^-$, corresponding to the loss of the side chain from C(20) to C(27), 1187.5 [M$_{Na}$−Na−C$_8$H$_{13}$O$_2$−C$_6$H$_{10}$O$_5$ (Glc)]$^-$, 1025.4 [M$_{Na}$−Na−C$_8$H$_{13}$O$_2$−2C$_6$H$_{10}$O$_5$ (Glc)]$^-$, 879.4 [M$_{Na}$−Na−C$_8$H$_{13}$O$_2$−2C$_6$H$_{10}$O$_5$ (Glc)−C$_6$H$_{10}$O$_4$ (Qui)]$^-$ and 565.1 [M$_{Na}$−Na−C$_{30}$H$_{45}$O$_3$ (Agl)−2C$_6$H$_{10}$O$_5$ (Glc)−C$_6$H$_{10}$O$_4$ (Qui)−H]$^-$, which confirmed the aglycone structure and the sugar units sequence in the carbohydrate chain of **4**.

All these data indicated that kuriloside D (**4**) is 3β-O-{β-D-glucopyranosyl-(1→3)-β-D-glucopyranosyl-(1→4)-β-D-quinovopyranosyl-(1→2)-[3-O-methyl-β-D-glucopyranosyl-(1→3)-6-O-sodium sulfate-β-D-glucopyranosyl-(1→4)]-β-D-xylopyranosyl}-16,22-dioxo-lanosta-9(11),25-diene.

The molecular formula of kuriloside E (**5**) was determined to be C$_{54}$H$_{87}$O$_{29}$SNa from the [M$_{Na}$−Na]$^-$ ion peak at an *m/z* of 1231.5082 (calc. 1231.5059) in the (−)HR-ESI-MS.

In the ^{1}H and ^{13}C NMR spectra of the carbohydrate part of kuriloside E (**5**) (Table 7), five signals of anomeric doublets at δ_H = 4.71–5.27 (d, J = 7.0–7.8 Hz) and corresponding to them signals of the anomeric carbons at δ_C = 104.0–105.4 deduced from the HSQC spectrum were observed. This indicated the presence of a pentasaccharide chain in **5**. The comparison of the ^{13}C NMR spectra of the sugar parts of kuriloside A$_1$ (**1**) and E (**5**) revealed the differences among the signals of the second monosaccharide residue, attached to C(2)Xyl1. The analysis of the ^{1}H,^{1}H-COSY, HSQC and 1D TOCSY spectra of **5** showed this residue is a glucose. The signals of the rest of the monosaccharide units were close in the ^{13}C NMR spectra of **1** and **5**. The only sulfate group is attached to C(6)Glc4 (δ_C 67.5), as in all other glycosides from *T. kurilensis*. The positions of the interglycosidic linkages elucidated by the ROESY and HMBC correlations (Table 7) were the same as in the kurilosides of group A. Thus, kuriloside E (**5**) is a branched monosulfated pentaoside with three glucose residues in the oligosaccharide chain—one of them occupying the second position—instead of the quinovose residue in the carbohydrate chains of compounds **1**–**4** and **7** and the majority of the other glycosides from sea cucumbers.

The ^{1}H and ^{13}C NMR spectra of the aglycone part of kuriloside E (**5**) demonstrated the presence of a hexa-*nor*-lanostane aglycone, having a 9(11) double bond and lacking a γ-lactone, as with the other kurilosides A$_1$–D (**1**–**6**) (Table 8). The oxo-group (signal at δ_C 208.8) was positioned as C(20) based on the correlations H(17)/C(20) and H(21)/C(20) in the HMBC spectrum of **5**. The comparison of the ^{13}C NMR spectra of the aglycone parts of kurilosides A$_2$ (**2**) and E (**5**) showed the similarity of the signals from C(1) to C(11) as well as the signals of the methyl groups C(30), C(31) and C(32) and the differences of the signals of the carbons assigned to ring D. This was explained by the absence of the second double bond in the aglycone of **5** in comparison with **2**. So, the aglycone of kuriloside E (**5**) was identical to that of isokoreoside A isolated first from *Cucumaria conicospermium* [12] and then found in *C. frondosa* [13].

Table 5. ^{13}C and ^{1}H NMR chemical shifts and HMBC and ROESY correlations of the carbohydrate moiety of kuriloside D (**4**).

Atom	δ_C mult. ^{a,b,c}	δ_H mult. (J in Hz) ^{d}	HMBC	ROESY
Xyl1 (1→C-3)				
1	105.0 CH	4.70 d (7.6)	C: 3	H-3; H-3, 5 Xyl1
2	83.3 CH ^{b}	3.95 t (8.3)	C: 3 Xyl1	H-1 Qui2
3	75.4 CH	4.14 t (8.3)	C: 2 Xyl1	H-1 Xyl1
4	79.7 CH ^{b}	4.07 m		H-1 Glc5
5	63.8 CH$_2$	4.30 dd (6.1; 12.1)		
		3.59 dd (9.1; 12.1)		H-1 Xyl1
Qui2 (1→2Xyl1)				
1	105.3 CH	5.02 d (7.6)	C: 2 Xyl1	H-2 Xyl1; H-3, 5 Qui2
2	75.8 CH	3.95 t (8.3)		H-4 Qui2
3	75.3 CH	4.05 t (8.3)	C: 2, 4 Qui2	H-1 Qui2
4	87.1 CH ^{b}	3.56 t (8.3)	C: 1 Glc3; C: 5 Qui2	H-3 Glc3; H-2 Qui2
5	71.6 CH	3.76 dd (6.1; 9.7)		H-1, 3 Qui2
6	17.9 CH$_3$	1.71 d (6.1)	C: 4, 5 Qui2	
Glc3 (1→4Qui2)				
1	104.8 CH	4.90 d (7.5)	C: 4 Qui2	H-4 Qui2
2	73.6 CH	4.03 t (8.2)	C: 1, 3 Glc3	
3	88.1 CH ^{b}	4.20 m	C: 4 Glc3	H-1 Glc4; H-1 Glc3
4	69.7 CH	4.00 m	C: 3, 5 Glc3	
5	78.5 CH	4.00 m		
6	62.1 CH$_2$	4.47 d (12.3)		
		4.13 m		
Glc4 (1→3Glc3)				
1	105.7 CH	5.28 d (8.2)	C: 3 Glc3	H-3 Glc3; H-3, 5 Glc4
2	75.3 CH	4.06 t (9.1)	C: 1, 3 Glc4	
3	77.9 CH	4.22 t (9.1)	C: 2, 4 Glc4	
4	71.5 CH	4.15 t (9.1)	C: 5, 6 Glc4	
5	78.1 CH	4.00 m		H-1 Glc4
6	62.4 CH$_2$	4.51 dd (3.0; 11.5)		
		4.28 dd (5.4; 11.5)		
Glc5 (1→4Xyl1)				
1	103.7 CH	4.86 d (7.8)	C: 4 Xyl1	H-4 Xyl1; H-3 Glc5
2	73.2 CH	3.88 t (7.8)	C: 1, 3 Glc5	
3	87.0 CH ^{b}	4.14 t (9.2)	C: 1 MeGlc6; C: 2, 4 Glc5	H-1 MeGlc6; H-1 Glc5
4	69.6 CH	3.92 t (9.2)	C: 3, 5, 6 Glc5	
5	76.1 CH	4.11 m		
6	67.2 CH$_2$ ^{c}	5.18 d (9.9)		
		4.76 dd (6.6; 11.2)	C: 5 Glc5	
MeGlc6 (1→3Glc4)				
1	105.3 CH	5.24 d (7.9)	C: 3 Glc5	H-3 Glc5; H-3, 5 MeGlc6
2	74.9 CH	3.95 t (8.6)	C: 1, 3 MeGlc6	
3	87.8 CH	3.68 t (8.6)	C: 2, 4 MeGlc6; OMe	H-1, 5 MeGlc6; OMe
4	70.4 CH	4.13 t (8.6)	C: 3, 6 MeGlc6	H-6 MeGlc6
5	78.2 CH	3.92 t (8.6)		H-1, 3 MeGlc6
6	61.9 CH$_2$	4.44 dd (2.6; 11.8)	C: 4 MeGlc6	
		4.26 dd (5.3; 11.8)	C: 5 MeGlc6	
OMe	60.5 CH$_3$	3.85 s	C: 3 MeGlc6	

^{a} Recorded at 176.04 MHz in C$_5$D$_5$N/D$_2$O (4/1). ^{b} Bold = interglycosidic positions. ^{c} Italic = sulfate position.
^{d} Recorded at 700.13 MHz in C$_5$D$_5$N/D$_2$O (4/1). Multiplicity by 1D TOCSY.

The (−)ESI-MS/MS of **5** demonstrated the fragmentation of the [M$_{Na}$−Na]$^−$ ion at an *m/z* of 1231.5. The peaks of the ion fragments were observed at an *m/z* of 1069.5 [M$_{Na}$−Na−C$_6$H$_{10}$O$_5$ (Glc)]$^−$, 1055.4 [M$_{Na}$−Na−C$_7$H$_{12}$O$_5$ (MeGlc)]$^−$, 907.4 [M$_{Na}$−Na−2C$_6$H$_{10}$O$_5$ (Glc)]$^−$ and 565.1 [M$_{Na}$−Na−C$_{24}$H$_{37}$O (Agl)−2C$_6$H$_{10}$O$_5$ (Glc)−H]$^−$, which confirmed the presence of glucose as the second sugar unit in the carbohydrate chain of kuriloside E (**5**).

All these data indicated that kuriloside E (**5**) is 3β-O-{β-D-glucopyranosyl-(1→4)-β-D-glucopyranosyl-(1→2)-[3-O-methyl-β-D-glucopyranosyl-(1→3)-6-O-sodium sulfate-β-D-glucopyranosyl-(1→4)]-β-D-xylopyranosyl}-22,23,24,25,26,27-hexa-*nor*-20-oxo-lanost-9(11)-ene.

Table 6. ^{13}C and ^{1}H NMR chemical shifts and HMBC and ROESY correlations of the aglycone moiety of kuriloside D (**4**).

Position	δ_C mult. [a]	δ_H mult. (J in Hz) [b]	HMBC	ROESY
1	36.1 CH$_2$	1.76 m		H-11, H-19
		1.39 m		H-3, H-11
2	26.9 CH$_2$	2.19 m		
		1.92 m		H-19, H-30
3	88.4 CH	3.19 dd (4.0; 12.0)	C: 30, C: 1 Xyl1	H-1, H-5, H-31, H1-Xyl1
4	39.7 C			
5	52.7 CH	0.88 m		H-1, H-3, H-7
6	21.0 CH$_2$	1.70 m		
		1.45 m		H-19
7	28.2 CH$_2$	1.49 m		
		1.28 m		H-32
8	40.2 CH	2.33 m		H-18, H-19
9	149.0 C			
10	39.4 C			
11	115.0 CH	5.35 brd (6.2)	C: 10, 13	H-1
12	36.5 CH$_2$	2.44 brd (16.4)		H-17, H-32
		2.20 dd (4.0; 16.8)	C: 9, 14	
13	43.7 C			
14	41.9 C			
15	48.1 CH$_2$	2.27 d (17.7)	C: 14, 16, 32	H-18
		2.03 d (17.7)	C: 13, 16, 32	H-7, H-32
16	216.6 C			
17	63.9 CH	3.67 s	C: 12, 13, 16, 18, 20	H-12, H-21, H-32
18	16.9 CH$_3$	1.28 s	C: 12, 13, 14, 17	H-8, H-19, H-21
19	22.2 CH$_3$	1.11 s	C: 1, 5, 9, 10	H-1, H-2, H-6, H-8
20	80.9 C			
21	24.5 CH$_3$	1.59 s	C: 17, 20, 22	H-12, H-17, H-18, H-23
22	216.5 C			
23	35.2 CH$_2$	3.55 dd (5.8; 9.8)	C: 22	
		3.24 ddd (6.2; 9.3; 18.2)	C: 22, 24, 25	
24	31.8 CH$_2$	2.59 m	C: 23, 25, 26, 27	
25	145.5 C			
26	110.0 CH$_2$	4.87 brs	C: 24, 27	
		4.79 brs	C: 24, 27	
27	22.6 CH$_3$	1.73 s	C: 24, 25, 26	H-23, H-24, H-26
30	16.5 CH$_3$	1.06 s	C: 3, 4, 5, 31	H-2, H-6, H-31
31	27.9 CH$_3$	1.25 s	C: 3, 4, 5, 30	H-3, H-5, H-6, H-30, H-1 Xyl1
32	18.7 CH$_3$	0.90 s	C: 8, 13, 14, 15	H-7, H-12, H-15, H-17

[a] Recorded at 176.03 MHz in C$_5$D$_5$N/D$_2$O (4/1). [b] Recorded at 700.00 MHz in C$_5$D$_5$N/D$_2$O (4/1).

The molecular formula of kuriloside F (**6**) was determined to be C$_{61}$H$_{99}$O$_{34}$SNa from the [M$_{Na}$–Na]$^-$ ion peak at an m/z of 1407.5778 (calc. 1407.5744) in the (–)HR-ESI-MS.

In the ^{1}H and ^{13}C NMR spectra corresponding to the carbohydrate part of kuriloside F (**6**) (Table 9), six signals of anomeric doublets at δ_H = 4.70–5.26 (d, J = 7.2–8.6 Hz) along with the signals of the corresponding anomeric carbons at δ_C = 103.7–105.5 were observed. This indicated the presence of a hexasaccharide chain in **6**. The comparison of the ^{13}C NMR spectra of the sugar moieties of kurilosides D (**4**) and F (**6**) showed the coincidence of the signals of the five monosaccharide units, except for the signals of the terminal (fourth) residue. The analysis of the ROESY, ^{1}H,^{1}H-COSY, HSQC and 1D TOCSY spectra of **6** revealed the residue, attached to C(3)Glc3, to be 3-O-methylglucose, instead of a glucose in this position of the carbohydrate chain of **4**. The presence of two signals of the O-methyl groups at δ_C = 60.5 and 60.6 and at δ_H = 3.85 (s) and 3.86 (s) in the ^{13}C and ^{1}H NMR spectra of **6** as well as the shifting of the signal of C(3)MeGlc4 to 87.8 due to the attachment of OMe-group confirmed the presence of two residues of 3-O-methylglucose as the terminal units in the chain of kuriloside F (**6**). The positions of the interglycosidic linkages were elucidated based on the ROESY and HMBC correlations (Table 9).

Table 7. ^{13}C and ^{1}H NMR chemical shifts and HMBC and ROESY correlations of the carbohydrate moiety of kuriloside E (5).

Atom	δ_C mult. [a,b,c]	δ_H mult. (J in Hz) [d]	HMBC	ROESY
Xyl1 (1→C-3)				
1	105.1 CH	4.71 d (7.4)	C: 3	H-3; H-3, 5 Xyl1
2	82.7 CH [b]	4.02 t (9.7)	C: 1 Xyl1	H-1 Glc2
3	75.6 CH	4.16 t (9.7)	C: 4 Xyl1	H-1, 5 Xyl1
4	80.8 CH [b]	4.09 m		H-1 Glc4
5	63.7 CH$_2$	4.29 dd (5.9; 12.6)	C: 3 Xyl1	
		3.60 dd (9.7; 12.2)		H-1, 3 Xyl1
Glc2 (1→2Xyl1)				
1	105.4 CH	5.10 d (7.7)	C: 2 Xyl1	H-2 Xyl1; H-3, 5 Glc2
2	76.1 CH	4.00 t (8.6)		
3	75.2 CH	4.30 t (8.6)		H-1, 5 Glc2
4	81.0 CH [b]	4.30 t (8.6)	C: 1 Glc3	H-1 Glc3
5	76.5 CH	3.85 m		H-1, 3 Glc2
6	61.5 CH$_2$	4.55 brd (12.2)		
		4.34 dd (3.2; 12.2)		
Glc3 (1→4Glc2)				
1	104.8 CH	5.11 d (7.0)	C: 4 Glc2	H-4 Glc2; H-3, 5 Glc3
2	74.6 CH	4.04 t (8.9)	C: 1, 3 Glc3	
3	77.9 CH	4.18 t (8.9)	C: 2, 4 Glc3	H-1 MeGlc5; H-1, 5 Glc3
4	71.3 CH	4.12 t (8.9)	C: 5, 6 Glc3	
5	78.3 CH	4.00 m		H-1, 3 Glc3
6	62.1 CH$_2$	4.48 d (12.2)		
		4.22 dd (7.0; 12.2)		
Glc4 (1→4Xyl1)				
1	104.0 CH	4.90 d (7.8)	C: 4 Xyl1	H-4 Xyl1; H-3 Glc4
2	73.3 CH	3.94 t (8.6)	C: 1, 3 Glc4	
3	87.0 CH [b]	4.18 t (8.6)	C: 1 MeGlc5; C: 2, 4 Glc4	H-1 Glc4
4	69.8 CH	3.88 t (8.6)		H-6 Glc4
5	75.7 CH	4.20 m		
6	67.5 CH$_2$ [c]	5.23 d (10.9)		
		4.72 t (10.1)		H-4 Glc4
MeGlc5 (1→3Glc4)				
1	105.4 CH	5.27 d (7.8)	C: 3 Glc4	H-3 Glc4; H-3, 5 MeGlc5
2	74.9 CH	3.96 t (8.6)	C: 1, 3 MeGlc5	H-4 MeGlc5
3	87.8 CH	3.69 t (8.6)	C: 2, 4 MeGlc5; OMe	H-1, 5 MeGlc5; OMe
4	70.3 CH	4.15 t (8.6)	C: 3, 5, 6 MeGlc5	
5	78.2 CH	3.94 m		H-1, 3 MeGlc5
6	61.9 CH$_2$	4.45 brd (9.4)		
		4.27 dd (5.5; 11.7)	C: 5 MeGlc5	
OMe	60.5 CH$_3$	3.86 s	C: 3 MeGlc5	H-3 MeGlc5

[a] Recorded at 176.04 MHz in C$_5$D$_5$N/D$_2$O (4/1). [b] Bold = interglycosidic positions. [c] Italic – sulfate position. [d] Recorded at 700.13 MHz in C$_5$D$_5$N/D$_2$O (4/1). Multiplicity by 1D TOCSY.

The carbohydrate chain of kuriloside F (6) is a new for the sea cucumber glycosides. This is the fifth representative of the sulfated hexaosides along with kuriloside D (4) found in the sea cucumbers.

The analysis of the ^{13}C and ^{1}H NMR spectra of the aglycone part of 6 indicated the presence of 22,23,24,25,26,27-hexa-*nor*-lanostane aglycone, with a 9(11) double bond (Table 10). The deshielding of C(16) to δ_C = 71.1 and H(16) to δ_H = 5.40 (brt, J = 7.8 Hz) indicated the presence of a hydroxyl group at C(16), which was confirmed by the correlations H(15)/C(16) and H(17)/C(16) in the HMBC spectrum of 6. The comparison of the NMR spectra of the aglycone parts of kuriloside F (6) and known kuriloside A (7) [10] showed their difference in the signals C(15), C(16) and C(17) due to the presence of different substituents (hydroxy or acetoxy group) at C(16). This was also corroborated by the (−)HR-ESI-MS spectra of 6 and 7, differing by 42 *amu*, corresponding to a C$_2$H$_2$O fragment.

Table 8. ^{13}C and ^{1}H NMR chemical shifts and HMBC and ROESY correlations of the aglycone moiety of kuriloside E (5).

Position	δ$_C$ mult. ^{a}	δ$_H$ mult. (J in Hz) ^{b}	HMBC	ROESY
1	36.3 CH$_2$	1.77 m		
		1.39 m		H-3, H-11
2	26.9 CH$_2$	2.19 m		
		2.00 m		
3	88.4 CH	3.18 dd (4.1; 11.9)	C: 30, C:1 Xyl1	H-1, H-5, H-31, H-1Xyl1
4	39.6 C			
5	52.8 CH	0.85d (11.9)		H-1, H-3, H-7, H-31
6	21.1 CH$_2$	1.61 m		H-31
		1.42 m		H-8
7	28.3 CH$_2$	1.60 m		H-5
		1.26 m		H-32
8	41.4 CH	2.15m		H-6, H-18, H-19
9	149.1 C			
10	39.2 C			
11	114.1 CH	5.29 brd (6.2)	C: 10, 14	H-1
12	36.0 CH$_2$	2.32 brdd (2.1; 16.2)		H-17, H-32
		1.96 dd (6.0; 16.2)	C: 9, 11, 13	H-18, H-21
13	47.5 C			
14	45.9 C			
15	33.9 CH$_2$	1.43 m		H-18
		1.37 m		H-32
16	21.9 CH$_2$	2.50 m		H-18
		1.68 m		H-32
17	59.7 CH	2.98t (9.0)	C: 14, 18, 20	H-12, H-21, H-32
18	16.4 CH$_3$	0.63 s	C: 12, 13, 14, 17	H-8, H-12, H-15, H-16, H-19
19	22.3 CH$_3$	1.10 s	C: 9	H-2, H-18
20	208.8 C			
21	30.7 CH$_3$	2.12 s	C: 17, 20	H-12, H-17, H-18
30	16.5 CH$_3$	1.05 s	C: 3, 4, 5, 31	H-2, H-6, H-31
31	27.9 CH$_3$	1.18 s	C: 3, 4, 5, 30	H-3, H-5, H-6, H-30, H-1 Xyl1
32	18.6 CH$_3$	0.81 s	C: 8, 13, 14, 15	H-7, H-12, H-15, H-16, H-17

^{a} Recorded at 176.03 MHz in C$_5$D$_5$N/D$_2$O (4/1). ^{b} Recorded at 700.00 MHz in C$_5$D$_5$N/D$_2$O (4/1).

The ROE correlations H(16)/H(15β) and H(16)/H(18) indicated a 16α-OH orientation in the aglycone of kuriloside F (6). The comparison of the coupling patterns of the protons of ring D in kuriloside F (6) and the known earlier kuriloside A (7), having an α-oriented O-acetic group at C(16) [10], showed their closeness. Hence, the aglycone of 6 having an α-hydroxylated C(16) can be considered as the biosynthetic precursor of the aglycone of 7 characterized by the O-acetic group at this position. Moreover, the glycosides with the 16-hydroxy groups have never been isolated earlier from the sea cucumbers. It probably may be related to the unusual α-OH orientation at C(16) in the glycoside from *T. kurilensis* while the other known glycosides are characterized by the β-oriented 16-acetoxy group. Apparently, their biosynthetic 16β-hydroxylated precursors are quickly transformed in order to "protect" the aglycone against 18(16) lactonization (it is known that the simultaneous presence of hydroxyls at C-16 and C-20 in 18-carboxylated precursor preferably leads to formation of an 18(16) lactone [1]) for the holostane-type aglycones (having 18(20)-lactone) to be formed.

So, all these data indicated that the aglycone of kuriloside F (6) is 22,23,24,25,26,27-hexa-*nor*-16α-hydroxy-20-oxo-lanost-9(11)-ene, first discovered in the glycosides from the sea cucumbers, and can be considered as a "hot metabolite", which is usually quickly metabolized into other derivatives and is the biosynthetic precursor of the 16-O-acetylated glycosides, particularly, kuriloside A (7).

Table 9. ^{13}C and ^{1}H NMR chemical shifts and HMBC and ROESY correlations of the carbohydrate moiety of kuriloside F (**6**).

Atom	δ_C mult. ^{a,b,c}	δ_H mult. (J in Hz) ^{d}	HMBC	ROESY
Xyl1 (1→C-3)				
1	104.7 CH	4.70 d (7.2)	C: 3	H-3; H-3, 5 Xyl1
2	83.2 CH ^{b}	3.96 m	C: 1 Xyl1	H-1 Qui2
3	75.7 CH	4.13 t (8.8)	C: 2 Xyl1	
4	79.8 CH ^{b}	4.07 m		H-1 Glc5
5	63.8 CH$_2$	4.29 dd (5.3; 11.4)	C: 3 Xyl1	
		3.58 dd (9.7; 11.4)		H-1 Xyl1
Qui2 (1→2Xyl1)				
1	105.0 CH	5.02 d (7.3)	C: 2 Xyl1	H-2 Xyl1; H-5 Qui2
2	76.0 CH	3.97 t (9.4)	C: 1 Qui2	
3	75.3 CH	4.10 m		
4	86.9 CH ^{b}	3.56 t (9.4)	C: 1 Glc3; C: 3, 5 Qui2	H-1 Glc3
5	71.6 CH	3.76 m		H-1 Qui2
6	17.8 CH$_3$	1.70 d (5.9)	C: 4, 5 Qui2	
Glc3 (1→4Qui2)				
1	104.7 CH	4.90 d (7.4)	C: 4 Qui2	H-4 Qui2; H-3, 5 Glc3
2	73.5 CH	4.01 t (8.3)	C: 1, 3 Glc3	
3	87.8 CH	4.20 t (8.3)	C: 4 Glc3	H-1 MeGlc4; H-1, 5 Glc3
4	69.6 CH	4.00 m		
5	77.9 CH	4.00 t (8.3)		H-1, 3 Glc3
6	61.9 CH$_2$	4.45 m		
		4.14 dd (5.5; 12.0)		
MeGlc4 (1→3Glc3)				
1	105.5 CH	5.26 d (8.1)	C: 3 Glc3	H-3 Glc3; H-3, 5 MeGlc4
2	74.9 CH	3.99 t (8.1)	C: 1, 3 MeGlc4	
3	87.8 CH	3.70 t (8.1)	C: 2, 4 MeGlc4; OMe	H-1 MeGlc4; OMe
4	70.5 CH	4.13 t (8.5)	C: 3, 5, 6 MeGlc4	
5	78.2 CH	3.95 m		H-1 MeGlc4
6	62.1 CH$_2$	4.46 dd (4.1; 12.2)	C: 4 MeGlc4	
		4.26 dd (6.1; 11.2)	C: 5 MeGlc4	
OMe	60.5 CH$_3$	3.85 s	C: 3 MeGlc4	H-3 MeGlc4
Glc5 (1→4Xyl1)				
1	103.7 CH	4.86 d (8.1)	C: 4 Xyl1	H-4 Xyl1; H-3 Glc5
2	73.2 CH	3.86 t (8.1)	C: 1 Glc5	
3	86.9 CH	4.15 t (9.1)	C: 1 MeGlc6; C: 2, 4 Glc5	H-1 MeGlc6
4	69.6 CH	3.91 m	C: 3 Glc5	
5	75.7 CH	4.13 m		H-1 Glc5
6	67.2 CH$_2$ ^{c}	5.19 d (11.2)		
		4.77 dd (5.1; 11.2)		
MeGlc6 (1→3Glc5)				
1	105.3 CH	5.25 d (8.6)	C: 3 Glc5	H-3 Glc5; H-3, 5 MeGlc6
2	74.8 CH	3.96 t (8.6)	C: 1, 3 MeGlc6	
3	87.9 CH	3.68 t (8.6)	C: 2, 4 MeGlc6; OMe	H-1, 5 MeGlc6; OMe
4	70.3 CH	4.14 t (8.6)	C: 3, 5, 6 MeGlc6	
5	78.2 CH	3.93 m		H-1, 3 MeGlc6
6	61.9 CH$_2$	4.44 brd (11.8)	C: 4 MeGlc6	
		4.27 dd (5.5; 11.8)	C: 5 MeGlc6	
OMe	60.6 CH$_3$	3.86 s	C: 3 MeGlc6	H-3 MeGlc6

^{a} Recorded at 176.04 MHz in C$_5$D$_5$N/D$_2$O (4/1). ^{b} Bold = interglycosidic positions. ^{c} Italic = sulfate position. ^{d} Recorded at 700.13 MHz in C$_5$D$_5$N/D$_2$O (4/1). Multiplicity by 1D TOCSY.

The (−)-ESI-MS/MS of **6** demonstrated the fragmentation of the [M$_{Na}$−Na]$^−$ ion at an *m/z* of 1407.5. The peaks of the ion fragments were observed at an *m/z* of 1231.5 [M$_{Na}$−Na−C$_7$H$_{12}$O$_5$ (MeGlc)]$^−$, 1069.4 [M$_{Na}$−Na−C$_7$H$_{12}$O$_5$ (MeGlc)−C$_6$H$_{10}$O$_5$ (Glc)]$^−$, 923.4 [M$_{Na}$−Na−C$_7$H$_{12}$O$_5$ (MeGlc)−C$_6$H$_{10}$O$_5$ (Glc)−C$_6$H$_{10}$O$_4$ (Qui)]$^−$ and 565.1 [M$_{Na}$−Na−C$_{24}$H$_{37}$O$_2$ (Agl)−C$_7$H$_{12}$O$_5$ (MeGlc)−C$_6$H$_{10}$O$_5$ (Glc)−C$_6$H$_{10}$O$_4$ (Qui)−H]$^−$, corroborating the structure elucidated by the NMR.

Table 10. ^{13}C and ^{1}H NMR chemical shifts and HMBC and ROESY correlations of the aglycone moiety of kuriloside F (6).

Position	δ_C mult. [a]	δ_H mult. (J in Hz) [b]	HMBC	ROESY
1	36.2 CH$_2$	1.77 m		H-11
		1.41 m		H-3, H-5, H-11, H-31
2	27.0 CH$_2$	2.19 m		
		1.94 m		
3	88.4 CH	3.19 dd (4.6; 12.5)	C: 4, 30, 31, C:1 Xyl1	H-1, H-5, H-31, H1-Xyl1
4	39.7 C			
5	52.8 CH	0.92 brd (12.5)	C: 4, 10, 19, 30	H-1, H-3, H-7, H-31
6	21.2 CH$_2$	1.70 m		H-31
		1.47 m		H-19
7	28.4 CH$_2$	1.64 m		
		1.36 m		
8	41.5 CH	2.16 m		H-18, H-19
9	149.0 C			
10	39.4 C			
11	114.2 CH	5.31 brd (6.3)	C: 8, 10, 12, 13	H-1
12	35.8 CH$_2$	2.48 brd (16.1)		H-17, H-32
		1.94 dd (6.3; 16.1)	C: 9, 11, 13, 18	H-8, H-18
13	46.9 C			
14	46.8 C			
15	45.2 CH$_2$	2.07 dd (9.2; 13.2) β	C: 8, 13, 32	H-16, H-18
		1.79 d (13.2) α	C: 14, 16, 32	H-32
16	71.1 CH	5.40 brt (7.5)	C: 13, 14, 20	H-15β, H-18
17	70.0 CH	3.40 d (6.4)	C: 12, 13, 14, 16, 18, 20	H-12, H-21, H-32
18	17.3 CH$_3$	0.71 s	C: 12, 13, 17	H-8, H-12, H-15β, H-16, H-19
19	22.3 CH$_3$	1.10 s	C: 1, 5, 9, 10	H-1, H-2, H-6, H-8, H-18
20	208.8 C			
21	31.2 CH$_3$	2.18 s	C: 17, 20	H-12, H-17
30	16.5 CH$_3$	1.05 s	C: 3, 4, 5, 31	H-2, H-6, H-31, H-6 Qui2
31	27.9 CH$_3$	1.24 s	C: 3, 4, 5, 30	H-3, H-5, H-6, H-30, H-1 Xyl1
32	20.0 CH$_3$	1.24 s	C: 8, 13, 15	H-7, H-12, H-15, H-17

[a] Recorded at 176.03 MHz in C$_5$D$_5$N/D$_2$O (4/1). [b] Recorded at 700.00 MHz in C$_5$D$_5$N/D$_2$O (4/1).

All these data indicated that kuriloside F (6) is 3β-O-{3-O-methyl-β-D-glucopyranosyl-(1→3)-β-D-glucopyranosyl-(1→4)-β-D-quinovopyranosyl-(1→2)-[3-O-methyl-β-D-glucopyranosyl-(1→3)-6-O-sodium sulfate-β-D-glucopyranosyl-(1→4)]-β-D-xylopyranosyl}-22,23,24,25,26,27-hexa-nor-16α-hydroxy-20-oxo-lanost-9(11)-ene.

Kuriloside A (7) was also isolated by us from the glycoside sum of *T. kurilensis* and identified with a known earlier compound [10] by the comparison of their ^{1}H and ^{13}C spectra. Moreover, extensive analysis of the 2D NMR spectra of 7 was made for the first time (Tables 1 and 11). The positions of the interglycosidic linkages in the carbohydrate chain were confirmed by the ROESY and HMBC spectra of 7 (Table 1). The ROE correlation H(16)/H(18) observed in the spectrum of 7 and the closeness of the coupling constants of the protons H(15α), H(15β), H(16) and H(17) to those in kuriloside A, isolated earlier, confirmed the 16α-OAc orientation, which was earlier established based on the different decoupling experiments performed with the protons of ring D followed by the comparison of the values of the experimental coupling constants of H(15α), H(15β), H(16) and H(17) in 7 with those calculated for the 16α- and 16β-substituted holostane derivatives [10].

The structure of kuriloside A (7) was also confirmed by the (−)HR-ESI-MS spectrum, in which the [M$_{Na}$−Na]$^-$ ion peak at an *m/z* of 1273.5196 (calc. 1273.5165) was observed, which corresponded to the molecular formula of C$_{56}$H$_{89}$O$_{30}$SNa.

As result of our investigation, six unknown earlier triterpene glycosides were isolated from the sea cucumber *Thyonidium* (= *Duasmodactyla*) *kurilensis*. The glycosides have five different carbohydrate chains (kurilosides of the groups A, C–F), including three novel ones. The sulfated hexasaccharide moieties of kurilosides D (4) and F (6) are the third and fourth findings, correspondingly, in additional to the carbohydrate chains of the cladolosides of the groups K and L [11] of such type sugar parts in the sea cucumber glycosides. They all differ from each other in monosaccharide composition and the sulfate position. Pentasaccharide, branched by C(4)Xyl1, the chain of kuriloside E (5) with glucose as the second unit, is also unique. The oligosaccharide chains of the kurilosides of groups A and C, characterized by the same position of branching, were also found only in the glycosides from *T. kurilensis*. Five non-holostane aglycones without a lactone and with a 9(11) double bond were discovered in glycosides 1–7. Four of them have shortened side chains (22,23,24,25,26,27-hexa-*nor*-lanostane aglycones) and one aglycone (in kuriloside D (4)) was characterized by a normal side chain and has never been found earlier. It should also be noted that only in the glycosides from *T. kurilensis* were the substituents at C(16) with an α-orientation found, while all the other glycosides with a 16-*O*-acetic group were characterized by their β-orientation [14,15].

Table 11. ^{13}C and ^{1}H NMR chemical shifts and HMBC and ROESY correlations of the aglycone moiety of kuriloside A (7).

Position	δ_C mult. [a]	δ_H mult. (J in Hz) [b]	HMBC	ROESY
1	36.1 CH$_2$	1.75 m		H-11, H-30
		1.40 m		H-5, H-11
2	27.0 CH$_2$	2.18 m		
		1.90 m		H-30
3	88.4 CH	3.19 dd (4.2; 11.9)	C: 4, 30, 31, C:1 Xyl1	H-1, H-5, H-31, H1-Xyl1
4	39.7 C			
5	52.8 CH	0.90 brd (11.9)	C: 4, 10, 19, 30	H-1, H-3, H-7, H-31
6	21.2 CH$_2$	1.68 m		H-31
		1.43 m		H-30
7	28.3 CH$_2$	1.59 m		
		1.32 m		H-5, H-32
8	41.3 CH	2.12 m		H-18, H-19
9	149.0 C			
10	39.4 C			
11	114.1 CH	5.29 brd (5.6)	C: 8, 10, 12, 13	H-1
12	35.6 CH$_2$	2.45 brd (17.3)	C: 9	H-17, H-21, H-32
		1.94 dd (6.5; 17.3)	C: 9, 11, 13	H-18
13	46.7 C			
14	46.2 C			
15	42.6 CH$_2$	2.07 brdd (10.0; 14.7) β	C: 8, 13, 32	
		1.58 d (14.8) α	C: 14, 16, 17, 32	H-32
16	75.4 CH	6.03 brt (7.5)	C: 13, 17, 20, OAc	H-18
17	65.8 CH	3.39 d (6.2)	C: 12, 13, 14, 16, 18, 20	H-12, H-21, H-32
18	17.1 CH$_3$	0.65 s	C: 12, 13, 17	H-8
19	22.2 CH$_3$	1.05 s	C: 1, 5, 9, 10	H-1, H-2, H-6, H-8, H-18
20	206.7 C			
21	30.7 CH$_3$	2.19 s	C: 17, 20	H-12, H-17, H-18
30	16.5 CH$_3$	1.05 s	C: 3, 4, 5, 31	H-2, H-6, H-31
31	27.9 CH$_3$	1.23 s	C: 3, 4, 5, 30	H-3, H-5, H-6, H-30, H-1 Xyl1
32	19.1 CH$_3$	1.02 s	C: 8, 13, 15	H-7, H-12, H-17
COOCH$_3$	170.4 C			
OCOCH$_3$	20.9 CH$_3$	2.00 s	C:16, OAc	

[a] Recorded at 176.03 MHz in C$_5$D$_5$N/D$_2$O (4/1). [b] Recorded at 700.00 MHz in C$_5$D$_5$N/D$_2$O (4/1).

2.2. Bioactivity of the Glycosides

The cytotoxic activities of compounds 1–7 against mouse neuroblastoma Neuro 2a, normal epithelial JB-6 cells and erythrocytes were studied (Table 12). Kuriloside A$_1$ (1) was the most active compound in the series, demonstrating strong cytotoxicity against erythrocytes and JB-6 cells and a moderate effect against Neuro 2a cells. While kurilosides A$_2$ (2) and A (7) were highly or moderately cytotoxic, respectively, against the erythrocytes and JB-6 cells, they were not effective against Neuro 2a cells, showing the influence of the aglycone structures on the activity of the glycosides. The presence of an *O*-acetic group at C(20) in 1 is apparently compensating for the absence of a normal side chain, resulting in its increasing cytotoxicity. The activity of kuriloside C$_1$ (3) was decreased in relation of all the tested cell lines in comparison with 1 due to the lack of a glucose unit attached to C(4)Qui2. Kuriloside E (5) was the less active compound in the series due to the presence of a glucose residue as the second unit of the carbohydrate chain. Hexaoside with a non-methylated terminal glucose residue, kuriloside D (**4**), demonstrated a stronger activity against erythrocytes and JB-6 cells when compared with kuriloside F (**6**), which has a hexasaccharide chain with methylated terminal sugar units. This influence can be explained also by the presence of a normal non-shortened side chain in the aglycone of **4**. It is interesting that the glycosides with branched pentasaccharide chains (the kurilosides of group A) possessed higher cytotoxicity than those with hexasaccharide chains (the kurilosides of groups D and F).

Table 12. The cytotoxic activities of glycosides **1–7** and cladoloside C (positive control) against mouse erythrocytes, neuroblastoma Neuro 2a cells and normal epithelial JB-6 cells.

Glycoside	ED_{50}, µM	Cytotoxicity EC_{50}, µM	
	Erythrocytes	JB-6	Neuro-2a
Kuriloside A_1 (**1**)	1.38 ± 0.07	2.81 ± 0.05	63.08 ± 2.42
Kuriloside A_2 (**2**)	4.62 ± 0.15	5.87 ± 0.05	>100.00
Kuriloside C_1 (**3**)	8.14 ± 0.01	45.24 ± 0.38	>100.00
Kuriloside D (**4**)	9.04 ± 0.54	11.58 ± 0.06	>100.00
Kuriloside E (**5**)	44.27 ± 0.80	96.80 ± 1.79	>100.00
Kuriloside F (**6**)	31.93 ± 0.44	49.81 ± 1.23	>100.00
Kuriloside A (**7**)	19.57 ± 0.32	23.02 ± 0.01	>100.00
Cladoloside C	0.31 ± 0.04	8.51 ± 0.12	11.92 ± 0.45

3. Materials and Methods

3.1. General Experimental Procedures

We used for specific rotation a Perkin-Elmer 343 Polarimeter (Perkin-Elmer, Waltham, MA, USA); for NMR, a Bruker Avance III 700 Bruker FT-NMR (Bruker BioSpin GmbH, Rheinstetten, Germany) (700.00/176.03 MHz) (^{1}H/^{13}C) spectrometer; for ESI MS (positive and negative ion modes), an Agilent 6510 Q-TOF apparatus (Agilent Technology, Santa Clara, CA, USA), sample concentration of 0.01 mg/mL; and for HPLC, an Agilent 1100 apparatus with a differential refractometer (Agilent Technology, Santa Clara, CA, USA). The column was a Supelco Discovery HS F5-5 (10 × 250 mm, 5 µm) (Supelco, inc., Bellefonte, PA, USA).

3.2. Animals and Cells

Specimens of the sea cucumber *Thyonidium* (= *Duasmodactyla*) *kurilensis* (Levin) (family Cucumariidae; order Dendrochirotida) were collected in August of 1990 using an industrial rake-type dredge in the waters of the Onekotan Island (Kurile islands, the Sea of Okhotsk) at a depth of 100 m by a middle fishing trawler "Breeze" with a rear scheme of trawling during scallop harvesting. The sea cucumbers were identified by Prof. V.S. Levin; voucher specimens are preserved in the A.V. Zhirmunsky National Scientific Center of Marine Biology, Vladivostok, Russia.

CD-1 mice, weighing 18–20 g, were purchased from the RAMS "Stolbovaya" nursery (Stolbovaya, Moscow District, Russia) and kept at the animal facility in standard conditions.

All experiments were performed following the protocol for animal study approved by the Ethics Committee of the Pacific Institute of Bioorganic Chemistry No. 0085.19.10.2020. All experiments were also conducted in compliance with all of the rules and international recommendations of the European Convention for the Protection of Vertebrate Animals Used for Experimental Studies.

Mouse epithelial JB-6 cells Cl 41-5a and mouse neuroblastoma cell line Neuro 2a (ATCC® CCL-131) were purchased from ATCC (Manassas, VA, USA).

3.3. Extraction and Isolation

The collected sea cucumbers were fixed by EtOH and then extracted twice with refluxing 60% EtOH. The extracts were evaporated to dryness and dissolved in water followed by chromatography on a Polychrom-1 column (powdered Teflon, Biolar, Latvia). The glycosides were eluted with 50% EtOH, and the fractions combined and evaporated. The first attempt to isolate the glycosides from another part of the sum was made in the early 1990s to obtain kurilosides A and C [10]. The remaining part of the crude glycosidic sum of *T. kurilensis* was stored at −18 °C. Then, it was separated by repeated chromatography on Si gel columns using $CHCl_3/EtOH/H_2O$ (100:100:17) and (100:125:25) as mobile phases to give five fractions (I–V). Fraction I was subsequently subjected to HPLC on a reversed-phase semipreparative Supelco Discovery HS F5-5 (10 × 250 mm) column with $MeOH/H_2O/NH_4OAc$ (1 M water solution) (70/29/1) as the mobile phase, resulting in the isolation of four subfractions (1–4) and an individual kuriloside C_1 (**3**) (2.6 mg). Each of the subfractions 1–4 was submitted to rechromatography on the same column but with different ratios of $MeOH/H_2O/NH_4OAc$ (1 M water solution) applied as the mobile phase. The use of the ratio (67/32/1) for subfraction 4 gave 12.6 mg of kuriloside A_1 (**1**); (61/38/1) applied for subfraction 3 gave 13 mg of kuriloside D (**4**) and 3.3 mg of kuriloside E (**5**); (60/39/1) applied for subfraction 2 gave 17 mg of kuriloside A_2 (**2**) and the same ratio used for the HPLC of subfraction 1 gave 42.4 mg of the known kuriloside A (**7**), as well as 4.5 mg of kuriloside F (**6**).

3.3.1. Kuriloside A_1 (**1**)

Colorless powder; $[\alpha]_D^{20}$ −5 (*c* 0.1, 50% MeOH). NMR: See Tables 1 and 2, Figures S1–S7. (−)HR-ESI-MS *m/z*: 1317.5449 (calc. 1317.5427) $[M_{Na}-Na]^-$; (−)ESI-MS/MS *m/z*: 1257.5 $[M_{Na}-Na-CH_3COOH]^-$, 1197.5 $[M_{Na}-Na-2CH_3COOH]^-$, 1035.4 $[M_{Na}-Na-2CH_3COOH-C_6H_{10}O_5 \text{ (Glc)}]^-$, 889.4 $[M_{Na}-Na-2CH_3COOH-C_6H_{10}O_5 \text{ (Glc)}-C_6H_{10}O_4 \text{ (Qui)}]^-$, 565.1 $[M_{Na}-Na-C_{28}H_{43}O_4 \text{ (Agl)}-C_6H_{10}O_5 \text{ (Glc)}-C_6H_{10}O_4 \text{ (Qui)}-H]^-$.

3.3.2. Kuriloside A_2 (**2**)

Colorless powder; $[\alpha]_D^{20}$ −4 (*c* 0.1, 50% MeOH). NMR: See Tables 1 and 3, Figures S8–S14. (−)HR-ESI-MS *m/z*: 1213.4964 (calc. 1213.4954) $[M_{Na}-Na]^-$; (−)ESI-MS/MS *m/z*: 1037.4 $[M_{Na}-Na-C_7H_{12}O_5 \text{ (MeGlc)}]^-$, 905.4 $[M_{Na}-Na-C_6H_{10}O_5 \text{ (Glc)}-C_6H_{10}O_4 \text{ (Qui)}]^-$, 565.1 $[M_{Na}-Na-C_{24}H_{35}O \text{ (Agl)}-C_6H_{10}O_5 \text{ (Glc)}-C_6H_{10}O_4 \text{ (Qui)}-H]^-$.

3.3.3. Kuriloside C_1 (**3**)

Colorless powder; $[\alpha]_D^{20}$ −4 (*c* 0.1, 50% MeOH). NMR: See Tables 2 and 4, Figures S15–S22. (−)HR-ESI-MS *m/z*: 1155.4923 (calc. 1155.4899) $[M_{Na}-Na]^-$; (−)ESI-MS/MS *m/z*: 1095.5 $[M_{Na}-Na-CH_3COOH]^-$, 1035.5 $[M_{Na}-Na-2CH_3COOH]^-$, 889.4 $[M_{Na}-Na-2CH_3COOH-C_6H_{10}O_4 \text{ (Qui)}]^-$, 565.1 $[M_{Na}-Na-C_{28}H_{43}O_4 \text{ (Agl)}-C_6H_{10}O_4 \text{ (Qui)}-H]^-$.

3.3.4. Kuriloside D (**4**)

Colorless powder; $[\alpha]_D^{20}$ −14 (*c* 0.1, 50% MeOH). NMR: See Tables 5 and 6, Figures S23–S31. (−)HR-ESI-MS *m/z*: 1489.6174 (calc. 1489.6163) $[M_{Na}-Na]^-$; (−)ESI-MS/MS *m/z*: 1349.5 $[M_{Na}-Na-C_8H_{13}O_2+H]^-$, 1187.5 $[M_{Na}-Na-C_8H_{13}O_2-C_6H_{10}O_5 \text{ (Glc)}]^-$, 1025.4 $[M_{Na}-Na-C_8H_{13}O_2-2C_6H_{10}O_5 \text{ (Glc)}]^-$, 879.4 $[M_{Na}-Na-C_8H_{13}O_2-2C_6H_{10}O_5 \text{ (Glc)}-C_6H_{10}O_4 \text{ (Qui)}]^-$, 565.1 $[M_{Na}-Na-C_{30}H_{45}O_3 \text{ (Agl)}-2C_6H_{10}O_5 \text{ (Glc)}-C_6H_{10}O_4 \text{ (Qui)}-H]^-$.

3.3.5. Kuriloside E (**5**)

Colorless powder; $[\alpha]_D^{20}$ −5 (*c* 0.1, 50% MeOH). NMR: See Tables 7 and 8, Figures S32–S40. (−)HR-ESI-MS *m/z*: 1231.5082 (calc. 1231.5059) $[M_{Na}-Na]^-$; (−)ESI-MS/MS *m/z*: 1069.5 $[M_{Na}-Na-C_6H_{10}O_5 \text{ (Glc)}]^-$, 1055.4 $[M_{Na}-Na-C_7H_{12}O_5 \text{ (MeGlc)}]^-$, 907.4 $[M_{Na}-Na-2C_6H_{10}O_5 \text{ (Glc)}]^-$, 565.1 $[M_{Na}-Na-C_{24}H_{37}O \text{ (Agl)}-2C_6H_{10}O_5 \text{ (Glc)}-H]^-$.

3.3.6. Kuriloside F (6)

Colorless powder; $[\alpha]_D^{20}$–1 (c 0.1, 50% MeOH). NMR: See Tables 9 and 10, Figures S41–S49. (−)HR-ESI-MS m/z: 1407.5778 (calc. 1407.5744) $[M_{Na}-Na]^-$; (−)ESI-MS/MS m/z: 1231.5 $[M_{Na}-Na-C_7H_{12}O_5$ (MeGlc)$]^-$, 1069.4 $[M_{Na}-Na-C_7H_{12}O_5$ (MeGlc)–$C_6H_{10}O_5$ (Glc)$]^-$, 923.4 $[M_{Na}-Na-C_7H_{12}O_5$ (MeGlc)–$C_6H_{10}O_5$ (Glc)–$C_6H_{10}O_4$ (Qui)$]^-$, 565.1 $[M_{Na}-Na-C_{24}H_{37}O_2$ (Agl)–$C_7H_{12}O_5$ (MeGlc)–$C_6H_{10}O_5$ (Glc)–$C_6H_{10}O_4$ (Qui)–H$]^-$.

3.3.7. Kuriloside A (7)

Colorless powder; See Tables 1 and 10, Figures S50–S58. (−)HR-ESI-MS m/z: 1273.5196 (calc. 1273.5165) $[M_{Na}-Na]^-$.

3.4. Cytotoxic Activity (MTT Assay)

All compounds were tested in concentrations from 1.5 µM to 100 µM using a two-fold dilution in dH$_2$O. The solutions (20 µL) of the tested substances in different concentrations and a cell suspension (180 µL) were added in the wells of 96-well plates (1 × 10^4 cells/well) and incubated for 24 h at 37 °C and at 5% CO$_2$. After incubation, the medium with the tested substances was replaced by 100 µL of fresh medium. Then, 10 µL of an MTT (thiazoyl blue tertrazolium bromide) stock solution (5 mg/mL) was added to each well and the microplate was incubated for 4 h. After that, 100 µL of sodium dodecyl sulfate (SDS)-HCl solution (1 g SDS/10 mL dH$_2$O/17 µL 6 N HCl) was added to each well followed by incubation for 18 h. The absorbance of the converted dye formazan was measured using a Multiskan FC microplate photometer (Thermo Fisher Scientific, Waltham, MA, USA) at a wavelength of 570 nm. The cytotoxic activity of the substances was calculated as the concentration that caused 50% metabolic cell activity inhibition (IC$_{50}$). All the experiments were made in triplicate, with a $p < 0.01$ indicating a significant difference.

3.5. Hemolytic Activity

Blood was taken from CD-1 mice (18–20 g). Erythrocytes were isolated from the blood of albino CD-1 mice by centrifugation with phosphate-buffered saline (pH 7.4) for 5 min at 4 °C and at 450× g (LABOFUGE 400R, Heraeus, Hanau, Germany), repeated three times. Then the residue of the erythrocytes was resuspended in an ice-cold phosphate saline buffer (pH 7.4) to a final optical density of 1.5 at 700 nm and kept on ice [16]. For the hemolytic assay, 180 µL of erythrocyte suspension was mixed with 20 µL of the test compound solution in V-bottom 96-well plates. After 1 h of incubation at 37 °C, the plates were exposed to centrifugation for 10 min at 900× g using a laboratory centrifuge (LMC-3000, Biosan, Riga, Latvia) [16]. Then, we carefully selected 100 µL of the supernatant and transferred it into new flat-plates, respectively. Lysis of erythrocytes was determined by measuring the concentration of hemoglobin in the supernatant with a microplate photometer (Multiskan FC, Themo Fisher Scientific, Waltham, MA, USA), with λ = 570 nm [17]. The effective dose causing 50% hemolysis of the erythrocytes (ED$_{50}$) was calculated using the computer program SigmaPlot 10.0. All the experiments were made in triplicate, with $p < 0.01$ indicating a significant difference.

4. Conclusions

It is known that triterpene glycosides of the sea cucumbers are formed by the mosaic type of biosynthesis [3,7]. From this viewpoint, the carbohydrate chains are biosynthesized independently from the aglycones by the stepwise glycosylation of the forming chain by individual monosaccharides, which bonded to certain positions only. Hence, the direction of the biosynthetic transformation of the sugar chains of compounds 1–7 is supposed to be as follows: the tetrasaccharide chain of the kurilosides of group C (known as kuriloside C [10] and C$_1$ (3)) is a precursor for the pentasaccharide chains of the kurilosides of group A (1, 2, 7); the subsequent glycosylation leads to the formation of a hexasaccharide chain of kuriloside D (4) and further attachment of the O-methyl group to C(3) of the terminal (fourth) residue, resulting in the formation of the chain of kuriloside F (6). The carbohydrate chain of kuriloside E (5) is obviously branching from the mainstream biosynthesis because the C(2)-position of the first (xylose) residue is glycosylated by the glucose residue instead of the quinovose residue, common for this position of kurilosides and attributed to the other groups. The rest of the monosaccharide units in the chain of 5 are the same as in the kurilosides of group A (1, 2, 7).

The biogenetic relationships of the aglycone parts of compounds 1–7 are presented in Figure 2. The precursor of the *nor*-lanostane aglycones is the derivative that has a normal side chain, with an oxygen-containing substituent at C(22), which is a necessary condition for the subsequent bond cleavage between 20 and 22 carbons with elimination of a side chain portion that leads to the formation of the 22,23,24,25,26,27-hexa-*nor*-lanostane (4,4,14-trimethyl-pregnane) aglycones without a lactone like in all glycosides of *T. kurilensis*, except for kuriloside D (4). In the process of forming of all the other aglycones of the kurilosides, side-chain cleavage occurs. The aglycone of kuriloside E (5) corresponds to this stage of biosynthesis. The introduction of an α-hydroxyl group to C(16) leads to the aglycone of kuriloside F (6). The introduction of a β-hydroxyl group to C(16) also occurs, but it quickly transformed to acetylated derivatives. The intermolecular dehydration of the 16-hydroxylated precursors leads to the aglycone of kuriloside A_2 (2). The acetylation of the 16α-hydroxy-group resulted in the synthesis of the aglycone of kuriloside A (7). The enzymatic 16β-O-acetylation followed by the reduction of the 20-keto group, with subsequent acetylation of this position, leads to the aglycones of kurilosides A_1 (1) and C_1 (3).

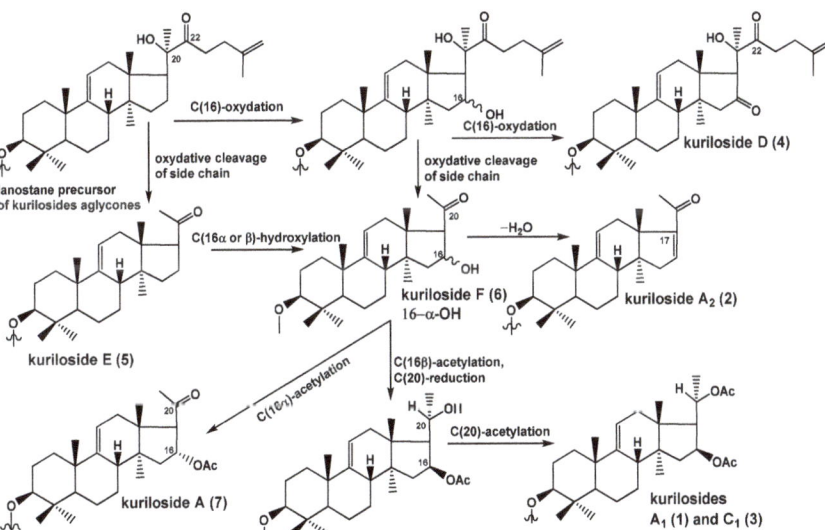

Figure 2. The biosynthetic pathways of the aglycones of the glycosides from *T. kurilensis*.

Supplementary Materials: The following are available online at http://www.mdpi.com/1660-3397/18/11/551/s1, Figure S1. The ^{13}C NMR (176.03 MHz) spectrum of kuriloside A_1 (1) in C_5D_5N/D_2O (4/1), Figure S2. The ^{1}H NMR (700.00 MHz) spectrum of kuriloside A_1 (1) in C_5D_5N/D_2O (4/1), Figure S3. The COSY (700.00 MHz) spectrum of the aglycone part of kuriloside A_1 (1) in C_5D_5N/D_2O (4/1), Figure S4. The HSQC (700.00 MHz) spectrum of the aglycone part of kuriloside A_1 (1) in C_5D_5N/D_2O (4/1), Figure S5. The ROESY (700.00 MHz) spectrum of the aglycone part of kuriloside A_1 (1) in C_5D_5N/D_2O (4/1), Figure S6. The HMBC (700.00 MHz) spectrum of the aglycone part of kuriloside A_1 (1) in C_5D_5N/D_2O (4/1), Figure S7. HR-ESI-MS and ESI-MS/MS spectra of kuriloside A_1 (1), Figure S8. The ^{13}C NMR (176.03 MHz) spectrum of kuriloside A_2 (2) in C_5D_5N/D_2O (4/1), Figure S9. The ^{1}H NMR (700.00 MHz) spectrum of kuriloside A_2 (2) in C_5D_5N/D_2O (4/1), Figure S10. The COSY (700.00 MHz) spectrum of the aglycone part of kuriloside A_2 (2) in C_5D_5N/D_2O (4/1), Figure S11. The HSQC (700.00 MHz) spectrum of the aglycone part of kuriloside A_2 (2) in C_5D_5N/D_2O (4/1), Figure S12. The HMBC (700.00 MHz) spectrum of the aglycone part of kuriloside A_2 (2) in C_5D_5N/D_2O (4/1), Figure S13. The ROESY

(700.00 MHz) spectrum of the aglycone part of kuriloside A$_2$ (2) in C$_5$D$_5$N/D$_2$O (4/1), Figure S14. HR-ESI-MS and ESI-MS/MS spectra of kuriloside A$_2$ (2), Figure S15. The ^{13}C NMR (176.03 MHz) spectrum of kuriloside C$_1$ (3) in C$_5$D$_5$N/D$_2$O (4/1), Figure S16. The ^{1}H NMR (700.00 MHz) spectrum of kuriloside C$_1$ (3) in C$_5$D$_5$N/D$_2$O (4/1), Figure S17. The COSY (700.00 MHz) spectrum of the carbohydrate part of kuriloside C$_1$ (3) in C$_5$D$_5$N/D$_2$O (4/1), Figure S18. The HSQC (700.00 MHz) spectrum of the carbohydrate part of kuriloside C$_1$ (3) in C$_5$D$_5$N/D$_2$O (4/1), Figure S19. The HMBC (700.00 MHz) spectrum of the carbohydrate part of kuriloside C$_1$ (3) in C$_5$D$_5$N/D$_2$O (4/1), Figure S20. The ROESY (700.00 MHz) spectrum of the carbohydrate part of kuriloside C$_1$ (3) in C$_5$D$_5$N/D$_2$O (4/1), Figure S21. 1 D TOCSY (700.00 MHz) spectra of the carbohydrate part of kuriloside C$_1$ (3) in C$_5$D$_5$N/D$_2$O (4/1), Figure S22. HR-ESI-MS and ESI-MS/MS spectra of kuriloside C$_1$ (3), Figure S23. The ^{13}C NMR (176.03 MHz) spectrum of kuriloside D (4) in C$_5$D$_5$N/D$_2$O (4/1), Figure S24. The ^{1}H NMR (700.00 MHz) spectrum of kuriloside D (4) in C$_5$D$_5$N/D$_2$O (4/1), Figure S25. The COSY (700.00 MHz) spectrum of kuriloside D (4) in C$_5$D$_5$N/D$_2$O (4/1), Figure S26. The HSQC (700.00 MHz) spectrum of kuriloside D (4) in C$_5$D$_5$N/D$_2$O (4/1), Figure S27. The ROESY (700.00 MHz) spectrum of kuriloside D (4) in C$_5$D$_5$N/D$_2$O (4/1), Figure S28. The HMBC (700.00 MHz) spectrum of kuriloside D (4) in C$_5$D$_5$N/D$_2$O (4/1), Figure S29. 1 D TOCSY (700.00 MHz) spectra of kuriloside D (4) in C$_5$D$_5$N/D$_2$O (4/1), Figure S30. 1 D TOCSY (700.00 MHz) spectra of kuriloside D (4) in C$_5$D$_5$N/D$_2$O (4/1), Figure S31. HR-ESI-MS and ESI-MS/MS spectra of kuriloside D (4), Figure S32. The ^{13}C NMR (176.03 MHz) spectrum of kuriloside E (5) in C$_5$D$_5$N/D$_2$O (4/1), Figure S33. The ^{1}H NMR (700.00 MHz) spectrum of kuriloside E (5) in C$_5$D$_5$N/D$_2$O (4/1), Figure S34. The COSY (700.00 MHz) spectrum of kuriloside E (5) in C$_5$D$_5$N/D$_2$O (4/1), Figure S35. The HSQC (700.00 MHz) spectrum of kuriloside E (5) in C$_5$D$_5$N/D$_2$O (4/1), Figure S36. The HMBC (700.00 MHz) spectrum of kuriloside E (5) in C$_5$D$_5$N/D$_2$O (4/1), Figure S37. The ROESY (700.00 MHz) spectrum of kuriloside E (5) in C$_5$D$_5$N/D$_2$O (4/1), Figure S38. 1D TOCSY (700.00 MHz) spectra of kuriloside E (5) in C$_5$D$_5$N/D$_2$O (4/1), Figure S39. 1D TOCSY (700.00 MHz) spectra of kuriloside E (5) in C$_5$D$_5$N/D$_2$O (4/1), Figure S40. HR-ESI-MS and ESI-MS/MS spectra of kuriloside E (5), Figure S41. The ^{13}C NMR (176.03 MHz) spectrum of kuriloside F (6) in C$_5$D$_5$N/D$_2$O (4/1), Figure S42. The ^{1}H NMR (700.00 MHz) spectrum of kuriloside F (6) in C$_5$D$_5$N/D$_2$O (4/1), Figure S43. The COSY (700.00 MHz) spectrum of kuriloside F (6) in C$_5$D$_5$N/D$_2$O (4/1), Figure S44. The HSQC (700.00 MHz) spectrum of kuriloside F (6) in C$_5$D$_5$N/D$_2$O (4/1), Figure S45. The ROESY (700.00 MHz) spectrum of kuriloside F (6) in C$_5$D$_5$N/D$_2$O (4/1), Figure S46. The HMBC (700.00 MHz) spectrum of kuriloside F (6) in C$_5$D$_5$N/D$_2$O (4/1), Figure S47. 1D TOCSY (700.00 MHz) spectra of the carbohydrate part of kuriloside F (6) in C$_5$D$_5$N/D$_2$O (4/1), Figure S48. 1D TOCSY (700.00 MHz) spectra of the carbohydrate part of kuriloside F (6) in C$_5$D$_5$N/D$_2$O (4/1), Figure S49. HR-ESI-MS and ESI-MS/MS spectra of kuriloside F (6), Figure S50. The ^{13}C NMR (176.03 MHz) spectrum of kuriloside A (7) in C$_5$D$_5$N/D$_2$O (4/1), Figure S51. The ^{1}H NMR (700.00 MHz) spectrum of kuriloside A (7) in C$_5$D$_5$N/D$_2$O (4/1), Figure S52. The COSY (700.00 MHz) spectrum of kuriloside A (7) in C$_5$D$_5$N/D$_2$O (4/1), Figure S53. The HSQC (700.00 MHz) spectrum of kuriloside A (7) in C$_5$D$_5$N/D$_2$O (4/1), Figure S54. The HMBC (700.00 MHz) spectrum of kuriloside A (7) in C$_5$D$_5$N/D$_2$O (4/1), Figure S55. The ROESY (700.00 MHz) spectrum of kuriloside A (7) in C$_5$D$_5$N/D$_2$O (4/1), Figure S56. 1 D TOCSY (700.00 MHz) spectra of kuriloside A (7) in C$_5$D$_5$N/D$_2$O (4/1), Figure S57. 1 D TOCSY (700.00 MHz) spectra of kuriloside A (7) in C$_5$D$_5$N/D$_2$O (4/1), Figure S58. HR-ESI-MS and ESI-MS/MS spectra of kuriloside A (7).

Author Contributions: Conceptualization, A.S.S., V.I.K.; methodology, A.S.S., S.A.A.; investigation, A.S.S., A.I.K., S.A.A., R.S.P., P.S.D., E.A.C., P.V.A.; writing—original draft preparation, A.S.S., V.I.K.; writing—review and editing, A.S.S., V.I.K. All authors have read and agreed to the published version of the manuscript.

Funding: The investigation was carried out with financial support from a grant of the Ministry of Science and Education, Russian Federation 13.1902.21.0012 (075-15-2020-796) (isolation of individual triterpene glycosides), and a grant of the Russian Foundation for Basic Research No. 19-04-000-14 (elucidation of structures of the glycosides and their biotesting).

Acknowledgments: The study was carried out with equipment of the Collective Facilities Center "The Far Eastern Center for Structural Molecular Research (NMR/MS) PIBOC FEB RAS". The authors are very appreciative to Valentin A. Stonik (PIBOC FEB RAS, Vladivostok, Russia) for reading and discussion of the manuscript.

Conflicts of Interest: The authors declare no conflict of interest.

References

1. Aminin, D.L.; Menchinskaya, E.S.; Pisliagin, E.A.; Silchenko, A.S.; Avilov, S.A.; Kalinin, V.I. Sea cucumber triterpene glycosides as anticancer agents. In *Studies in Natural Product Chemistry*; Atta-ur-Rahman, Ed.; Elsevier: Amsterdam, The Netherlands, 2016; Volume 49, pp. 55–105. [CrossRef]
2. Silchenko, A.S.; Kalinovsky, A.I.; Avilov, S.A.; Kalinin, V.I.; Andrijaschenko, P.V.; Dmitrenok, P.S.; Chingizova, E.A.; Ermakova, S.P.; Malyarenko, O.S.; Dautova, T.N. Nine new triterpene glycosides, magnumosides A1–A4, B2, C1, C2 and C4, from the Vietnamese sea cucumber Neothyonidium (=Massinum) magnum: Structures and activities against tumor cells independently and in synergy with radioactive irradiation. *Mar. Drugs* **2017**, *15*, 256. [CrossRef] [PubMed]

3. Kalinin, V.I.; Silchenko, A.S.; Avilov, S.A.; Stonik, V.A. Non-holostane aglycones of sea cucumber triterpene glycosides. Structure, biosynthesis, evolution. *Steroids* **2019**, *147*, 42–51. [CrossRef] [PubMed]
4. Silchenko, A.S.; Kalinovsky, A.I.; Avilov, S.A.; Dmitrenok, P.S.; Kalinin, V.I.; Berdyshev, D.V.; Chingizova, E.A.; Andryjaschenko, P.V.; Minin, K.V.; Stonik, V.A. Fallaxosides B_1 and D_3, triterpene glycosides with novel skeleton types of aglycones from the sea cucumber *Cucumaria fallax*. *Tetrahedron* **2017**, *73*, 2335–2341. [CrossRef]
5. Silchenko, A.S.; Kalinovsky, A.I.; Avilov, S.A.; Kalinin, V.I.; Andrijaschenko, P.V.; Dmitrenok, P.S.; Popov, R.S.; Chingizova, E.A. Structures and bioactivities of psolusosides B_1, B_2, J, K, L, M, N, O, P, and Q from the sea cucumber *Psolus fabricii*. The first finding of tetrasulfated marine low molecular weight metabolites. *Mar. Drugs* **2019**, *17*, 631. [CrossRef] [PubMed]
6. Silchenko, A.S.; Kalinovsky, A.I.; Avilov, S.A.; Kalinin, V.I.; Andrijaschenko, P.V.; Dmitrenok, P.S.; Chingizova, E.A.; Ermakova, S.P.; Malyarenko, O.S.; Dautova, T.N. Magnumosides B_3, B_4 and C_3, mono- and disulfated triterpene tetraosides from the Vietnamese sea cucumber *Neothyonidium* (=*Massinum*) *magnum*. *Nat. Prod. Commun.* **2017**, *12*, 1577–1582. [CrossRef]
7. Silchenko, A.S.; Kalinovsky, A.I.; Avilov, S.A.; Kalinin, V.I.; Andrijaschenko, P.V.; Dmitrenok, P.S.; Popov, R.S.; Chingizova, E.A.; Ermakova, S.P.; Malyarenko, O.S. Structures and bioactivities of six new triterpene glycosides, psolusosides E, F, G, H, H_1 and I and the corrected structure of psolusoside B from the sea cucumber *Psolus fabricii*. *Mar. Drugs* **2019**, *17*, 358. [CrossRef] [PubMed]
8. Kalinovskii, A.I.; Avilov, S.A.; Stepanov, V.R.; Stonik, V.A. Glycosides of marine invertebrates. XXIII. Kurilogenin—A new genin from the glycosides of the holothurian *Duasmodactyla kurilensis*. *Chem. Nat. Compd.* **1983**, *19*, 688–691. [CrossRef]
9. Avilov, S.A.; Kalinovskii, A.I. New triterpene aglycone from the holothurian *Duasmodactyla kurilensis*. *Chem. Nat. Compd.* **1989**, *25*, 309–311. [CrossRef]
10. Avilov, S.A.; Kalinovskii, A.I.; Stonik, V.A. Two new triterpene glycosides from the holothurian *Duasmodactyla kurilensis*. *Chem. Nat. Compd.* **1991**, *27*, 188–192. [CrossRef]
11. Silchenko, A.S.; Kalinovsky, A.I.; Avilov, S.A.; Andryjaschenko, P.V.; Dmitrenok, P.S.; Chingizova, E.A.; Dolmatov, I.Y.; Kalinin, V.I. Cladolosides I_1, I_2, J_1, K_1 and L_1, monosulfated triterpene glycosides with new carbohydrate chains from the sea cucumber *Cladolabes schmeltzii*. *Carbohydr. Res.* **2017**, *445*, 80–87. [CrossRef] [PubMed]
12. Avilov, S.A.; Antonov, A.S.; Silchenko, A.S.; Kalinin, V.I.; Kalinovsky, A.I.; Dmitrenok, P.S.; Stonik, V.A.; Riguera, R.; Jimenes, C. Triterpene glycosides from the Far Eastern sea cucumber *Cucumaria conicospermium*. *J. Nat. Prod.* **2003**, *66*, 910–916. [CrossRef] [PubMed]
13. Silchenko, A.S.; Avilov, S.A.; Kalinovsky, A.I.; Dmitrenok, P.S.; Kalinin, V.I.; Morre, J.; Deinzer, M.L.; Woodward, C.; Collin, P.D. Glycosides from the North Atlantic sea cucumber *Cucumaria frondosa* V—Structures of five new minor trisulfated triterpene oligoglycosides, frondosides A_7-1, A_7-3, A_7-4, and isofrondoside C. *Can. J. Chem.* **2007**, *85*, 626–636. [CrossRef]
14. Bahrami, Y.; Franko, C.M.M. Acetylated triterpene glycosides and their biological activity from Holothuroidea reported in the past six decades. *Mar. Drugs* **2016**, *14*, 147. [CrossRef] [PubMed]
15. Mondol, M.A.M.; Shin, H.J.; Rahman, M.A. Sea cucumber glycosides: Chemical structures, producing species and important biological properties. *Mar. Drugs* **2017**, *15*, 317. [CrossRef] [PubMed]
16. Taniyama, S.; Arakawa, O.; Terada, M.; Nishio, S.; Takatani, T.; Mahmud, Y.; Noguchi, T. *Ostreopsis* sp., a possible origin of palytoxin (PTX) in parrotfish *Scarus ovifrons*. *Toxicon* **2003**, *42*, 29–33. [CrossRef]
17. Malagoli, D. *A Full-Length Protocol to Test Hemolytic Activity of Palytoxin on Human Erythrocytes*; Technical Report; Department of Animal Biology, University of Modena and Reggio Emilia: Modena, Italy, 2007; pp. 92–94.

Publisher's Note: MDPI stays neutral with regard to jurisdictional claims in published maps and institutional affiliations.

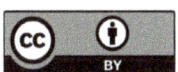

© 2020 by the authors. Licensee MDPI, Basel, Switzerland. This article is an open access article distributed under the terms and conditions of the Creative Commons Attribution (CC BY) license (http://creativecommons.org/licenses/by/4.0/).

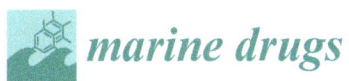

Article

New Conjugates of Polyhydroxysteroids with Long-Chain Fatty Acids from the Deep-Water Far Eastern Starfish *Ceramaster patagonicus* and Their Anticancer Activity

Timofey V. Malyarenko [1,2,*], Alla A. Kicha [1], Olesya S. Malyarenko [1], Viktor M. Zakharenko [2], Ivan P. Kotlyarov [2], Anatoly I. Kalinovsky [1], Roman S. Popov [1], Vasily I. Svetashev [3] and Natalia V. Ivanchina [1]

[1] G.B. Elyakov Pacific Institute of Bioorganic Chemistry, Far Eastern Branch of the Russian Academy of Sciences, Pr. 100-let Vladivostoku 159, Vladivostok 690022, Russia; kicha@piboc.dvo.ru (A.A.K.); malyarenko.os@gmail.com (O.S.M.); kaaniw@piboc.dvo.ru (A.I.K.); prs_90@mail.ru (R.S.P.); ivanchina@piboc.dvo.ru (N.V.I.)

[2] Department of Bioorganic Chemistry and Biotechnology, School of Natural Sciences, Far Eastern Federal University, Sukhanova Str. 8, Vladivostok 690000, Russia; rarf247@gmail.com (V.M.Z.); ivan_1999_19@icloud.com (I.P.K.)

[3] A.V. Zhirmunsky National Scientific Center of Marine Biology, Far Eastern Branch of the Russian Academy of Sciences, 17 Palchevsky St., Vladivostok 690041, Russia; vsvetashev@mail.ru

* Correspondence: malyarenko-tv@mail.ru; Tel.: +7-423-2312-360; Fax: +7-423-2314-050

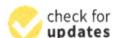

Received: 27 April 2020; Accepted: 13 May 2020; Published: 15 May 2020

Abstract: Four new conjugates, esters of polyhydroxysteroids with long-chain fatty acids (**1–4**), were isolated from the deep-water Far Eastern starfish *Ceramaster patagonicus*. The structures of **1–4** were established by NMR and ESIMS techniques as well as chemical transformations. Unusual compounds **1–4** contain the same 5α-cholestane-3β,6β,15α,16β,26-pentahydroxysteroidal moiety and differ from each other in the fatty acid units: 5′Z,11′Z-octadecadienoic (**1**), 11′Z-octadecenoic (**2**), 5′Z,11′Z-eicosadienoic (**3**), and 7′Z-eicosenoic (**4**) acids. Previously, only one such steroid conjugate with a fatty acid was known from starfish. After 72 h of cell incubation, using MTS assay it was found that the concentrations of compounds **1**, **2**, and **3** that caused 50% inhibition of growth (IC_{50}) of JB6 Cl41 cells were 81, 40, and 79 µM, respectively; for MDA-MB-231 cells, IC_{50} of compounds **1**, **2**, and **3** were 74, 33, and 73 µM, respectively; for HCT 116 cells, IC_{50} of compounds **1**, **2**, and **3** were 73, 31, and 71 µM, respectively. Compound **4** was non-toxic against tested cell lines even in three days of treatment. Compound **2** (20 µM) suppressed colony formation and migration of MDA-MB-231 and HCT 116 cells.

Keywords: polyhydroxysteroidal esters; NMR spectra; fatty acids; starfish; *Ceramaster patagonicus*; cytostatic activity; soft agar assay; wound healing assay

---

1. Introduction

Starfish (Echinodermata, Asteroidea) are a rich source of various secondary metabolites: peptides, fatty acids, polar steroids and their glycosides, carotenoids, quinone pigments, and also sphingolipids and their derivatives [1]. Polar steroid compounds are a major class of starfish secondary metabolites. They are polyhydroxysteroids; glycosides of polyhydroxysteroids (mono-, bi-, and triglycosides); cyclic glycosides; and asterosaponins –oligoglycosides containing 3β,6α-dihydroxysteroidal moieties with the a 9(11)-double bond and an O-sulfate group at C-3 [2–9]. Generally, polyhydroxysteroids have from four to nine hydroxyl groups: in the steroid nucleus at positions 3β (or more rarely 3α), 6α (or β), 8, 15α (or β), and 16β and, more rarely, at positions 4β, 5, 7α (or β), and 14; in the side chains at positions 26 and 24, or simultaneously in the side chain at 25 and 26 positions. The hydroxyl group can also be attached to C-28 or C-29 of the ergostane or stigmastane skeletons, respectively [2–9]. Starfish polyhydroxysteroids often occur in sulfated forms. Usually the sulfate group is located at C-3 or C-15 of the steroidal nucleus or at C-24 or C-26 of the side chain. Sometimes, starfish polyhydroxysteroids and related glycosides are found in the form of conjugates with amino acids. For example, several rare derivatives of starfish polyhydroxysteroids such as polyhydroxysteroid amides conjugated with taurine were isolated from the Arctic starfish *Asterias microdiscus* [10]. In addition, only one rare steroidal ester of polyhydroxysteroid with long-chain fatty acid, (25S)-5α-cholestane-3β,6α,7α,8,15α,16β-hexaol-26-yl 14′Z-eicosenoate, was isolated from the starfish *Asterina pectinifera* [11].

Starfish polar steroids have been reported to show a wide spectrum of biological activities, including cytotoxic, antiviral, antibacterial, neuritogenic, and anticancer effects [1–9]. Some starfish polyhydroxylated compounds have been shown to exhibit significant cytotoxicity. For example, certonardosterol D_2 revealed cytotoxic effects with effective doses that inhibited a viability of 50% cells (ED_{50}) against human lung cancer A549 (ED_{50} = 0.15 μg/mL), melanoma SK-MEL-2 (ED_{50} = 0.09 μg/mL), ovarian cancer SK-OV-3 (ED_{50} = 0.08 μg/mL), CNS cancer XF498 (ED_{50} = 0.07 μg/mL), and colon cancer HCT15 (ED_{50} = 0.01 μg/mL) cell lines [12]. However, (25S)-5α-cholestane-3β,6α,7α,8,15α,16β-hexaol-26-yl 14′Z-eicosenoate did not possess inhibitory activity against herpes simplex virus type 1 (HSV-1) and human liver carcinoma HepG2 cells in vitro [11].

Herein, we report the results of the structural elucidation of four new polyhydroxysteroidal esters (**1–4**) with fatty acids from the methanol chloroform ethanolic extract of the deep-water Far Eastern starfish *Ceramaster patagonicus* collected at the Sea of Okhotsk near Iturup Island. We examined the cytotoxic and cytostatic activities of **1–4** on mouse normal epidermal, human breast cancer, and colorectal carcinoma cells. In addition, the effects of these compounds on the colony formation and migration of human breast cancer and colorectal carcinoma cells were investigated using soft agar and wound healing assays.

2. Results and Discussion

2.1. The Isolation and Structure Elucidation of Compounds 1–4 from C. patagonicus

The concentrated methanol chloroform ethanolic extract of *C. patagonicus* was partitioned between H_2O and AcOEt/BuOH, and the organic layer was washed with cold acetone. The acetone-soluble part was subjected to separation by chromatography on silica gel column followed by HPLC on semi-preparative Diasfer-110-C18 column to obtain four new polyhydroxysteroidal compounds: (25S)-5α-cholestane-3β,6β,15α,16β-tetraol-26-yl 5′Z,11′Z-octadecadienoate (**1**), (25S)-5α-cholestane-3β,6β,15α,16β-tetraol-26-yl 11′Z-octadecenoate (**2**), (25S)-5α-cholestane-3β,6β,15α,16β-tetraol-26-yl 5′Z,11′Z-eicosadienoate (**3**), and (25S)-5α-cholestane- 3β,6β,15α,16β-tetraol-26-yl 7′Z-eicosenoate (**4**) (Figure 1).

The IR spectrum of compound **1** showed the presence of hydroxyl (3504 cm^{-1}), ester carbonyl (1723 cm^{-1}), and olefinic (1602 cm^{-1}) groups. The molecular formula of compound **1** was determined to be $C_{45}H_{78}O_6$ from the [M + Na]$^+$ sodiated adduct ion peak at *m/z* 737.5695 in the (+)HRESIMS, the [(M − H) + AcOH]$^-$ ion peak at *m/z* 773.5934, and the [M − H]$^-$ deprotonated ion peak at *m/z* 713.5726 in the (−)HRESIMS (Figures S1 and S2). The ^{1}H- and ^{13}C-NMR spectroscopic data belonging to the tetracyclic moiety of **1** showed the resonances of protons and carbons of two angular methyls, CH$_3$-18 and CH$_3$-19 (δ_H 1.27 s, 1.47 s; δ_C 14.9, 16.2), and four oxygenated methines, HC-3 (δ_H 3.99 m; δ_C 71.1), HC-6 (δ_H 4.15 brs; δ_C 71.2), HC-15 (δ_H 4.40 brd (*J* = 10.0); δ_C 84.7), and HC-16 (δ_H 4.66 brd (*J* = 7.3); δ_C 82.2) (Table 1, Figures S4–S12). The NMR spectra of steroidal side chain indicated the existence of two secondary methyls, CH$_3$-21 (δ_H 1.13 d (*J* = 6.8); δ_C 18.3) and CH$_3$-27 (δ_H 0.94 d (*J* = 6.8); δ_C 17.0), and one oxygenated methylene, H$_2$C-26 (δ_H 4.11 dd (*J* = 10.6, 5.4), 3.96 dd (*J* = 10.6, 6.8);

δ_C 69.1) (Table 1, Figures S4–S12). The ^{1}H-^{1}H COSY and HSQC correlations attributable to steroidal moiety revealed the corresponding sequences of protons at C-1 to C-8; C-8 to C-12 through C-9 and C-11; C-8 to C-17 through C-14; C-17 to C-21, and C-20 to the end of the side chain (Figure 2A, Figures S13–S16). The key HMBC cross-peaks, such as H-1/C-10, C-19; H-4/C-5, C-6; H-7/C-8; H-14/C-7, C-8, C-13, C-15, C-18; H-17/C-13, C-20; H$_3$-18/C-12, C-13, C-14, C-17; H$_3$-19/C-1, C-5, C-9, C-10; H$_3$-21/C-17, C-20, C-22; H$_2$-26/C-24, C-25, C-27; and H$_3$-27/C-24, C-25, C-26 confirmed the overall structure of the steroidal part of **1** (Figure 2A, Figures S17 and S18).

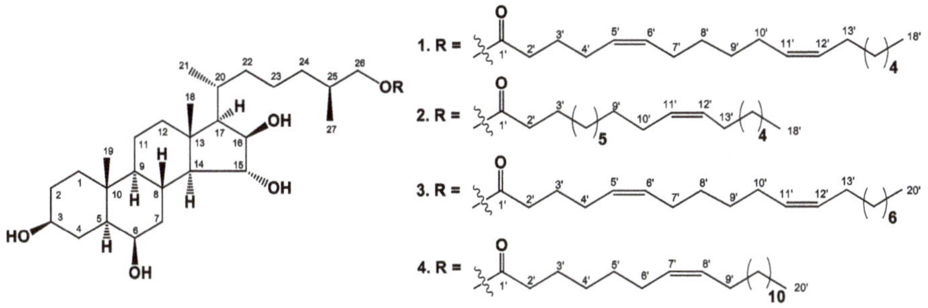

Figure 1. The structures of compounds **1–4** isolated from *C. patagonicus*.

Table 1. ^{1}H- (700.13 MHz) and ^{13}C- (176.04 MHz) NMR chemical shifts of the steroidal moiety of **1–4** in C$_5$D$_5$N at 30 °C, with δ in ppm and J values in Hz.

Position	δ_H	δ_C	Position	δ_H	δ_C
1	1.76 dt (11.4, 3.5) 1.10 m	39.1	15	4.40 brd (10.0)	84.7
2	2.13 m 1.86 m	32.5	16	4.66 brd (7.3)	82.2
3	3.99 m	71.1	17	1.55 dd (11.1, 7.3)	59.3
4	2.45 m 2.04 brd (12.2)	37.0	18	1.27 s	14.9
5	1.35 m	48.3	19	1.47 s	16.2
6	4.15 brd (2.6)	71.2	20	2.35 m	30.0
7	2.95 dt (14.2, 3.5) 1.82 m	41.2	21	1.13 d (6.8)	18.3
8	2.55 qd (11.1, 3.5)	30.8	22	1.92 m 1.28 m	36.4
9	0.96 m	54.9	23	1.60 m 1.39 m	23.9
10	–	36.0	24	1.41 m 1.17 m	34.0
11	1.64 m 1.59 m	21.2	25	1.82 m	32.8
12	2.10 m 1.36 m	41.1	26	4.11 dd (10.6, 5.4) 3.96 dd (10.6, 6.8)	69.1
13	–	43.9	27	0.94 d (6.8)	17.0
14	1.45 t (10.4)	61.0			

δ_H-chemical shift of proton (ppm); δ_C-chemical shift of carbon (ppm); s-singlet; d-doublet; t-triplet; m-multiplet; brd-broad doublet; dd-doublet of doublets; dt-doublet of triplets; qd-quartet of doublets.

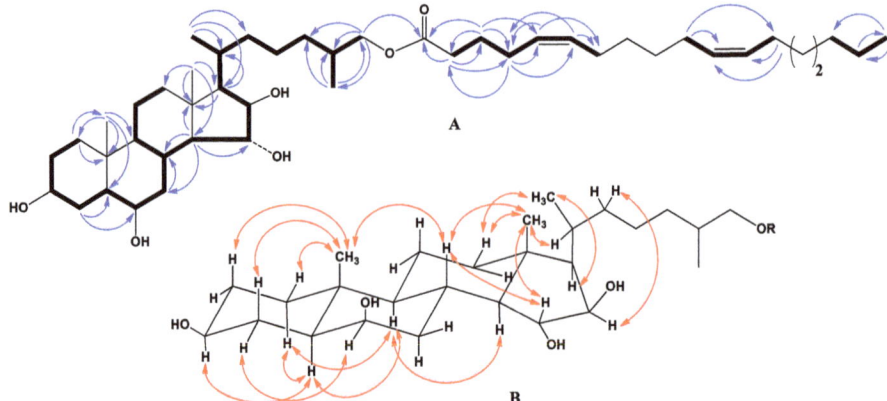

Figure 2. (**A**) ^{1}H-^{1}H COSY and key HMBC correlations for compound **1**. (**B**) Key ROESY correlations of steroidal moiety for compounds **1**–**4**.

The key ROESY cross-peaks showed the common 5α/9α/10β/13β stereochemistry of the steroidal nucleus, 3β,6β,15α,16β-configurations of oxygenated substituents and 26-hydroxycholestane side chain in **1** (Figure 2B, Figures S19 and S20). The 20*R*-configuration was assumed on the basis of ROESY correlations of H$_3$-18/H-20, H$_\beta$-16/H-22, and H$_3$-21/H$_\beta$-12 (Figure 2B, Figures S19 and S20). ^{1}H- and ^{13}C-NMR data of the steroidal part of compound **1** were practically identical to those of (25*S*)-5α-cholestane-3β,6β,15α,16β,26-pentaol, which was isolated for the first time from the starfish *Hacelia attenuata* [13] and later from the starfish *C. patagonicus* [14], which confirmed the identity of the steroid parts of these compounds and indicated the 25*S*-configuration of the side chain of **1**. Based on these data, the steroidal moiety of **1** was determined as (20*R*,25*S*)-5α-cholestane-3β,6β,15α,16β,26-pentaol.

In addition, the ^{1}H- and ^{13}C-NMR spectra of compound **1** indicated the presence of one primary methyl, CH$_3$-18' (δ_H 0.88 t (*J* = 6.9); δ_C 14.0); four olefinic methines, HC-5' (δ_H 5.44 m; δ_C 128.9), HC-6' (δ_H 5.51 m; δ_C 130.9), HC-11' (δ_H 5.48 m; δ_C 129.8), and HC-12' (δ_H 5.49 m; δ_C 130.1); two characteristic allyl methylenes, H$_2$C-4' (δ_H 2.17 m; δ_C 26.7) and H$_2$C-7' (δ_H 2.10 m; δ_C 27.4); one ester carbonyl (δ_C 173.3); and one characteristic methylene, H$_2$C-2' (δ_H 2.43 t (*J* = 7.4); δ_C 33.7), located at the α-position from ester carbonyl group (Table 2, Figures S4–S12). The (−)ESIMS/MS of the ion [M − H]$^-$ at *m/z* 713 contained the fragment ion peaks at *m/z* 449 [C$_{27}$H$_{45}$O$_5$]$^-$, corresponding to the loss of long-chain fatty acid residue, and at *m/z* 279 [C$_{18}$H$_{31}$O$_2$]$^-$, corresponding to the loss of steroidal moiety. The ^{1}H-^{1}H COSY and HSQC correlations attributable to fatty acid unit revealed the corresponding sequences of protons at C-2' to C-7', C-10' to C-13', and C-16' to C-18' (Figure 2A, Figures S13–S16), while the key HMBC cross-peaks, such as H-2'/C-1', C-3', C-4'; H-3'/C-1', C-2', C-4', C-5'; H-4'/C-2', C-5', C-6'; H-5'/C-4', C-7'; and H-6'/C-4', C-7', confirmed the localization of Δ$^{5(6)}$-double bound in the fatty acid unit of **1** (Figure 2A, Figures S17 and S18). The geometry of the double bond in the long-chain fatty acids can be determined on the basis of the ^{13}C-NMR chemical shift of the methylene carbon adjacent to the olefinic carbon (δ_C ≈ 27 for (*Z*) isomers and δ_C ≈ 32 for (*E*) isomers). ^{13}C-NMR spectrum of compound **1** indicated the presence of four characteristic allyl carbons: C-4' (δ_C 26.7), C-7' (δ_C 27.4), C-10' (δ_C 27.4), and C-13' (δ_C 27.1). Thus, the olefin groups in **1** were determined to have *cis* (*Z*) geometry. Compound **1** was methanolyzed with methanolic hydrochloric acid to give the fatty acid methyl esters (FAME-1) of **1**. Additionally, 4,4-dimethyloxazoline derivatives (DMOXs-1) of fatty acids of compound **1** were prepared from FAME-1 according to the procedure described previously [15]. This method allows for determining double bond in polyunsaturated fatty acids. Fatty acids were identified by equivalent chain length (ECL) values in GC analysis and mass spectra of FAME-1 and DMOXs-1 derivatives in GC-MS [15,16]. GC-MS analysis showed the existence of one major component, which was characterized as methyl 5′Z,11′Z-octadecadienoate. Minor components and their percentage are shown in Table 3. On the basis of all the above-mentioned data, the structure of **1** was determined to be (25S)-5α-cholestane-3β,6β,15α,16β-tetraol-26-yl 5′Z,11′Z-octadecadienoate. It should be noted that NMR, MS, TLC, and HPLC analyses indicated the homogeneity of compounds **1–4**; however, GLC-MS analysis of methyl ester of fatty acids **1–4** showed the presence of other fatty acids.

Table 2. ^{1}H- (700.13 MHz) and ^{13}C- (176.04 MHz) NMR chemical shifts of the fatty acid units of **1–4** in C$_5$D$_5$N at 30 °C, with δ in ppm and J values in Hz.

Position	1		2		3		4	
	δ$_H$	δ$_C$	δ$_H$	δ$_C$	δ$_H$	δ$_C$	δ$_H$	δ$_C$
1′	–	173.3	–	173.3	–	173.1	–	173.3
2′	2.43 t (7.4)	33.7	2.40 t (7.5)	34.3	2.43 t (7.2)	33.6	2.40 t (7.5)	34.2
3′	1.80 m	25.2	1.70 m	25.1	1.80 m	25.2	1.71 m	25.1
4′	2.17 m	26.7			2.17 q (7.2)	26.7		
5′	5.44 m	128.9			5.46 m	128.9		
6′	5.51 m	130.9			5.51 m	130.9	2.11 m	27.3
7′	2.10 m	27.4			2.10 m	27.4	5.50 m	130.2
10′	2.11 m	27.4	2.11 m	27.3	2.11 m	27.4	5.48 m	129.7
11′	5.48 m	129.8	5.49 m	130.0	5.49 m	129.8	2.11 m	27.1
12′	5.49 m	130.1	5.49 m	130.0	5.50 m	130.1		
13′	2.11 m	27.1	2.11 m	27.1	2.11 m	27.1		
16′ or 18′	1.25 m	31.7	1.25 m	31.8	1.25 m	31.9	1.25 m	31.8
17′ or 19′	1.28 m	22.7	1.28 m	22.8	1.28 m	22.7	1.28 m	22.8
18′ or 20′	0.88 t (6.9)	14.0	0.87 t (6.9)	14.0	0.88 t (7.0)	14.0	0.89 t (6.9)	14.0

Table 3. Fatty acid composition of compounds **1–4** based on GC-MS analysis.

Fatty Acids	Content, %			
	1	2	3	4
16:0	14.91	9.36	11.83	5.88
Δ^7-16:1	5.11	0.75	5.06	1.07
18:0	11.23	8.92	8.13	8.03
Δ^5-18:1	1.62	4.62	17.05	0.57
Δ^9-18:1	5.97	6.53	6.65	4.83
Δ^{11}-18:1	4.06	51.16	3.92	2.05
Δ^{5,11}-18:2	53.31		3.73	6.14
Δ^7-20:1		8.86	3.50	66.67
Δ^9-20:1			0.63	3.88
Δ^{5,11}-20:2	3.78	9.79	39.51	0.87
Total	100.00	100.00	100.00	100.00

The IR spectrum of compound **2** showed the presence of hydroxyl (3504 cm^{-1}), ester carbonyl (1723 cm^{-1}), and olefinic (1602 cm^{-1}) groups. The molecular formula of compound **2** was determined to be C$_{45}$H$_{80}$O$_6$ from the [M + Na]$^+$ sodiated adduct ion peak at m/z 739.5852 in the (+)HRESIMS, the [(M − H) + AcOH]$^-$ ion peak at m/z 775.6096, and the [M − H]$^-$ deprotonated ion peak at m/z 715.5889 in the (−)HRESIMS (Figures S21 and S22). The comparison of the molecular masses of **1** and **2** showed that the difference between **1** and **2** is 2 atomic mass units (amu). The comparison of ^{1}H- and

^{13}C-NMR spectra and application of extensive 2D NMR analysis of compounds **1** and **2–4** exhibited that steroidal moieties of **2–4** are identical to that of compound **1**, while long-chain fatty acid residues of **1–4** differ from each other by the length of the hydrocarbon chains and the number and positions of double bonds (Figure 1, Tables 1 and 2).

The ^{1}H- and ^{13}C-NMR spectra of fatty acid residue of compound **2** indicated the existence of one primary methyl, CH$_3$-18' (δ_H 0.87 t (J = 6.9); δ_C 14.0); two olefinic methines, HC-11' and HC-12' (2H, each δ_H 5.49 m; δ_C 130.0); two characteristic allyl methylenes, H$_2$C-10' (δ_H 2.11 m; δ_C 27.3) and H$_2$C-13' (δ_H 2.11 m; δ_C 27.1); one ester carbonyl (δ_C 173.3); and one characteristic methylene, H$_2$C-2' (δ_H 2.40 t (J = 7.5); δ_C 34.3), located at the α-position from ester carbonyl group (Table 2, Figures S24 and S25). The (−)ESIMS/MS of the ion [M − H]$^-$ at m/z 715 contained the fragment ion peaks at m/z 449 [C$_{27}$H$_{45}$O$_5$]$^-$, corresponding to the loss of long-chain fatty acid, and m/z 281 [C$_{18}$H$_{33}$O$_2$]$^-$, corresponding to the loss of steroidal moiety. Difference of 2 amu between fragment ion peaks at m/z 281 [C$_{18}$H$_{33}$O$_2$]$^-$ and 279 [C$_{18}$H$_{31}$O$_2$]$^-$ in the (−)ESIMS/MS mass spectra of compounds **2** and **1** indicated the absence of one double bond in the fatty acid moiety of compound **2** compared to **1** (Figures S3 and S23). The comparison of ^{1}H- and ^{13}C-NMR data of **2** and **1** also confirmed this conclusion (Table 2, Figures S4–S12 and S24, S25). The *cis* (Z) geometry of the double bond in the long-chain fatty acid moiety of **2** can be determined on the basis of the ^{13}C-NMR chemical shift of the C-10' (δ_C 27.3) and C-13' (δ_C 27.1).

Fatty acid units in **2** were identified by ECL values of fatty acids in GC analysis and mass spectra of FAME-2 and DMOXs-2 derivatives in GC-MS [16] similar to compound **1**. GC-MS analysis showed the existence of one major component, which was identified as methyl 11'Z-octadecenoate. Minor components and their percentage are shown in Table 3. Thereby, the structure of **2** was established to be (25S)-5α-cholestane-3β,6β,15α,16β-tetraol-26-yl 11'Z-octadecenoate.

The IR spectrum of compound **3** showed the presence of hydroxyl (3510 cm^{-1}), ester carbonyl (1723 cm^{-1}), and olefinic (1603 cm^{-1}) groups. The molecular formula of compound **3** was determined to be C$_{47}$H$_{82}$O$_6$ from the [M + Na]$^+$ sodiated adduct ion peak at m/z 765.6008 in the (+)HRESIMS, the [(M − H) + AcOH]$^-$ ion peak at m/z 801.6254, and the [M − H]$^-$ deprotonated ion peak at m/z 741.6044 in the (−)HRESIMS (Figures S30 and S31). The comparison of the molecular masses of **1** and **3** showed that the difference between them is 28 amu. At the same time, the ^{1}H- and ^{13}C-NMR spectra of compounds **1** and **3** were almost identical (Tables 1 and 2, Figures S4–S12 and S33, S34). The (−)ESIMS/MS of the ion [M − H]$^-$ at m/z 741 contained the fragment ion peaks at m/z 449 [C$_{27}$H$_{45}$O$_5$]$^-$, corresponding to the loss of long-chain fatty acid, and m/z 307 [C$_{20}$H$_{35}$O$_2$]$^-$, corresponding to the loss of steroidal moiety. Fatty acid units in **3** were identified by ECL values of fatty acids in GC analysis and mass spectra of FAME-3 and DMOXs-3 derivatives in GC-MS [15,16]. GC-MS analysis showed the existence of one major component, which was identified as methyl 5'Z,11'Z-eicosadienoate. Accordingly, the structure of **3** was determined to be (25S)-5α-cholestane-3β,6β,15α,16β-tetraol-26-yl 5'Z,11'Z-eicosadienoate. The *cis* (Z) geometry of the double bond in the long-chain fatty acid moiety of **3** can be determined on the basis of the ^{13}C-NMR chemical shift of the C-10' (δ_C 27.3) and C-13' (δ_C 27.1).

The IR spectrum of compound **4** showed the presence of hydroxyl (3515 cm^{-1}), ester carbonyl (1723 cm^{-1}), and olefinic (1602 cm^{-1}) groups. The molecular formula of compound **4** was determined to be C$_{47}$H$_{84}$O$_6$ from the [M + Na]$^+$ sodiated adduct ion peak at m/z 767.6157 in the (+)HRESIMS, the [(M − H) + AcOH]$^-$ ion peak at m/z 803.6409, and the [M − H]$^-$ deprotonated ion peak at m/z 743.6199 in the (−)HRESIMS (Figures S39 and S40). The comparison of the molecular masses of **3** and **4** showed the difference of 2 amu between **3** and **4**. The (−)ESIMS/MS of the ion [M − H]$^-$ at m/z 743 contained the fragment ion peaks at m/z 449 [C$_{27}$H$_{45}$O$_5$]$^-$, corresponding to the loss of long-chain fatty acid, and m/z 309 [C$_{20}$H$_{37}$O$_2$]$^-$, corresponding to the loss of steroidal moiety. Fatty acids were identified in the same manner as for other compounds [15,16]. GC-MS analysis showed the existence of one major component, which was characterized as methyl 7'Z-eicosenoat. On the basis of these results, the structure of **4** was determined to be (25S)-5α-cholestane-3β,6β,15α,16β-tetraol-26-yl 7'Z-eicosenoate.

2.2. In Vitro Anticancer Activity of Compounds 1–4

2.2.1. The Cytotoxic Activity of Compounds 1–4 against Normal and Cancer Cells

At the first stage of biological activity evaluation, the cytotoxicity of compounds 1–4 against mouse normal epidermal JB6 Cl41 cells, human breast cancer MDA-MB-231 cells, and colorectal carcinoma HCT 116 cells was determined by MTS assay, which is based on the cleavage of (3-(4,5-dimethylthiazol-2-yl)-5-(3-carboxymethoxyphenyl)-2-(4-sulfophenyl)-2H-tetrazolium) (MTS reagent) into a formazan product soluble in tissue culture medium. It was found that compounds 1–4 suppressed the cell viability by less than 15% at 100 µM after 24 h of incubation (Figure S48).

Many natural compounds do not possess direct cytotoxic activity but are able to suppress cell viability time-dependently [17]. That is why the cytostatic activity of compounds 1–4 was determined against JB6 Cl41, MDA-MB-231, and HCT 116 cell lines for 24, 48, and 72 h. After 72 h cell incubation, it was shown that the concentrations of compounds 1, 2, and 3 that caused 50% inhibition of growth (IC_{50}) of JB6 Cl41 cells were 81, 40, and 79 µM, respectively (Figure 3A); for MDA-MB-231 cells, IC_{50} concentrations of compounds 1, 2, and 3 were 74, 33, and 73 µM, respectively; for HCT 116 cells, IC_{50} concentrations of compounds 1, 2, and 3 were 73, 31, and 71 µM, respectively (Figure 3). The cytostatic effect of 2 was more prominent in colorectal carcinoma HCT 116 cells.

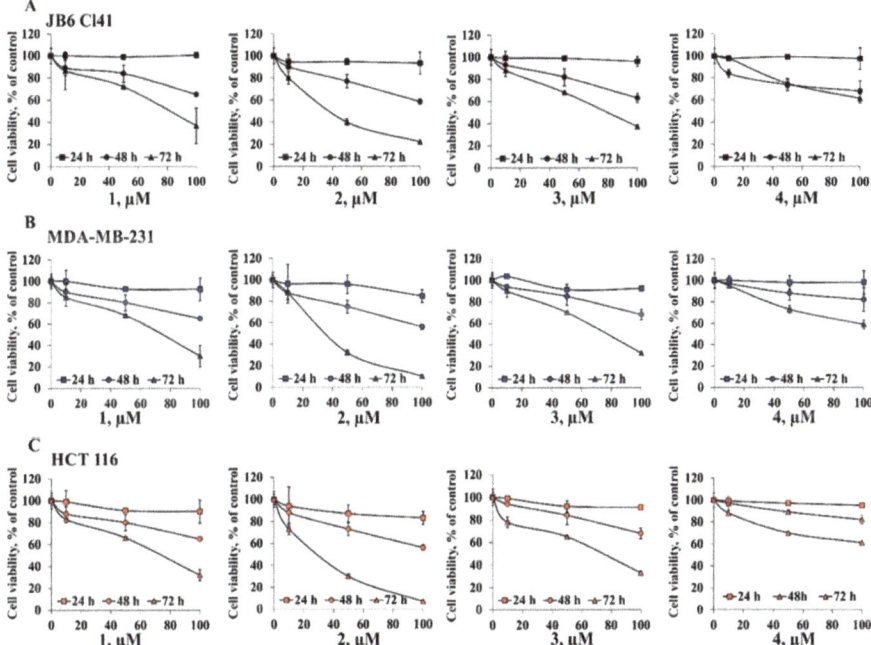

Figure 3. The cytostatic activity of compounds 1–4 against normal epidermal JB6 Cl41 cells, breast cancer MDA-MB-231 cells, and colorectal carcinoma HCT 116 cells. (**A**) JB6 Cl41, (**B**) MDA-MB-231, or (**C**) HCT 116 cells were treated with compounds 1–4 at concentrations of 1–100 µM for 24, 48, and 72 h. Cell viability was estimated using the MTS assay. Data are represented as the mean ± SD as determined from triplicate experiments.

It should be noted that investigated compounds did not exert a selective effect on cancer cells, because the viability of normal cells was suppressed as well. Therefore we checked the assumption whether compounds 1–4 were able to influence the process of carcinogenesis (colony formation, growth, and migration of cancer cells) at the non-toxic concentration of 20 µM.

2.2.2. The Effect of Compounds 1–4 on the Colony Formation and Growth of Human Cancer Cells

The formation of colonies is one of the most stringent characteristics for malignant transformation in cells [18]. In the present study the soft agar assay was used to investigate the effect of compounds 1–4 on capability of cancer cells to form colonies.

It was found that compounds 1, 2, 3, and 4 inhibited colony formation in MDA-MB-231 cells by 17%, 26%, 15%, and 10%, respectively. Meanwhile, compounds 1, 2, 3, and 4 inhibited colony formation in HCT 116 cells by 20%, 27%, 18%, and 16%, respectively. Compound 2 possessed comparable inhibitory activity against colony formation of both types of cancer cell lines (Figure 4).

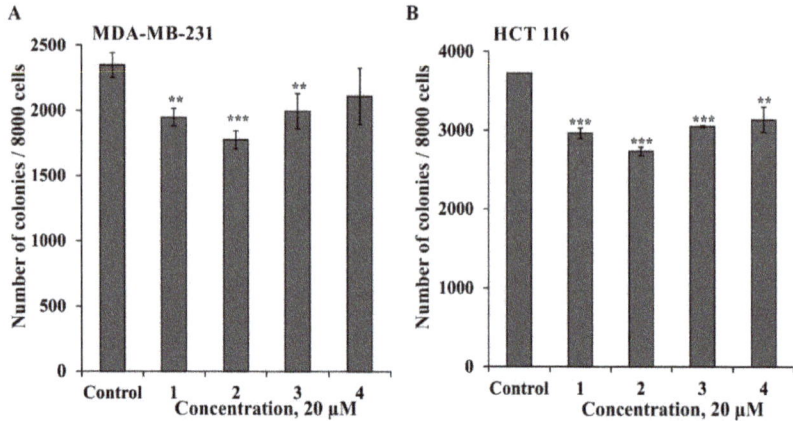

Figure 4. The effect of compounds 1–4 on colony formation in human cancer cells. MDA-MB-231 (**A**) or HCT 116 cells (**B**) (2.4×10^4) were treated with or without investigated compounds (20 µM) and applied onto 0.3% Basal Medium Eagle (BME) agar containing 10% FBS, 2 mM L-glutamine, and 25 µg/mL gentamicin. After 14 days of incubation, the number of colonies was evaluated under a microscope with the aid of the ImageJ software program. Results are expressed as the mean ± standard deviation (SD). The asterisks (** $p < 0.01$, *** $p < 0.001$) indicate a significant decrease in colony number of cancer cells treated by compounds compared with control.

2.2.3. The Effect of Compounds 1–4 on Migration of Human Cancer Cells

The metastasis process is proven to be the leading cause of cancer-related death. Metastasis is a multistep process that includes migration and invasion of cancer cells, hallmarks of malignancy [19]. Therefore, we investigated the ability of compounds 1–4 to inhibit the migration of breast cancer MDA-MB-231 cells and colorectal carcinoma HCT 116 cells with high metastatic potential. It was demonstrated that compounds 1 and 2 (at concentration 20 µM) were able to prevent migration of MDA-MB-231 cells by 42% and 50%, respectively, compared to control after 48 h of incubation (Figure 5). Compounds 3 and 4 possessed moderate inhibitory activity against migration of MDA-MB-231 cells. On the other hand, the migration of HCT 116 cells was almost completely inhibited by compound 2 (with the percentage of migration prevention being 73%). Compounds 1, 3, and 4 prevented HCT 116 cell migration by 36%, 30%, and 24%, respectively (Figure 5). Compounds 1, 3, and 4 prevented HCT 116 cell migration by 36%, 30%, and 24%, respectively (Figure 5).

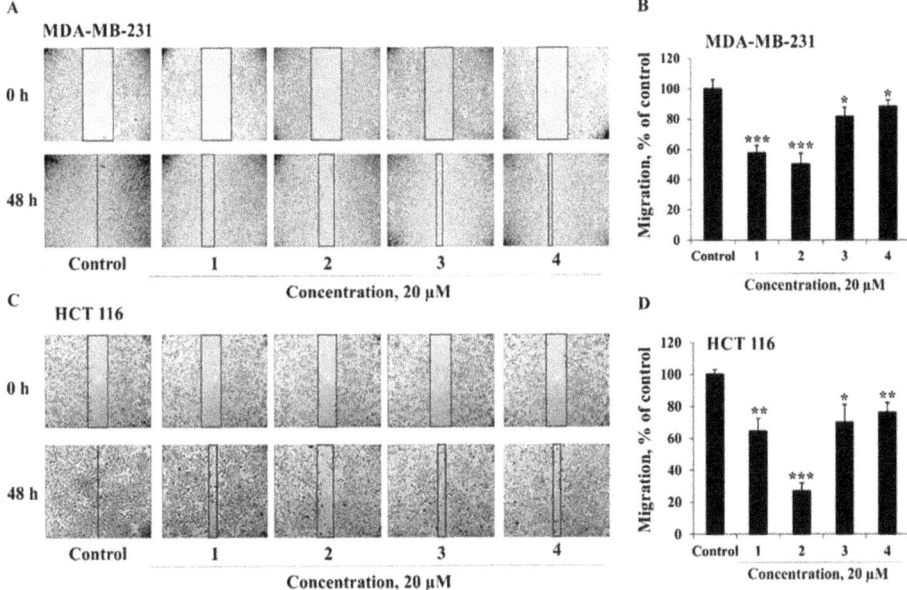

Figure 5. The effect of compounds 1–4 on migration of human cancer cells. MDA-MB-231 (**A**,**B**) and HCT 116 (**C**,**D**) cells migration distance was estimated by measuring the width of the wound and expressed as a percentage of each control for the mean of wound closure area. All experiments were repeated at least three times in each group (n = 18 for control and each compound, n—quantity of photos). The magnification of representative photos is ×10. Results are expressed as the mean ± standard deviation (SD). The asterisks (* $p < 0.05$, ** $p < 0.01$, *** $p < 0.001$) indicate a significant decrease in migration of cells treated with compounds compared with the control.

3. Materials and Methods

3.1. General Procedures

Optical rotations were determined on a PerkinElmer 343 polarimeter (Waltham, MA, USA). IR spectra were determined on a Bruker OPUS Vector-22 infrared spectrophotometer in CDCl$_3$. The ^{1}H- and ^{13}C-NMR spectra were recorded on Bruker Avance III 700 spectrometer (Bruker, Germany) at 700.13 and 176.04 MHz, respectively, and chemical shifts were referenced to the corresponding residual solvent signal (δ_H 3.30/δ_C 49.0 for CD$_3$OD). The HRESIMS spectra were recorded on a Bruker Impact II Q-TOF mass spectrometer (Bruker, Germany); the samples were dissolved in MeOH (c 0.001 mg/mL). HPLC separations were carried out on an Agilent 1100 Series chromatograph (Agilent Technologies, Santa Clara, CA, USA) equipped with a differential refractometer; Discovery C18 (5 μm, 250 × 10 mm, Supelco, Bellefonte, PA, USA) column was used. GC and GC-MS analyses were performed on a GC 2010 chromatograph with a flame ionization detector and a gas chromatograph couple to a mass spectrometer GCMS-QP5050, both from Shimadzu (Japan). Fused silica capillary columns Supelcowax 10 and MDN-5S (both columns 30 m, 0.25 mm ID, 0.25 μm film, Supelco, PA, USA) were used in the apparatus. Low-pressure liquid column chromatography was carried out with the Si gel KSK (50–160 μm, Sorbpolimer, Krasnodar, Russia). Sorbfil Si gel plates (4.5 × 6.0 cm, 5–17 μm, Sorbpolimer, Krasnodar, Russia) were used for thin-layer chromatography.

3.2. Animal Material

Specimens of *Ceramaster patagonicus* Sladen, 1889 (order Valvatida, family Goniasteridae), were collected at a depth of 150–300 m in the Sea of Okhotsk near Iturup Island during 42nd scientific cruise of the research vessel *Akademik Oparin*, in August 2012. Species identification was carried out by B. B. Grebnev (G. B. Elyakov Pacific Institute of Bioorganic Chemistry FEB RAS, Vladivostok, Russia). A voucher specimen (No. 042-67) is on deposit at the marine specimen collection of the G. B. Elyakov Pacific Institute of Bioorganic Chemistry FEB RAS, Vladivostok, Russia.

3.3. Extraction and Isolation

The fresh animals of *C. patagonicus* (3 kg, crude weight) were chopped into small pieces and extracted with $CHCl_3$:MeOH (2:1) followed by further extraction with $CHCl_3$:MeOH (1:1) and EtOH. The combined extracts were concentrated in vacuo to give a residue of 159.5 g. This residue was partitioned between H_2O (1.5 L) and AcOEt:BuOH (2:1) (4.5 L), and the organic layer was concentrated in vacuo to give the less polar fraction (51.5 g), which was washed with cold acetone (1 L). The acetone-soluble part (28.5 g) was chromatographed over a silica gel column (19 × 4.5 cm) using $CHCl_3$, $CHCl_3$:MeOH (97:3), and $CHCl_3$:MeOH (9:1) to yield four fractions: 1 (932 mg), 2 (486 mg), 3 (735 mg), and 4 (1.04 g). Fractions 1–4 were further chromatographed over a Si gel column (10 × 4 cm) using *n*-hexane:AcOEt:MeOH (stepwise gradient, 6:3:0.1→6:3:0.7, *v/v/v*) to yield six subfractions: 21 (123 mg), 31 (475 mg), 32 (231 mg), 41 (55 mg), 42 (212 mg), and 43 (570 mg), which were then analyzed by TLC in the eluent system $CHCl_3$:MeOH:H_2O (8:1:0.1, *v/v/v*). Subfractions 21–43 mainly contained the ceramides, cerebrosides, admixtures of pigments, and concomitant other lipids. HPLC separation of subfraction 32 (231 mg) on a Diasfer-110-C18 column (2.5 mL/min) with MeOH as an eluent yielded pure **1** (4.4 mg, R_t 42.3 min), **2** (2.5 mg, R_t 51.9 min), **3** (3.9 mg, R_t 55.7 min), and **4** (2.9 mg, R_t 72.5 min).

3.4. Compound Characterization Data

(25*S*)-5α-Cholestane-3β,6β,15α,16β-tetraol-26-yl 5′*Z*,11′*Z*-octadecadienoate (**1**): Amorphous powder; $[\alpha]_D^{25}$: +8.1 (*c* 0.44, MeOH); IR (CDCl$_3$) ν_{max} 3504, 2929, 2856, 1723, 1602, 1459, 1379, 1216, 1042 cm^{-1}; (+)HRESIMS *m/z* 737.5695 [M + Na]$^+$ (calcd for $C_{45}H_{78}O_6Na$, 737.5695); (−)HRESIMS *m/z* 773.5934 [(M − H) + AcOH]$^-$ (calcd for $C_{47}H_{81}O_8$, 773.5937), 713.5726 [M − H]$^-$ (calcd for $C_{45}H_{77}O_6$, 713.5729); (−)ESIMS/MS of the ion at *m/z* 713: *m/z* 449 $[C_{27}H_{45}O_5]^-$, 279 $[C_{18}H_{31}O_2]^-$; ^{1}H- and ^{13}C-NMR data, see Tables 1 and 2.

(25*S*)-5α-Cholestane-3β,6β,15α,16β-tetraol-26-yl 11′*Z*-octadecenoate (**2**): Amorphous powder; $[\alpha]_D^{25}$: +14.1 (*c* 0.25, MeOH); IR (CDCl$_3$) ν_{max} 3504, 2929, 2856, 1723, 1602, 1465, 1379, 1260, 1216, 1043 cm^{-1}; (+)HRESIMS *m/z* 739.5852 [M + Na]$^+$ (calcd for $C_{45}H_{80}O_6Na$, 739.5847); (−)HRESIMS *m/z* 775.6096 [(M − H) + AcOH]$^-$ (calcd for $C_{47}H_{83}O_8$, 775.6093); *m/z* 715.5889 [M − H]$^-$ (calcd for $C_{45}H_{79}O_6$, 715.5882); (−)ESIMS/MS of the ion at *m/z* 715: *m/z* 449 $[C_{27}H_{45}O_5]^-$, 281 $[C_{18}H_{33}O_2]^-$; ^{1}H- and ^{13}C-NMR data, see Tables 1 and 2.

(25*S*)-5α-Cholestane-3β,6β,15α,16β-tetraol-26-yl 5′*Z*,11′*Z*-eicosadienoate (**3**): Amorphous powder; $[\alpha]_D^{25}$: +9.5 (*c* 0.39, MeOH); IR (CDCl$_3$) ν_{max} 3510, 2929, 2856, 1723, 1603, 1493, 1465, 1379, 1365, 1248, 1216, 1189, 1080, 1042 cm^{-1}; (+)HRESIMS *m/z* 765.6008 [M + Na]$^+$ (calcd for $C_{47}H_{82}O_6Na$, 765.6004); (−)HRESIMS *m/z* 801.6254 [(M − H) + AcOH]$^-$ (calcd for $C_{49}H_{85}O_8$, 801.6250); *m/z* 741.6044 [M − H]$^-$ (calcd for $C_{47}H_{81}O_6$, 741.6039); (−)ESIMS/MS of the ion at *m/z* 741: *m/z* 449 $[C_{27}H_{45}O_5]^-$, 307 $[C_{20}H_{35}O_2]^-$; ^{1}H- and ^{13}C-NMR data, see Tables 1 and 2.

(25*S*)-5α-Cholestane-3β,6β,15α,16β-tetraol-26-yl 7′*Z*-eicosenoate (**4**): Amorphous powder; $[\alpha]_D^{25}$: +15.4 (*c* 0.29, MeOH); IR (CDCl$_3$) ν_{max} 3515, 2929, 2856, 1723, 1602, 1466, 1378, 1261, 1204, 1043 cm^{-1}; (+)HRESIMS *m/z* 767.6157 [M + Na]$^+$ (calcd for $C_{47}H_{84}O_6Na$, 767.6160); (−)HRESIMS *m/z* 803.6409 [(M − H) + AcOH]$^-$ (calcd for $C_{49}H_{87}O_8$, 803.6406); *m/z* 743.6199 [M − H]$^-$ (calcd for $C_{47}H_{83}O_6$, 743.6195); (−)ESIMS/MS of the ion at *m/z* 743: *m/z* 449 $[C_{27}H_{45}O_5]^-$, 309 $[C_{20}H_{37}O_2]^-$; ^{1}H- and ^{13}C-NMR data, see Tables 1 and 2.

3.5. Methanolysis and Preparation of 4,4-Dimethyloxazoline Derivatives of Fatty Acids

Compounds **1–4** (1 mg) were heated with 1 N HCl in 80% aq MeOH (1.0 mL) at 80 °C for 4 h. The reaction mixtures were then extracted with *n*-hexane, and the extracts were concentrated in vacuo to yield FAME-1–FAME-4. The 4,4-Dimethyloxazoline derivatives of fatty acids of compounds **1** and **4** were prepared from FAME-1 and FAME-4 according to the procedure described previously [15].

3.6. FAME and DMOX Analysis.

FAMEs were analyzed on Supelcowax 10 columns at 200 °C. DMOX derivatives analyzed on a nonpolar MDN-5S column, where the temperature program ranged from 200 to 260 °C at 2 °C/min. Helium was used as the carrier gas at a linear velocity of 30 cm/s. Mass spectra were recorded at 70 eV. Mass spectra were compared with the NIST library and internet fatty acid mass spectra archive site.

3.7. Bioactivity Assay

3.7.1. Reagents

Phosphate buffered saline (PBS), L-glutamine, penicillin–streptomycin solution (10,000 U/mL, 10 µg/mL) were from Sigma-Aldrich (St. Louis, MO, USA). MTS reagent (3-(4,5-dimethylthiazol-2-yl)-5-(3-carboxymethoxyphenyl)-2-(4-sulfophenyl)-2H-tetrazolium) was purchased from Promega (Madison, WI, USA). The Basal Medium Eagle (BME), Minimum Essential Medium Eagle (MEM), Dulbecco's Modified Eagle's Medium (DMEM), McCoy's 5A Modified Medium (McCoy's 5A), trypsin, fetal bovine serum (FBS), and agar were purchased from Thermo Fisher Scientific (Waltham, MA, USA).

3.7.2. Cell Cultures

Mouse epidermal JB6 Cl41 (ATCC No. CRL-2010), human breast cancer MDA-MB-231 (ATCC HTB-26), and colorectal carcinoma HCT 116 (ATCC CCL-247) cell lines were cultured in MEM, DMEM, and McCoy's 5A medium supplemented with 5%, 10%, and 10% FBS, respectively, and 1% penicillin–streptomycin solution. The cell cultures were maintained at 37 °C in humidified atmosphere containing 5% CO_2.

3.7.3. Compounds Preparation

Compounds **1–4** were dissolved in DMSO to prepare stock concentrations of 20 mM. Cells were treated with serially diluted compounds (culture medium used as diluent) to give the intended final concentrations (1, 10, 20, 50, and 100 µM). Solvent tolerance testing up to 0.5% of DMSO in control cells under identical conditions confirmed that the viability of all cell lines was unaffected. The vehicle control was the cells treated with equivalent volume of DMSO for all presented experiments.

3.7.4. Cell Viability Assay

To determine the cytotoxicity of compounds **1–4**, JB6 Cl41, MDA-MB-231, and HCT 116 cells (1.0×10^4) were seeded in 200 µL of complete MEM/5% FBS, DMEM/10% FBS, and McCoy's 5A/10% FBS medium, respectively, and incubated for 24 h at 37 °C in 5% CO_2 incubator. The attached cells were incubated with fresh medium containing various concentrations of **1–4** (0–100 µM) or equivalent volume of DMSO (control) for additional 24 h. Subsequently, the cells were incubated with 15 µL MTS reagent for 3 h, and the absorbance of each well was measured at 490/630 nm using Power Wave XS microplate reader (BioTek, Winooski, VT, USA). All experimental conditions were assessed in triplicate.

To determine the effect of compounds **1–4** on cell proliferation, the tested cell lines (8×10^3 cells/200 µL) were treated with tested compounds at concentrations of 1, 10, 50, and 100 µM or equivalent volume of DMSO (control) and incubated for additional 24, 48, and 72 h at 37 °C in 5% CO_2. MTS reagent (20 µL) was added to each well, and the cells were incubated for additional 3 h in 5% CO_2

incubator. Absorbance was measured at 490/630 nm by microplate reader. All experimental conditions were assessed in triplicate.

3.7.5. Soft Agar Assay

To estimate the effects of **1–4** on colony formation (phenotype expression), MDA-MB-231 and HCT 116 cells (2.4×10^4 cells/200 µL) were treated equivalent volume of DMSO (control) or with compounds **1–4** (20 µM) in 1 mL of 0.3% Basal Medium Eagle (BME) agar containing 10% FBS, 2 mM L-glutamine, and 25 µg/mL gentamicin. The cultures were maintained in a 37 °C, 5% CO_2 incubator for 14 days, and the cell colonies were scored using a Motic AE 20 microscope (XiangAn, Xiamen, China) and ImageJ software bundled with 64-bit Java 1.8.0_112 (NIH, Bethesda, MD, USA).

3.7.6. Wound Healing Assay

MDA-MB-231 and HCT 116 cells (3×10^5 cells/mL) were seeded into six-well plates and grown to 80% confluence for 24 h. After removing the culture medium, the cells' monolayer was scraped with a 200 µL sterile pipette tip to create a straight scratch. Then, MDA-MB-231 and HCT 116 cells were treated with equivalent volume of DMSO (control) or **1–4** at concentration of 20 µM and incubated for 48 h. All experiments were conducted in triplicate for each group. For the image analysis, cell migration into the wound area was photographed at the stages of 0 and 48 h using a Motic AE 20 microscope and ImageJ software. The cell migration distance was estimated by measuring the width of the wound and expressed as a percentage of each control for the mean wound closure area.

3.7.7. Statistical Analysis

All assays were performed using least three independent experiments. Results are expressed as the mean ± standard deviation (SD). Student's *t*-test was used to evaluate the data with the following significance levels: * $p < 0.05$, ** $p < 0.01$, *** $p < 0.001$.

4. Conclusions

Four new steroidal conjugates, esters of polyhydroxysteroids with long-chain fatty acids (**1–4**), were isolated from the Far Eastern starfish *C. patagonicus*. Unusual compounds **1–4** contain the same 5α-cholestane-3β,6β,15α,16β,26-pentahydroxysteroidal moiety and differ from each other in fatty acid residues: 5′Z,11′Z-octadecadienoic (**1**), 11′Z-octadecenoic (**2**), 5′Z,11′Z-eicosadienoic (**3**), and 7′Z-eicosenoic (**4**) acid units. It should be noted that the isolated conjugates **1–4** have a shared steroidal part and differ in the composition of fatty acid residues. The question arises about the biological role of the extracted compounds. Previously we have been found that starfish polyhydroxylated steroids were presented mainly in digestive organs of starfishes during the whole year, and their maximum concentration coincided with periods of active nutrition of these animals [20,21]. Recently, we confirmed the digestive function of polyhydroxysteroids, when studying the distribution of polar steroids in various organs of the starfish *Lethasterias fusca* using the nLC/CSI–QTOF–MS method, and the highest level of polar steroids was found in the stomach and the pyloric caeca [22] Thus, it can be assumed that polyhydroxysteroids can bind food fatty acids and participate in their transport to peripheral tissues, like cholesterol of vertebrates and humans. This assumption is partially confirmed by the heterogeneous composition of fatty acids in compounds **1–4**, since saturated, mono- and di-unsaturated C16, C18, and C20 fatty acids were found together with the main components. The isolation of conjugates of polyhydroxysteroids and fatty acids from the Far Eastern starfish *C. patagonicus* is a very interesting finding; to the best of our knowledge, hypotheses about the possible transport role of polyhydroxysteroids have not been put forward. At the same time, this assumption requires confirmation by experimental data.

We have expanded the data on the biological activity of these unique compounds—conjugates of polyhydroxysteroids and fatty acids. It was shown that tested compounds **1–4** possessed cytostatic activity against normal JB6 Cl41 cells and cancer MDA-MB-231 and HCT 116 cell lines. The compounds

1–4 at low concentration of 20 µM were able to suppress the colony formation in MDA-MB-231 and HCT 116 cells and almost completely prevent the migration of human breast and colorectal cancer cells. It should be noted that compound **2** was the most active in all experiments performed. This is likely due to the presence of an 11′Z-octadecenoic acid residue in its structure. Unfortunately, the lack of selectivity of the investigated compounds against normal and cancer cells was determined, which can be limit their possible practical use. However, the identification of these novel compounds and an initial characterization of their biological activity, performed for the first time, might be helpful to other researchers working on the development of conjugates of polyhydroxysteroids and fatty acids.

Supplementary Materials: The following are available online at http://www.mdpi.com/1660-3397/18/5/260/s1. Copies (+)HRESIMS (Figures S1, S21, S30, and S39), (−)HRESIMS (Figures S2, S22, S31, and S40), (−)ESIMS/MS (Figures S3, S23, S32, and S41), ^{1}H-NMR (Figures S4–S8, S24, S33, and S42), ^{13}C-NMR (Figures S9–S12, S25, S34, and S43), COSY (Figures S13, S14, S26, S35, and S44), HSQC (Figures S15, S16, S27, S36, and S45), HMBC (Figures S17, S18, S28, S37, and S46), and ROESY (Figures S19, S20, S29, S38, and S47) spectra of compounds **1**, **2**, **3**, and **4**, respectively.

Author Contributions: T.V.M., the isolation and structure elucidation of metabolites, and manuscript preparation; A.A.K. and N.V.I., the analysis of the compounds and manuscript editing; V.M.Z. and I.P.K., the isolation and structure elucidation of metabolites; A.I.K., the acquisition and interpretation of NMR spectra; V.I.S., the analysis and identification of fatty acids; O.S.M., the determination of the metabolites' effects on the viability, proliferation, colony formation, and migration of tested cells; R.S.P., the acquisition and interpretation of mass spectra. All authors have read and agreed to the published version of the manuscript.

Funding: The isolation and establishment of chemical structures were partially supported by Grant No. 20-03-00014 from the RFBR (Russian Foundation for Basic Research). The study on the anticancer activity of starfish metabolites was supported by Grant No. 18-74-10028 from the RSF (Russian Science Foundation).

Acknowledgments: The study was carried out on the equipment of the Collective Facilities Center "The Far Eastern Center for Structural Molecular Research (NMR/MS) of PIBOC FEB RAS". We are grateful to B.B. Grebnev (G.B. Elyakov Pacific Institute of Bioorganic Chemistry FEB RAS, Vladivostok, Russia) for species identification of the starfish and V.A. Stonik for the manuscript editing.

Conflicts of Interest: The authors declare no conflict of interest.

References

1. Gomes, A.R.; Freitas, A.C.; Rocha-Santos, T.A.P.; Duarte, A.C. Bioactive compounds derived from echinoderms. *RSC Adv.* **2014**, *4*, 29365–29382. [CrossRef]
2. Minale, L.; Riccio, R.; Zollo, F. Steroidal oligoglycosides and polyhydroxysteroids from Echinoderms. *Fortschr. Chem. Org. Nat.* **1993**, *62*, 75–308.
3. Stonik, V.A. Marine polar steroids. *Russ. Chem. Rev.* **2001**, *70*, 673–715. [CrossRef]
4. Iorizzi, M.; De Marino, S.; Zollo, F. Steroidal oligoglycosides from the Asteroidea. *Curr. Org. Chem.* **2001**, *5*, 951–973. [CrossRef]
5. Stonik, V.A.; Ivanchina, N.V.; Kicha, A.A. New polar steroids from starfish. *Nat. Prod. Commun.* **2008**, *3*, 1587–1610. [CrossRef]
6. Dong, G.; Xu, T.H.; Yang, B.; Lin, X.P.; Zhou, X.F.; Yang, X.W.; Liu, Y.H. Chemical constituents and bioactivities of starfish. *Chem. Biodivers.* **2011**, *8*, 740–791. [CrossRef]
7. Ivanchina, N.V.; Kicha, A.A.; Stonik, V.A. Steroid glycosides from marine organisms. *Steroids* **2011**, *76*, 425–454. [CrossRef]
8. Ivanchina, N.V.; Kicha, A.A.; Malyarenko, T.V.; Stonik, V.A. *Advances in Natural Products Discovery*; Gomes, A.R., Rocha-Santos, T., Duarte, A., Eds.; Nova Science Publishers: Hauppauge, NY, USA, 2017; Volume 6, pp. 191–224.
9. Xia, J.M.; Miao, Z.; Xie, C.L.; Zhang, J.W.; Yang, X.W. Chemical constituents and bioactivities of starfishes: An update. *Chem. Biodivers.* **2020**, *17*, e1900638. [CrossRef]
10. Kicha, A.A.; Ivanchina, N.V.; Malyarenko, T.V.; Kalinovsky, A.I.; Popov, R.S.; Stonik, V.A. Six new polyhydroxylated steroid taurine conjugates, microdiscusols A–F, from the Arctic starfish *Asterias microdiscus*. *Steroids* **2019**, *150*, 108458. [CrossRef]

11. Peng, Y.; Zheng, J.; Huang, R.; Wang, Y.; Xu, T.; Zhou, X.; Liu, Q.; Zeng, F.; Ju, H.; Yang, X.; et al. Polyhydroxy steroids and saponins from China sea starfish *Asterina pectinifera* and their biological activities. *Chem. Pharm. Bull.* **2010**, *58*, 856–858. [CrossRef]
12. Wang, W.; Hong, J.; Lee, C.-O.; Im, K.S.; Choi, J.S.; Jung, J.H. Cytotoxic sterols and saponins from the starfish *Certonardoa semiregularis*. *J. Nat. Prod.* **2004**, *67*, 584–591. [CrossRef] [PubMed]
13. Minale, L.; Pizza, C.; Zollo, F. 5α-cholestane-3β,6β,15α,16β,26-pentaol: A polyhydroxylated sterol from the starfish *Hacelia attenuata*. *Tetrahedron Lett.* **1982**, *23*, 1841–1844. [CrossRef]
14. Kicha, A.A.; Kalinovsky, A.I.; Stonik, V.A. New polyhydroxysteroids and steroid glycosides from the Far East starfish *Ceramaster patagonicus*. *Russ. Chem. Bull.* **1997**, *46*, 186–191. [CrossRef]
15. Svetashev, V.I. Mild method for preparation of 4,4-dimethyloxazoline derivatives of polyunsaturated fatty acids for GC–MS. *Lipids* **2011**, *46*, 463–467. [CrossRef]
16. Stransky, K.; Jursik, T.; Vitek, A. Standard equivalent chain length values of monoenic and polyenic (methylene interrupted) fatty acids. *J. High Resolut. Chromatogr.* **1997**, *20*, 143–158. [CrossRef]
17. Ling, T.; Lang, W.H.; Maier, J.; Centurion, M.Q.; Rivas, F. Cytostatic and cytotoxic natural products against cancer cell models. *Molecules* **2019**, *24*, 2012. [CrossRef]
18. Borowicz, S.; Van Scoyk, M.; Avasarala, S. The soft agar colony formation assay. *J. Vis. Exp.* **2014**, *92*, e51998. [CrossRef]
19. Tahtamouni, L.; Ahram, M.; Koblinski, J.; Rolfo, C. Molecular regulation of cancer cell migration, invasion, and metastasis. *Anal. Cell. Pathol.* **2019**, *2019*, 1356508. [CrossRef]
20. Kicha, A.A.; Ivanchina, N.V.; Gorshkova, I.A.; Ponomarenko, L.P.; Likhatskaya, G.N.; Stonik, V.A. The distribution of free sterols, polyhydroxysteroids and steroid glycosides in various body components of the starfish *Patiria (=Asterina) pectinifera*. *Comp. Biochem. Physiol.* **2001**, *128*, 43–52. [CrossRef]
21. Kicha, A.A.; Ivanchina, N.V.; Stonik, V.A. Seasonal variations in the levels of polyhydroxysteroids and related glycosides in the digestive tissues of the starfish *Patiria (=Asterina) pectinifera*. *Comp. Biochem. Physiol.* **2003**, *136*, 897–903. [CrossRef]
22. Popov, R.S.; Ivanchina, N.V.; Kicha, A.A.; Malyarenko, T.V.; Grebnev, B.B.; Stonik, V.A.; Dmitrenok, P.S. The distribution of asterosaponins, polyhydroxysteroids and related glycosides in different body components of the Far Eastern starfish *Lethasterias fusca*. *Mar. Drugs* **2019**, *17*, 523. [CrossRef] [PubMed]

Sample Availability: Samples of all compounds in the manuscripts are available from the authors.

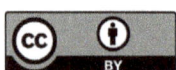

© 2020 by the authors. Licensee MDPI, Basel, Switzerland. This article is an open access article distributed under the terms and conditions of the Creative Commons Attribution (CC BY) license (http://creativecommons.org/licenses/by/4.0/).

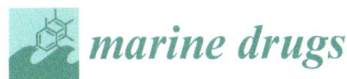

Article

Sterol Composition of Sponges, Cnidarians, Arthropods, Mollusks, and Echinoderms from the Deep Northwest Atlantic: A Comparison with Shallow Coastal Gulf of Mexico

Laura Carreón-Palau [1,2,*], Nurgül Şen Özdemir [1,3], Christopher C. Parrish [1] and Camilla Parzanini [1,4]

1. Department of Ocean Sciences, Memorial University of Newfoundland, Marine Lab Rd., St. John's, NL A1C 5S7, Canada; nsozdemir@bingol.edu.tr (N.Ş.Ö.); cparrish@mun.ca (C.C.P.); cparzanini@ryerson.ca (C.P.)
2. Centro de Investigaciones Biológicas del Noroeste (CIBNOR), El Comitán, La Paz, Baja California Sur 23205, Mexico
3. Department of Veterinary Medicine, Vocational School of Food, Agriculture and Livestock, Bingöl University, Bingöl 12000, Turkey
4. Department of Chemistry and Biolog, Ryerson University, Toronto, ON M5B 2K3, Canada
* Correspondence: lcarreon@cibnor.mx

Received: 21 October 2020; Accepted: 23 November 2020; Published: 27 November 2020

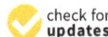

Abstract: Triterpenoid biosynthesis is generally anaerobic in bacteria and aerobic in Eukarya. The major class of triterpenoids in bacteria, the hopanoids, is different to that in Eukarya, the lanostanoids, and their 4,4,14-demethylated derivatives, sterols. In the deep sea, the prokaryotic contribution to primary productivity has been suggested to be higher because local environmental conditions prevent classic photosynthetic processes from occurring. Sterols have been used as trophic biomarkers because primary producers have different compositions, and they are incorporated in primary consumer tissues. In the present study, we inferred food supply to deep sea, sponges, cnidarians, mollusks, crustaceans, and echinoderms from euphotic zone production which is driven by phytoplankton eukaryotic autotrophy. Sterol composition was obtained by gas chromatography and mass spectrometry. Moreover, we compared the sterol composition of three phyla (i.e., Porifera, Cnidaria, and Echinodermata) collected between a deep and cold-water region and a shallow tropical area. We hypothesized that the sterol composition of shallow tropical benthic organisms would better reflect their photoautotrophic sources independently of the taxonomy. Shallow tropical sponges and cnidarians from environments showed plant and zooxanthellae sterols in their tissues, while their deep-sea counterparts showed phytoplankton and zooplankton sterols. In contrast, echinoids, a class of echinoderms, the most complex phylum along with hemichordates and chordates (deuterostomes), did not show significant differences in their sterol profile, suggesting that cholesterol synthesis is present in deuterostomes other than chordates.

Keywords: *Thenea muricata*; *Aplysina* sp.; *Pseudoanthomastus agaricus*; *Montastraea cavernosa*; *Buccinum* sp.; *Pasiphaea tarda*; *Phormosoma placenta*; *Echinometra lucunter*; sterols; gas chromatography; mass spectrometry

1. Introduction

In the deep sea (i.e., below 200 m depth), light and temperature diminish while pressure increases with depth [1]. In addition, both food quantity and quality decrease along the depth gradient [2].

However, there is evidence that the abyssal food web is supported by a flux of phytodetritus from the euphotic zone, and the abundance of some populations fluctuates interannually in concert with changes in this food supply [3].

Euphotic zone primary production is driven by eukaryotic autotrophy by phytoplankton and, to a lesser extent, by macroalgae and vascular plants from marine and terrestrial sources. In the deep sea, the prokaryotic contribution to primary productivity has been suggested to be higher because local environmental conditions prevent classic photosynthetic processes from occurring [4]. In reducing environments, for example, chemoautotrophic bacteria are responsible for converting inorganic energy sources (e.g., H_2S) into organic products that can be utilized by the rest of the community [4]. Furthermore, methanotrophic bacteria can use methane as a carbon source to synthesis macromolecules, and they can usually be discriminated from other sources with the stable isotopes of carbon with a $\delta^{13}C$ of −50‰ to −100‰ [5].

The lipid signature approach, including lipid class, fatty acid, and sterol composition has been used successfully to help understand marine trophodynamics [6,7]. Typically, energy flows from lower to higher trophic levels of food webs. This energy flow is accomplished by trophic interactions within biological communities. These communities, hence, have the potential to play a major role in the flux of organic matter and may be an important food source to vertebrate consumers, including humans. However, organic matter transfer can be difficult to elucidate. In this context, lipids are important biochemical compounds in marine food webs because they are rich in carbon and are energy-dense [8]. Lipids can also be used as biomarkers in ecological studies [9,10]. The sterol composition of lower trophic levels can provide useful biogeochemical information [11,12], leading to a better understanding of ecosystem functioning. Sterols can be used in trophic ecology as they play an important role in marine organisms. They are key constituents of animal cell membranes [13] and are present in all eukaryotic taxa [14,15]; they are also precursors of steroid hormones [16] and represent essential dietary nutrients for marine organisms [17,18]. For instance, diets with limited cholesterol content (<1%) significantly decreased the growth and survival rates of early stages in the crustacean *Panaeus monodon* [18,19].

As triterpenoid biosynthesis is generally anaerobic in bacteria and aerobic in Eukarya, the major class of triterpenoids in bacteria, the hopanoids, is different to that in Eukarya, the lanostanoids, and their 4,4,14-demethylated derivatives, sterols. There is a further bifurcation in the pathway of sterol biosynthesis in that photosynthetic organisms (e.g., algae and plants) form primarily cycloartenol as the first cyclization product, whereas nonphotosynthetic organisms (animals and fungi) form mostly lanosterol. There are exceptions to this general pattern of triterpenoid distribution, with hopanoids being found in some Eukarya (e.g., ferns and lichens) and sterols being found in certain methanotrophic bacteria and in cyanobacteria. It is possible that the two pathways are very primitive and that one or other of these pathways has, for functional reasons, been subsequently selected in different groups of organisms [20]. However, none of the bacteria that were identified to have an oxidosqualenecyclase (Osc) homolog in their genome are anaerobes, providing strong evidence that sterol synthesis is an aerobic biosynthetic pathway in bacteria as it is in eukaryotes [21].

The pathway of sterol synthesis has been thoroughly studied in vertebrates, fungi, and terrestrial plants, with cholesterol and ergosterol at the end of the synthesis pathway in vertebrates and fungi, respectively, and a higher variety of sterols in plants such as campesterol, sitosterol, and stigmasterol [22]. In contrast, knowledge of sterols in invertebrates, which comprise at least 16 phyla with important phylogeny differences (Figure 1), is lagging behind. The phylum Porifera is the simplest metazoan alive, and poriferans or sponges have one germ layer and lack true tissue organization. In the phylum Cnidaria, there are two germ layers in the blastula, endoderm and ectoderm; therefore, they are diploblastic organisms. The endoderm allows them to develop true tissue, including tissue associated with the gut and associated glands. The ectoderm, on the other hand, gives rise to the epidermis, the nervous tissue, and, if present, nephridia. Species of Mollusca, Arthropoda, and Echinodermata are triploblasts which emerged within the diploblasts, with gastrulation forming three primary germ layers: the ectoderm, mesoderm, and endoderm. Among them, Mollusca and Arthropoda are protostomes, and Echinodermata, the most complex phylum along with those of Hemichordata and Chordata (which include vertebrates), are deuterostomes [23]. Cholesterol biosynthesis pathway (CBP) genes in the basal metazoans were inherited from their last common eukaryotic ancestor and evolutionarily conserved for cholesterol biosynthesis. The genomes of the basal metazoans and deuterostomes retain almost the full set of CBP genes, while Cnidaria and many protostomes have independently experienced multiple massive losses of CBP genes that might have been due the appearance of an exogenous sterol supply and the frequent perturbation of ocean oxygenation [24].

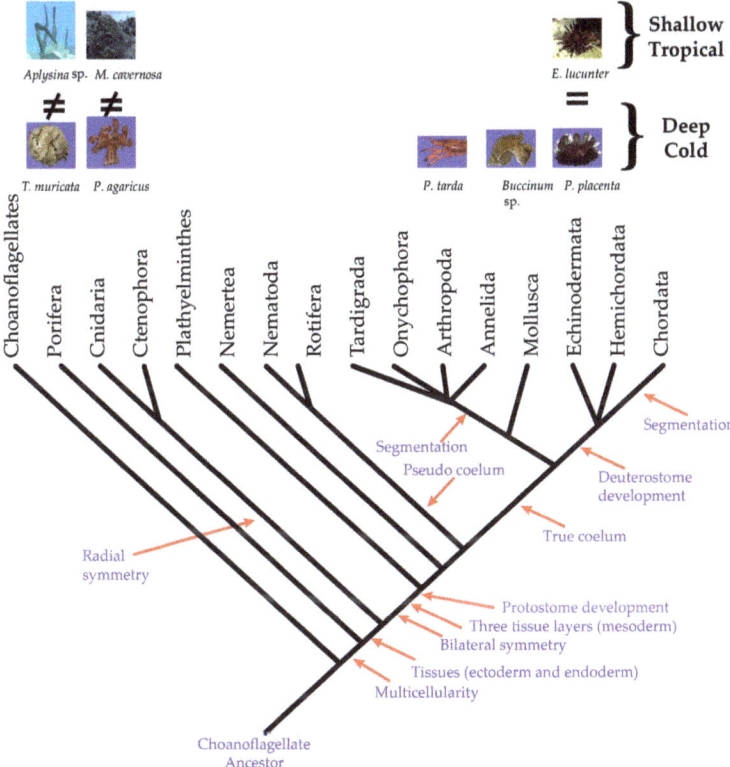

Figure 1. Phylogenetic position of Porifera, Cnidaria, Mollusca, Arthropoda, and Echinodermata in the tree of life of the kingdom Animalia in contrasting geographical zones.

To assess the euphotic contribution from phytodetritus to deep-sea sponges, corals, gastropods, decapods, and echinoids, we used sterols, most of which are absent in prokaryotes, with the exception of modified lanosterol products [21] probably acquired via horizontal gene transfer from eukaryotes [22]. Although photoautotrophs are a rich source of sterols, some have to be altered before they suit metazoan needs, for example, the exchangeable use of cholesterol and stigmasterol [25].

Sterol biosynthesis in invertebrates does not take place or else proceeds at a slow rate; therefore, they should be provided by diet [26]. Certain phytosterols were more efficient in supporting somatic growth of the crustacean *Daphnia magna* than cholesterol (e.g., fucosterol and brassicasterol), while others were less efficient (e.g., dihydrocholesterol and lathosterol), indicating substantial differences in the assimilation efficiency and further processing within the body for these dietary sterols [27]. Therefore, phytosterols detected in consumers which have no bioconversion capacity can be used as biomarkers.

Here, we evaluated sterol composition of five phyla, Porifera, Cnidaria, Mollusca, Arthropoda, and Echinodermata, from the deep and cold northeast Atlantic Ocean to infer their food sources. We then compared three phyla, Porifera, Cnidaria [28], and Echinoidea, from Echinodermata [29] with published data to investigate if their sterol composition was affected by temperature and depth. We hypothesized that the tissues of shallow, tropical benthic organisms would better represent photoautotrophic sources, such as phytoplankton, zooxanthellae, macroalgae, and plants, than tissues in their deep-water counterparts, independently of the phylogenetic relationships (phyla) [30]. To test our hypothesis, we compared sterol profiles of Porifera, Cnidaria, and Echinoidea from two contrasting sites: the Northwest Atlantic continental slope and southwest Gulf of Mexico shallow tropical coral reefs.

2. Results

2.1. Sterol Composition of Five Benthic Phyla, Porifera, Cnidaria, Mollusca, Arthropoda, and Echinodermata, from the Cold and Deep Northeast Atlantic

Species systematics, sample size, depth, and water temperature of animals collected in the deep Northwest Atlantic off Newfoundland and in the coral reef system of Veracruz are shown in Table 1. Total sterol concentrations ranged from 1.2 ± 1 mg·g^{-1} wet weight in Porifera to 37.7 ± 12.1 mg·g^{-1} in Echinodermata. While the number of sterols ranged from five, in the arthropod *Pasiphaea. tarda*, to 17, in the sponge *Thenea muricata*, no hopanoids were detected. Porifera had the lowest proportion of cholesterol (22.8% ± 1.8%), but significantly higher proportions of phytoplankton sterols, such as 24-methylencholesterol (12.2% ± 0.4%) and episterol (11.4% ± 1.6%), the phytoplankton and red algae sterol brassicasterol (12.1% ± 0.5%), the terrestrial plant sterol β-sitosterol (8.9% ± 0.8%), and a zooplankton sterol 24-nordehydrocholesterol (6.1% ± 0.8%). Furthermore, from the deep, cold-water site, Porifera was the only phylum showing sterols previously reported in diatoms and brown algae such as poriferasterol (2.0% ± 0.6%) and fucosterol (3.5% ± 0.7%), and specifically in brown algae such as 4-24 dimethyl 5,7-dien-3β-ol (2.0% ± 0.6%), compared to the other phyla studied. The cnidarian *Pseudoanthomastus agaricus* had more cholesterol than sponges with 68.8% ± 0.3%; in second place was occelasterol (11.6% ± 0.7%) probably from zooplankton, followed by brassicasterol (8.0% ± 2.6%) from phytoplankton and red algae. The mollusk *Buccinum* sp. and the arthropod *P. tarda* had similar sterol composition with cholesterol at 91.7% ± 1.0% and 95.3% ± 2.0%, respectively, with low contributions of occelasterol from zooplankton at 1.9% ± 0.9% and 2.2% ± 0.9%, respectively, and a detritus contribution detected with stigmasterol at 0.6% ± 0.2% and 1.5% ± 0.6%, respectively. The echinoid *Phormosoma placenta* had cholesterol at 73.9% ± 11.0%, similar to cnidarians, with sterols previously reported in zooplankton [31] such as 24-nordehydrocholesterol (2.5% ± 1.3%) and occelasterol (7.2% ± 3.1%), as well as plant-derived sterols such as β-sitosterol (2.1% ± 1.3%), along with characteristic sterols such as 9-10 secocholesta-5(10), 6, 8 trien β-ol, an analogue of vitamin D (1.0% ± 0.2%), and lathosterol (1.5% ± 0.5%), a cholesterol precursor (Table 2).

Table 1. Species systematics, sample size, water temperature, and depth of animals collected in the Northwest deep Atlantic off Newfoundland, Canada, and in the coral reef system of Veracruz, Mexico.

Scientific Name	Phylum	Class	Order	Family	n	Depth (m)	Temperature (°C)
Thenea muricata	Porifera	Desmospongiae	Astrophorida	Pachastrellidae	4	353	4.0 ± 0.3
Aplysina sp.			Verongida	Aplysinidae	2	20	25.3 ± 0.9
Pseudoanthomastus agaricus	Cnidaria	Anthozoa	Alcyonacea	Alcyoniidae	3	1027	4.0 ± 0.3
Montastraea cavernosa			Scleractinia	Montastreidae	4	20	25.3 ± 0.4
Buccinum sp.	Mollusca	Gastropoda	Neogastropoda	Buccinidae	3	759	4.0 ± 0.3
Pasiphaea tarda	Arthropoda	Malacostraca	Decapoda	Pasiphaeidae	21	1321	4.0 ± 0.3
Phormosoma placenta	Echinodermata	Echinoidea	Echinothurioida	Phormosomatidae	3	889	4.0 ± 0.3
Echinometra lucunter			Echinoida	Echinometridae	4	20	25.3 ± 0.4

Table 2. Sterol composition (percent of total sterols) and total concentration (mg·g^{-1} wet weight) of deep cold-water sponge, cnidarian, mollusk, arthropod, and echinoid representatives. Values are means ± intervals at 95% confidence.

Sterol Composition (%)	Sponge Thenea muricata	Cnidaria Pseudoanthomastus agaricus	Mollusk Buccinum sp.	Arthropod Pasiphaea terda	Echinoderm Phormosoma placenta	F	p
24-Nordehydrocholesterol	6.1 ± 0.8 [a]	0.9 ± 0.7 [b]	0.9 ± 0.1 [b]	0.3 ± 0.3 [b]	2.5 ± 1.3 [b]	23.23	<0.001
24-Nordehydrocholestanol	1.3 ± 0.3	-	-	-	-		
24-Nor-22, 23 methylenecholest-5-en-3-β-ol	-	-	-	-	1.4 ± 0.3		
Occelasterol	3.2 ± 0.5 [a]	11.6 ± 0.7 [b]	1.9 ± 0.9 [a]	2.2 ± 0.9 [a]	7.2 ± 3.1 [a,b]	18.77	<0.001
Cholesterol	22.8 ± 1.8 [a]	68.8 ± 0.3 [b]	91.7 ± 1.0 [c]	95.3 ± 2.0 [c]	73.9 ± 11.0 [b,c]	49.82	<0.001
Cholestanol	2.0 ± 0.3 [a]	3.6 ± 2.6 [a]	1.5 ± 0.5 [a]	-	1.5 ± 1.0 [a]	2.92	0.067
9-10 Secocholesta-5(10), 6, 8 trien-3-βol (analogue of vitamin D)	-	-	-	-	1.0 ± 0.2		
Brassicasterol	12.1 ± 0.5 [a]	8.0 ± 2.6 [a,b]	0.8 ± 0.4 [c]	0.7 ± 0.9 [c]	2.9 ± 0.9 [b,c]	57.18	<0.001
Brassicastanol	1.5 ± 0.6	-	-	-	-		
Stellasterol	3.9 ± 0.4 [a]	-	-	-	0.3 ± 0.04 [b]	41.13	<0.001
24-Methylenecholesterol	12.2 ± 0.4 [a]	1.3 ± 0.3 [b]	1.7 ± 0.8 [b]	-	1.1 ± 0.3 [b]	65.67	<0.001
Campesterol	2.6 ± 1.4 [a]	2.0 ± 0.4 [a]	-	-	2.5 ± 1.6 [a]	0.24	0.827
Lathosterol	-	-	-	-	1.5 ± 0.9		
Stigmasterol	2.6 ± 0.3 [a]	-	0.6 ± 0.2 [b]	1.5 ± 0.6 [a,b]	0.4 ± 0.1 [b]	22.56	<0.001
Episterol	11.4 ± 1.6 [a]	-	-	-	1.8 ± 1.4 [b]	79.29	<0.001
4-24 Dimethyl 5, 7-dien-3-β-ol	2.9 ± 1.9	-	-	-	-		

Table 2. Cont.

Sterol Composition (%)	Sponge *Thenea muricata*	Cnidaria *Pseudoanthomastus agaricus*	Mollusk *Buccinum sp.*	Arthropod *Pasiphaea terda*	Echinoderm *Phormosoma placenta*	F	p
Poriferasterol	2.0 ± 0.6	-	-	-	-		
Spinasterol	1.2 ± 0.4	-	-	-	-		
β-Sitosterol	8.9 ± 0.8 [a]	3.8 ± 0.7 [b]	0.9 ± 0.4 [c]	-	2.1 ± 1.3 [b,c]	69.47	<0.001
Fucosterol	3.5 ± 0.7	-	-	-	-		
Total sterols (GC-MS) Concentration (mg·g^{-1} wet weight) [1]	0.6 ± 0.5 [a]	0.59 ± 0.56 [a]	0.5 ± 0.4 [a]	1.6 ± 0.5 [b]	3.8 ± 1.2 [c]	15.39	<0.001
Total free sterols (Iatroscan) concentration (mg·g^{-1} wet weight)	0.6 ± 0.2	0.5 ± 0.2	1.4 ± 0.4	1.5 ± 1.2	0.9 ± 0.2	17.53	<0.001
Organic carbon source using sterols	Phytoplankton macroalgae, and higher plants (?)	Phytoplankton and zooplankton	Zooplankton	Zooplankton and detritus	Phytodetritus		

[1] Quantification of sterols (µg·mL^{-1} of hexane) of samples was achieved by dividing the areas from integrated chromatographic peaks by their respective slope obtained with the calibration curve [29] (pp. 18–19). Sum of sterol concentration (µg·mL^{-1}) was normalized to wet tissue biomass, multiplying the concentration by hexane volume (mL) added to each sample and dividing by lipid extracted wet biomass (mg), to obtain total sterols expressed as µg·mg^{-1}, equivalent to mg·g^{-1}. To obtain mg per 100 g, it was multiplied by 100. [a-c] Different superscript letters denote significant differences among columns ($p < 0.001$).

2.2. Comparison of Sterol Composition of Benthic Invertebrates from the Deep, Cold Sea Northwest Atlantic and Shallow, Tropical Coastal Gulf of Mexico

As hypothesized, we found significant dissimilarity in sterol profiles between shallow tropical and deep cold-water organisms (Figure 2a). In addition, phylogeny had a significant effect on the sterol profile; however, there was a significant interaction effect between depth/temperature and phylogeny (Figure 2b). Some tropical benthic organisms had significantly more campesterol, gorgosterol, and β-sitosterol from photoautotrophic sources such as zooxanthellae and plants, independent of phylum (t = 8.68, Markov chain probability (p(MC)) = 0.001, Figure 3a). Among them, the cnidarian *Montastraea cavernosa* had significantly higher proportions of campesterol and gorgosterol from zooxanthellae, while the deep-water cnidarian *P. agaricus* had a higher proportion of cholesterol, occelasterol, and brassicasterol, thus indicating zooplankton and phytoplankton sources (t = 11.86, p(MC) = 0.001, Figure 3b). Similarly, the sponge *Aplysina* sp., from the shallow, tropical site, showed high proportions of plant related sterols β-sitosterol and stigmasterol, as well as campesterol and cholesterol. On the other hand, the deep-water sponge *T. muricata* showed significantly higher proportions of phytoplankton sterols such as 24-methylenecholesterol and episterol (t = 9.43, p(MC) = 0.001, Figure 4a). In contrast to sponges and cnidarians, echinoids did not show significant differences in their sterol profiles (t = 2.09, p(MC) = 0.082, Figure 4b). In quantitative terms, lipids in shallow, tropical benthic organisms were significantly higher than in deep cold-sea organisms. The sponge *Aplysina* sp. had 15.4 ± 5.4 mg·g^{-1} wet weight, around fivefold more lipids than *T. muricata* with 2.6 ± 1.2 mg·g^{-1}, while the cnidarian *M. cavernosa* had 7.2 ± 3.6 mg·g^{-1}, almost twice the content of *P. agaricus* (4.1 ± 2.2 mg·g^{-1}). A similar pattern was detected in echinoids, with *Echinometra lucunter* having 12.6 ± 1.2 mg·g^{-1} of lipids and *P. placenta* having 6.0 ± 3.1 mg·g^{-1} (Table 3).

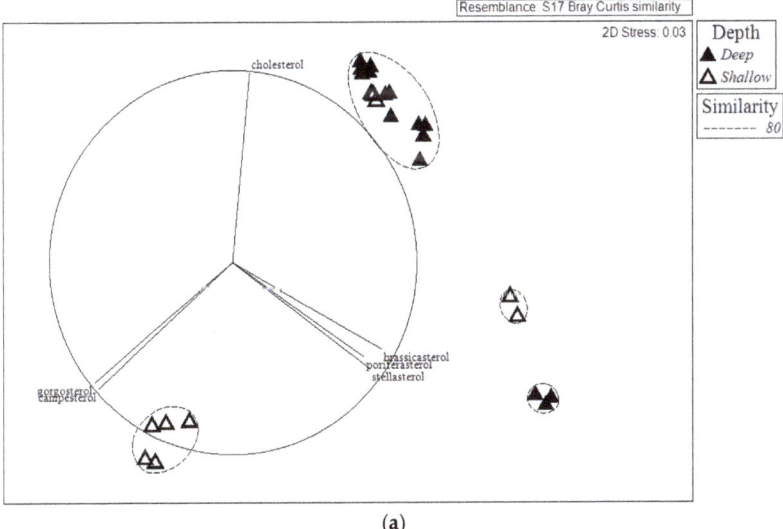

(a)

Figure 2. *Cont.*

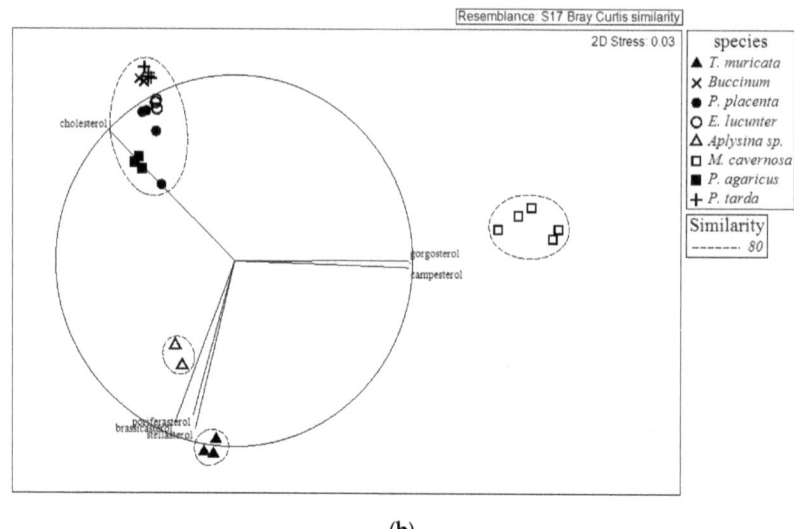

(b)

Figure 2. Scatter plot of nonmetric multidimensional scaling (nMDS) using Bray–Curtis similarity matrix for sterols (expressed as percentage of total sterols) of sponges *T. muricata* and *Aplysina* sp., cnidarians *A. agaricus* and *M. cavernosa*, the mollusk *Buccinum* sp., the arthropod *P. tarda*, and echinoids *P. placenta* and *E. lucunter* from deep, cold (filled symbols) and shallow, tropical (open symbols) waters. Axis scales are arbitrary in nMDS. (**a**) Sterol composition depending on depth ($F_{1,26}$ = 75.22, p(MC) = 0.001), and (**b**) interaction among depth and phyla ($F_{2,26}$ = 80.20, p(MC) = 0.001). Only variables with Pearson's correlations with MDS 1 and MDS 2 >0.86 are plotted. Contours grouped with 80% similarity on the basis of hierarchical cluster analysis.

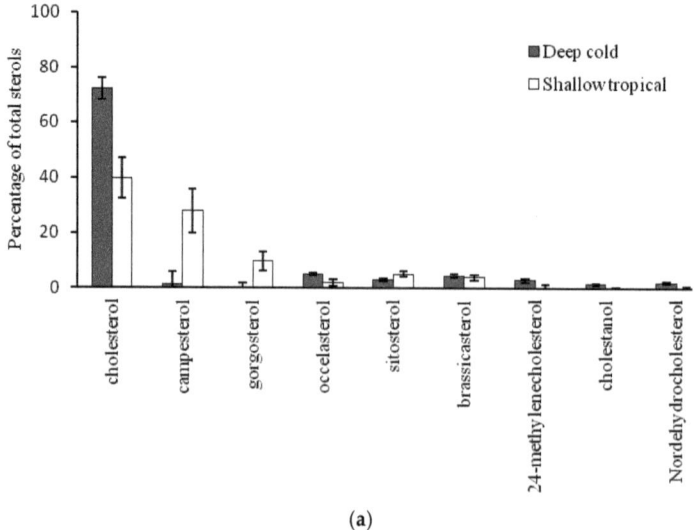

(a)

Figure 3. *Cont.*

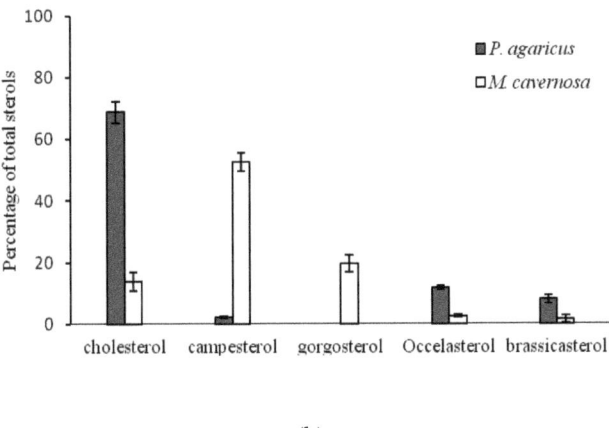

(b)

Figure 3. Average contribution of sterols primarily providing the discrimination between (**a**) deep, cold and shallow, tropical environments considering the three phyla studied. Sterols showed a significant similarity percentages (SIMPER) dissimilarity of 48.76% (t = 8.67 and p(MC) = 0.001). (**b**) Cnidaria *P. agaricus* (deep, cold) and *M. cavernosa* (shallow, tropical) with a significant dissimilarity of 78.76% (t = 11.86 and p(MC) = 0.001). Error bars denote 95% of the confidence interval.

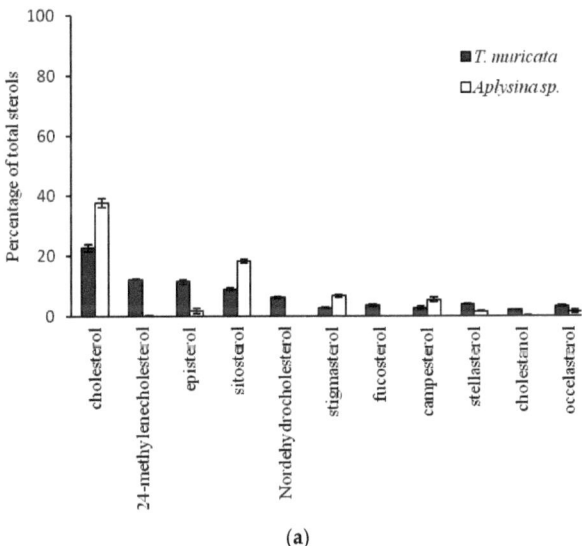

(a)

Figure 4. *Cont.*

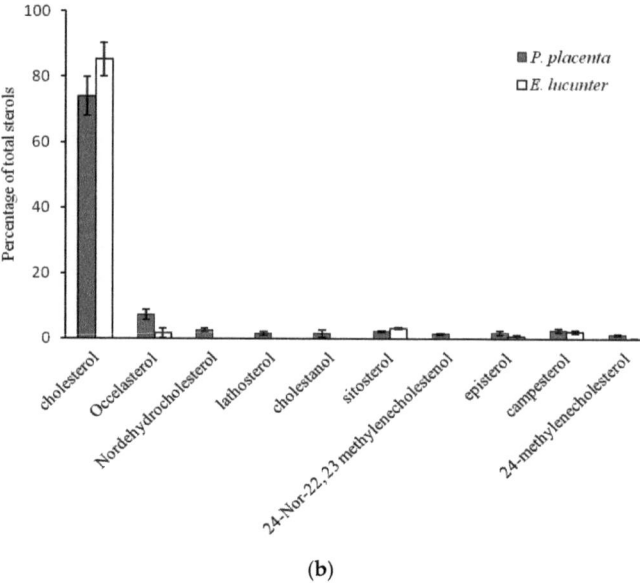

(b)

Figure 4. Average contribution of sterols primarily providing the discrimination between deep, cold and shallow, tropical waters. Error bars denote 95% of the confidence interval of (**a**) Porifera of factor phyla *T. muricata* (deep, cold) and *Aplysina* sp. (shallow, tropical) with a significant dissimilarity of 39.30% (t = 9.43 and p(MC) = 0.001), and (**b**) echinoids of factor phyla *P. placenta* (deep, cold) and *E. lucunter* (shallow, tropical) with no significant dissimilarity of 15.99% (t = 2.09 and p(MC) = 0.082).

Table 3. Wet weight (WW) per organism, total lipids, stable isotopes, and C:N molar ratio of animals collected in the deep Northwest Atlantic off Newfoundland. Values are mean ± 95% confidence interval. Information obtained from [28]. The sponge *Aplysina* sp., coral *M. cavernosa*, and sea urchin *E. lucunter* were collected in the shallow, tropical coral reef system of Veracruz [31]. TAG, triacylglycerol; ST, sterol.

Scientific Name	Wet Weight (g)	Lipid Content (mg·g^{-1} WW)	TAG:ST Ratio	δ^{13}C	Organic Carbon Source	δ^{15}N	C:N Molar Ratio	Functional Group
Thenea muricata	16.2 ± 2.1 [b]	2.6 ± 1.2 [a]	0.3	−17.4 ± 0.4 [b]	Pelagic	14.2 ± 0.3 [a]	5.4 ± 0.3 [b]	Filter feeder zooplanktivore
Pseudoanthomastus agaricus	12.2 ± 8.0 [a,b]	4.1 ± 2.2 [a]	0.4	−13.8 ± 4.9 [b]	Bentho-pelagic	11.0 ± 1.4 [b,c]	6.5 ± 3.1 [a,b,c]	Omnivore detritivore
Buccinum sp.	5.8 ± 2.9 [c]	6.9 ± 0.3 [b]	0.02	−17.0 ± 1.0 [b]	Pelagic	12.6 ± 0.6 [b]	4.2 ± 0.1 [a]	Carnivore scavenger
Pasiphaea tarda	29.2 ± 6.6 [a]	8.7 ± 2.3 [b]	0.5	−19.2 ± 0.1 [a]	Pelagic	11.4 ± 0.1 [c]	3.8 ± 0.04 [a]	Zooplanktivore
Phormosoma placenta	19.6 ± 8.4 [a,b]	6.0 ± 3.1 [a,b]	0.5	−14.3 ± 0.9 [c]	Bentho-pelagic	12.3 ± 0.3 [b]	5.3 ± 0.5 [b]	Omnivore carnivore
Aplysina sp.	28 ± 11 [a]	15.4 ± 5.4 [b,c]	0.4 ± 0.1		Pelagic			Filter feeder
Montastraea cavernosa	9.8 ± 3.8 [c]	7.2 ± 3.6 [b,c]	1.4 ± 0.5	−11.1 ± 2.5 [c,d]	Symbiont	4.0 ± 1.9 [d]	16.9 ± 9.5 [c,1]	Zooxanthellae and zooplankton
Echinometra. lucunter	6.9 ± 1.6 [c]	12.6 ± 1.2 [c]	25 ± 14	−10 ± 0.1 [d]	Macroalgae	3.3 ± 0.3 [d]	8.5 ± 0.4 [c]	Herbivore

[1] The high variation was probably due to carbonate residuals. [a–d] Different superscript letters denote significant differences among columns ($p < 0.05$).

3. Discussion

3.1. Food Supply to Deep Cold Ocean Invertebrates Using Sterols, C:N Ratios, and Stable Isotopes of Carbon and Nitrogen

Sterol composition of the sponge *T. muricata* suggests apportionment from phytoplankton, brown algae, and perhaps terrestrial vascular plants (Table 2); however, its $\delta^{13}C$ at $-17.4‰ \pm 4.9‰$ is indicative of phytoplankton sources more than macroalgae or higher plants [31]. Moreover, its $\delta^{15}N$ of $14.2‰ \pm 0.3‰$ [30] suggests a higher trophic level more related to zooplanktivore and detritivore food habits (Table 3). The zooplankton and recent detritus diet is more likely because its C:N ratio of 5.4 ± 0.3 is low compared to C:N values as high as 10 with increasing organic matter decomposition, which is more common in old detritus [32].

Similarly, the Cnidaria *P. agaricus* reflects a phytoplankton supply due the presence of 24-methylenecholesterol and occelasterol characteristic of phytoplankton. They were probably trophically transferred by zooplankton, coinciding with the high proportion of cholesterol [29]. The latter is coincident with a lower trophic level indicated by its $\delta^{15}N$ mean value of $11.0‰ \pm 1.4‰$, a wide $\delta^{13}C$ value of $-13.8‰ \pm 4.9‰$, and a C:N ratio of 6.5 ± 3.1 [30].

The mollusk *Buccinum* sp. and the arthropod *P. tarda* had the highest proportion of cholesterol, and a low or zero proportion of the phytosterol β-sitosterol. Cholesterol is probably provided by carnivore and scavenger food habits, since crustaceans with no or limited cholesterol content (<1%) have significantly decreased growth and survival rates in early stages [18]. There is consistency with the lowest C:N ratios of 4.2 ± 0.1 and 3.8 ± 0.04, respectively (Table 3), suggesting high apportionment of nitrogen from proteins characteristic of carnivores.

Lastly, the echinoid *P. placenta* had a greater variety of sterols including phytoplankton sterols such as occelasterol and zooplankton-related sterols such as 24-nordehydrocholesterol [29], a lower proportion of cholesterol, and a higher C:N ratio of 5.3 ± 0.5, suggesting that they are omnivores. Absence of hopanoids and C stable isotopes values far from metanothropic bacteria with a $\delta^{13}C$ of $-50‰$ to $-100‰$ [5] suggest that the principal food supply is eukaryotic photoautotrophic in origin.

3.2. Comparison of Sterol Composition of Benthic Invertebrates from the Cold, Deep Northwest Atlantic and Tropical, Shallow Coastal Gulf of Mexico

Small sample sizes were not a statistical issue due to small variation and clear differences among species and sites. Permutational multivariate analysis of variance (PERMANOVA) allows multivariate comparisons of compositional data such as sterol profiles with data with or without a normal distribution of residuals. Here, 996 permutations were performed in the main test, and, in those species with small sample sizes such as sponges, 10 permutations allowed detecting significant differences ($p = 0.001$). Furthermore, between cnidarians there were 56 permutations allowing detection of significant differences ($p = 0.001$). In contrast, echinoids with 35 permutations did not show a significant difference ($p = 0.082$) because sterol profiles of echinoids from shallow and deep sites were quite similar.

Tropical, shallow benthic organisms with a lower complexity such as Porifera and Cnidaria reflected the available food supply in their sterol composition. The most obvious difference was detected in cnidarians because *M. cavernosa* reflected zooxanthellae sterols such as gorgosterol. Zooxanthellae contribution in deep, cold-water cnidarians is limited by light. In locations with clear water, the reduced light is enough to maintain hermatypic corals deeper than 50 m; for example, in the Atlantic Ocean, *Agaricia grahamae* grows at 119 m in the Bahamas [33], whereas, in the Red Sea, *Leptoseris fragilis* grows at 145 m [34]. The deepest record in the Pacific Ocean is for *Leptoseris hawaiiensis* at 165 m in Johnston Atoll [35]. However, *P. agaricus* was collected at 1027 m; thus, even a zooplankton supply revealed by 24-methylenecholesterol, occelasterol and brasicasterol is surprising. Similarly, tropical, shallow sponges had higher proportions of macroalgae and vascular plant sterols, in contrast to deep, sea sponges, also reflecting phytoplankton sterols such as 24-methylenecholesterol and episterol.

These probably were trophically transferred by zooplankton, detected with nordehydrocholesterol [29]. We did not expect to see brown algae sterol, 4-24 dimethyl 5, 7-dien-3-β-ol, in deep-water sponges. Moreover, stellasterol (cholesta-7, 22E-dien-3β-ol), poriferasterol (24-ethylcholesta-5, 22Z-dien-3β-ol), and fucosterol (24-ethylcholesta-5,24(28) E-dien-3β-ol) were present in sponges from both environments, suggesting they could be synthesized by sponges [36] or their symbionts; however, they should be from fungi or other eukaryotic symbionts at this depth of 353 m since light is not available. Five dominant end products of sterol biosynthesis (cholesterol, ergosterol, 24-methyl cholesterol, 24-ethyl cholesterol, and brassicasterol) and intermediates in the formation of 24-ethyl cholesterol are major sterols in 175 species of Fungi [37].

Echinoids from the tropical, shallow site were herbivores, as their $\delta^{13}C$ of −10‰ ± 0.1‰ from macroalgae and their $\delta^{15}N$ of 3.3‰ ± 0.3‰ [31] suggest a low trophic level (Table 3). In contrast, the echinoids from the cold, deep site had a more depleted $\delta^{13}C$ of −14.3‰ ± 0.9‰, indicating bentho-pelagic carbon sources, and higher $\delta^{15}N$ ratios of 12.3‰ ± 0.3‰ [30], indicating higher tropic levels, such as those of omnivores or even carnivores (Table 3). However, echinoid sterol profiles did not show significant differences between tropical, shallow and cold, deep sites. There are two possible explanations. The first is that echinoids can select cholesterol rich macroalgae, which could explain why the sea urchin *E. lucunter* had a high contribution of red algae *Galaxaura* sp. [31], coincident with the high proportion of cholesterol in *Galaxaura* sp. [29]. The second is that echinoids can modify phytosterols via dealkylation or synthesize cholesterol similarly to vertebrates among the chordates. The presence of lathosterol, a precursor of cholesterol, in *P. placenta* suggests that echinoderms can actually synthesize cholesterol. Lathosterol has been recorded in other cold, deep-water echinoderms such as the holoturian *Cucumaria japonica* [38]. This suggests that the maintenance of the complete set of CBP genes in vertebrates [24] is also maintained in echinoids.

Lastly, as lipids are the storage reservoir of energy in animals [19], the ratio between triacylglycerols and sterols (TAG:ST) can be used as an indicator of nutritional condition in fish larvae [39] and invertebrates [40]. Tropical, shallow sponges, cnidarians, and echinoids showed a significantly higher concentration of lipids and higher TAG:ST ratios, suggesting a better nutritional condition than deep, cold-water invertebrates, even if primary productivity was slightly higher in the Newfoundland offshore with a chlorophyll concentration of 1.24 mg·m^{-3} [41] in comparison with the Parque Nacional Sistema Arrecifal Veracruzano (PNSAV) with a chlorophyll concentration of 1.0 mg·m^{-3} [42] in similar seasons. Further investigation comparing essential fatty acids would provide more information about food quality.

4. Materials and Methods

4.1. Study Area

The geographical location and depth profile of the northwest Atlantic and southwest Gulf of Mexico sites are shown for comparison in Figures 5 and 6. The cold, deep study area was located in zone 3K, which represents the marine area located off the northern coasts of Newfoundland, according to the Northwest Atlantic Fisheries Organization (NAFO) division of the North Atlantic Ocean (Figure 6; more details in [43]). Mean daily bottom temperature during the sampling period at the sampling site ranged between 3.2 and 4.5 °C, with a slight decrease with depth. This region of the Northwest Atlantic is characterized by high productivity levels and is affected by seasonal blooms of large-celled phytoplankton; for instance, in 2012, chlorophyll *a* ranged from 1.24 mg·m^{-3} in November to 2.23 mg·m^{-3} in April [41], and there are strong lateral food inputs [44–46]. Due to its well-known productivity, the area has been heavily exploited and fished.

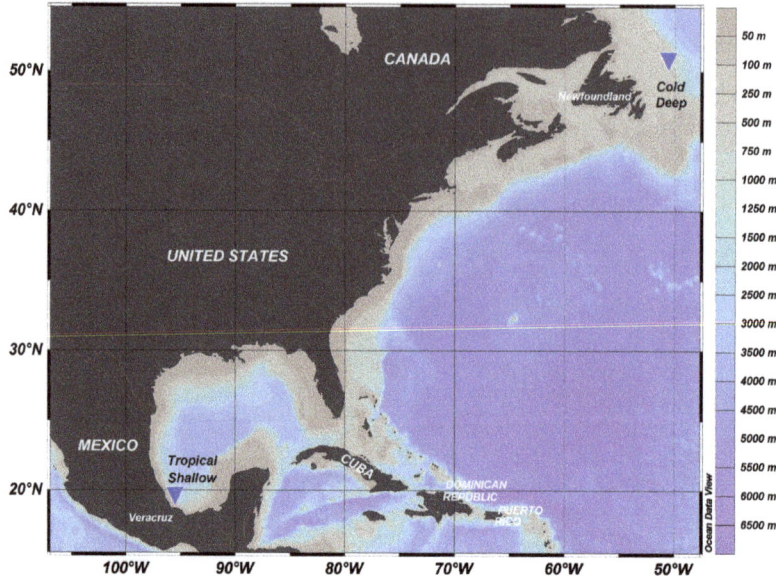

Figure 5. Map of sampling sites off the northeastern coast of the Province of Newfoundland and Labrador, Canada, in the Northwest Atlantic (cold, deep) and off the coast of Veracruz, Mexico in the southwest Gulf of Mexico (tropical, shallow).

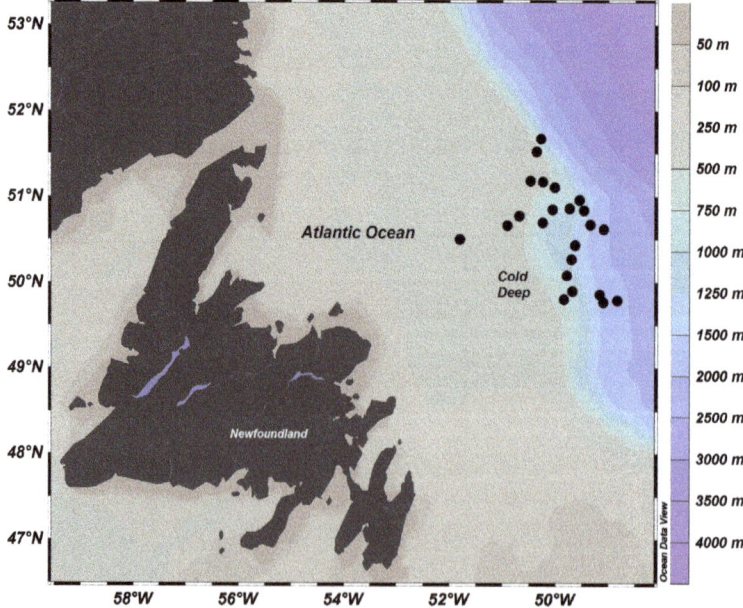

Figure 6. Map of sampling sites off the northeastern coast of the Canadian province of Newfoundland and Labrador (Northwest Atlantic). Dots (•) represent the locations of the sampling tows.

In contrast, the tropical shallow samples were collected in the Veracruz reef system national park (Parque Nacional Sistema Arrecifal Veracruzano; PNSAV), which is located off the State of Veracruz,

Mexico, adjacent to the cities of Boca del Rio and Anton Lizardo (19°02′24″ to 19°15′27″ north (N), 96°12′01″ to 95°46′46″ west (W)). It is part of a larger coral reef system in the Caribbean and Gulf of Mexico. A group of 13 reefs is located near Veracruz and Boca del Rio, and another group of 15 reefs with larger structures is located near Antón Lizardo; the two reefs are separated by the Río Jamapa and delimited to the north by Río La Antigua and to the south by the Río Papaloapan. During the summer, under sustained southward winds, a cyclonic eddy develops off Veracruz Port, which enhances productivity in the area reaching 2.3 ± 1.1 g·m^{-3} total plankton wet biomass [47] and a chlorophyll concentration of 1 mg·m^{-3} [42].

4.2. Sampling

In the cold, deep site, animals belonging to five phyla were opportunistically collected within 7 days in November–December 2013, during one of the annual multispecies bottom-trawl surveys conducted by Fisheries and Oceans (DFO), Canada. Individuals were sampled onboard the CCGS Teleost, from a total of 23 tows inside a 100 km radius and a depth range of 313 to 1407 m. The gear used to collect the samples (Campelen 1800 shrimp trawl) included a 16.9 m wide net with four panels of polyethylene twine. Once on board, individuals were immediately vacuum-packed and frozen at −20 °C to minimize lipid oxidation and hydrolysis. Individuals were identified to the lowest possible taxonomic level, from direct observation and through photo-identification. A total of 34 deep-sea organisms, belonging to five species from different phyla, were weighed, and samples of 0.7 ± 0.2 g wet weight were collected from each individual and processed for lipid analysis at the Core Research Equipment and Instrument Training Aquatic Research Cluster (CREAIT-ARC) Facility at Memorial University (Table 1). The following were sampled: pieces of sponges, body walls from cnidarians, foot muscle from gastropods, dorsal abdominal muscle from crustaceans, and wall and tube feet from echinoids.

Sponges, cnidarians, and echinoids sterols from the deep, cold-water site were compared to sterols of sponges and cnidarians [28] and echinoderms [29] from shallow tropical coral reefs. Sponges and echinoderms were collected in September 2007 and coral was collected in October 2009 in the Cabezo and Blanca reefs at depths from 18 to 20 m (Figure 7).

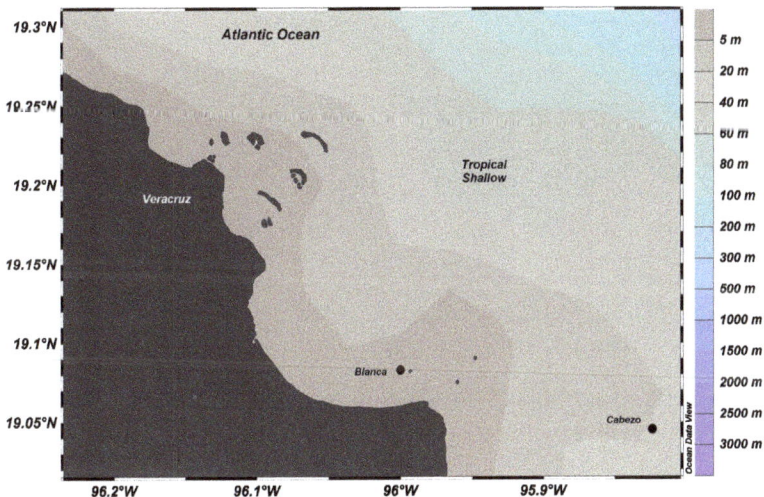

Figure 7. Map of sampling sites off Veracruz harbor in the coral reef system of Veracruz, Mexico. Dots (•) represent the locations of the sampling by scuba diving.

4.3. Laboratory Analysis

Samples were weighed wet, and around 0.7 ± 0.2 g was immersed in 4 mL of chloroform, sealed under nitrogen gas, and stored in a freezer (-20 °C). Lipids were extracted by adding 2 mL of methanol and 1.8 mL of distilled water, mixed with a vortex, and centrifuged to separate polar and nonpolar phases. The lower phase was recovered in a lipid-cleaned tube; an aliquot was separated into lipid classes by Chromarod thin-layer chromatography (TLC) [48]. Chromarod TLC and Iatroscan flame ionization detection (FID) were used to quantify the lipid classes in the extracts. TLC/FID was performed with Chromarods SIII and an Iatroscan MK VI (Iatron Laboratories, Tokyo, Japan). Concentrations of triacylglycerols (TAG), steryl esters, and free sterols were obtained by interpolation with a calibration curve constructed with five amounts, ranging between 0.5 and 4.0 µg, of the following standards: cholesteryl stearate, triplamitin, and cholesterol (Sigma-Aldrich, Toronto, Canada). The remainder of the extract was separated by a solid-phase extraction column (Strata SI-1 Silica 55 mm, 70 A; Phenomenex, Torrance, CA, USA). Neutral lipid fractions were recovered with 6 mL of chloroform/methanol/formic acid (98:1:0.05); then, galactoglycerolipids were recovered with 6 mL of 100% acetone, and phosphoglycerolipids were recovered with 9 mL of chloroform/methanol (5:4) as a modification of [49]. Quantification of lipids, stable isotopes, and C:N molar ratios for cold, deep samples were obtained from [30], and lipids and stable isotopes of tropical shallow echinoids were obtained from [31]. Stable isotopes and C:N molar ratios were used to assign functional group and possible organic carbon source (Table 3).

Neutral lipid, galactoglycerolipid, and phosphoglycerolipid fractions were transmethyl esterified with Hilditch reagent, and then silylated with bis trimethylsilyl trifluoroacetamide (BSTFA) (Supelco: 3-2024) [49]. Sterols from all samples were recovered in hexane and analyzed in a gas chromatograph coupled to a mass spectrometer (GC–MS (EI): Agilent 6890N GC-5973 MSD (quadrupole) with a DB-5 column 30 m × 0.32 mm × 0.25 µm, Agilent Technologies, Santa Clara, CA, USA). The quadrupole was set at 150 °C, and the mass spectrophotometer ion source was set at 270 °C and 70 eV. The positive ionization voltage on the repeller pushed the positive ions into several electrostatic lenses, producing a positive ionization mode. Peaks were identified by the retention time of standards and mass spectra interpretation. Sterols were identified by reference to [20] and [50] (p. 235). Positions of peaks were useful for identification of sterols with the same molecular ion, and the list provided by [20] was used to infer position relative to cholesterol. Mass spectra were searched with Wsearch 32 software (Wsearch 2008; version 1.6 2005, Sidney, Australia) and the NIST Mass Spectral Search Program for the NIST/EPA/NIH Mass Spectral Library (Demo version 2.0 f. build Apr 1 2009, USA). Sterol identity was confirmed by mass spectrum interpretation using the molecular weight (MW) ion (M$^+$) which provides information on number of carbons and double bonds [29,50]. Some important fragments for interpretation of the whole structure were (M-R)$^+$, (M-R-2H)$^+$, (M-H$_2$O)$^+$, (MR-H$_2$O)$^+$, (M-R-2H-H$_2$O)$^+$, and (M-CH$_3$-H$_2$O)$^+$. Other fragments indicated the position of double bonds. For instance, the lathosterol–TMS ether has a MW = 458, suggesting that the molecule has 27 carbons and one double bond. We should expect a signal at $m/z = 213$ indicating a double bond at C$_7$. For the stigmasterol–TMS ether, double bonds at C$_5$ and C$_{22}$ are shown by ions with $m/z = 129$ and $m/z = 255$ [29] (p. 15), [50] (p. 235). Finally, three standards were injected to build calibration curves for cholesterol, campesterol, and β-sitosterol (Sigma-Aldrich). Areas under the chromatographic peak (Figure 8) were integrated with Wsearch 32 software (Wsearch 2008; version 1.6 2005), and quantification was performed by interpolation of a calibration curve [29] (pp. 17–19). No peaks were detected in the galactoglycerolipid or phosphoglycerolipid fractions; therefore, all results refer to the neutral lipid fraction.

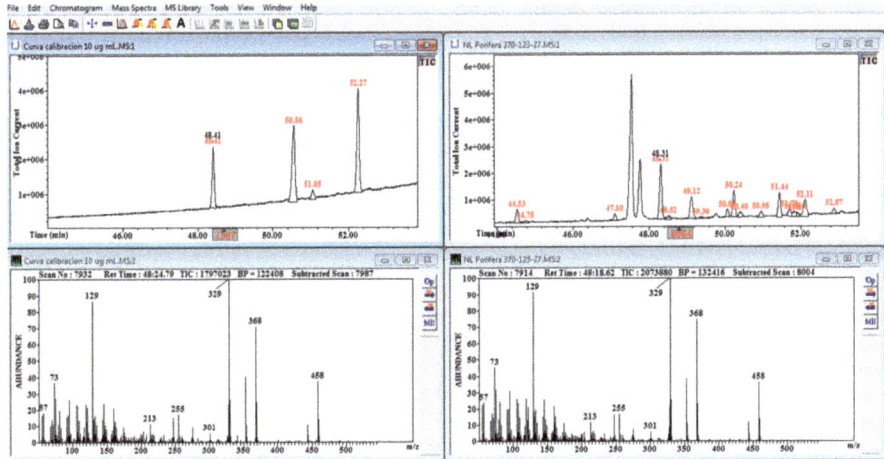

Figure 8. Total ion current (TIC) chromatogram and retention time (RT) of standards mix (upper left panel) including cholesterol (48.41), campesterol (50.56), stigmasterol (51.05), and β-sitosterol (52.27). The black number indicates the mass spectrum for cholesterol in the calibration curve (lower left panel). Identified chromatogram peaks of sponge *T. muricata* (upper right panel) were 24-nordehydrocholesterol (44.53), 24-nordehydrocholestanol (44.75), occelasterol (47.10), cholesterol (48.31), cholestanol (48.52), brassicasterol (49.12), brassicastanol (49.36), stellasterol (50.01), 24-methylenecholesterol (50.24), campesterol (50.40), stigmasterol (50.95), episterol (51.44), 4-24 dimethyl 5, 7-dien-3-β-ol (51.70), poriferasterol (51.81), spinasterol (51.89), β-sitosterol (52.11), and fucosterol (52.87). The black number indicates the mass spectrum for cholesterol in the sponge (lower right panel) for comparison with the standard.

4.4. Data Analysis

Species differences of individual (univariate) sterols were tested with one-way ANOVA using the Fisher statistic (F). Residual analyses were used to test assumptions of normality and equal variance. The effect of tropical shallow vs. cold deep waters on sponge, cnidarian, and echinoderm sterols was tested with multivariate analyses of sterol profile (>2% in a least one sample) using PRIMER 6.1.16 software and PERMANOVA + 1.0.6 (PRIMER-E, Plymouth, UK). Nonmetric multidimensional scaling was conducted on the basis of the Bray–Curtis similarity coefficient.

No transformation was used to avoid artificial weighting of sterols that gave only trace contributions to their respective profiles. Similarities among species and depth were investigated using the similarity percentages function (SIMPER), and statistical differences were tested with two-way analysis, for depth and phyla, using permutational multivariate analysis of variance (PERMANOVA), which allows multivariate comparisons with data with or without a normal distribution of residuals. The method of permutation of residuals under a reduced model was used, and significant differences were tested with Markov chain probability p(MC) values because the sample size was $n < 30$.

5. Conclusions

In the deep cold sites, gastropods and arthropods had cholesterol as their main sterol. Other extraction systems such as acetic acid and methanol could facilitate finding bioactive sterol metabolites for use against diabetes and oxidative stress-induced inflammatory diseases [51]. Sponges and cnidarians from shallow, tropical environments had plants such as mangrove or seagrass and zooxanthellae sterols, respectively, while cold, deep sponges had 24-ethyl sterols probably synthesized themselves [36], and cnidarians had phytoplankton, zooplankton, and probably fungal sterols. In contrast, echinoids, belonging to Echinodermata, the most complex phylum along with hemichordates and chordates (deuterostomes), did not show significant differences in their sterol profiles, suggesting that cholesterol synthesis is present in deuterostomes other than chordates. Tropical, shallow sponges, cnidarians, and echinoids showed a significantly higher concentration of lipids, as well as higher TAG:ST ratios, suggesting a better nutritional condition than deep, cold invertebrates. However, other echinoderm groups should be studied such as holothurians which did not have cholesterol as the main sterol, but rather diatomsterol, probably because supercritical fluid extraction was used [38]. Sex was the main factor affecting sterol amount in the gonads (intact, spawned) and gametes of echinoderm *A. dufresnii*, with differences in their total concentration from intact to spawned states explained by gamete concentrations [52]. As gonads are a good functional food for diabetes mellitus treatment in mice [53], sex and gonad composition of echinoderms should be recorded in future surveys.

Author Contributions: Conceptualization, L.C.-P., C.C.P., N.Ş.Ö., and C.P. methodology, C.P. and N.Ş.Ö.; software, L.C.-P.; validation, L.C.-P.; formal analysis, L.C.-P.; investigation, L.C.-P., N.Ş.Ö., and C.P.; resources, C.C.P.; data curation, L.C.-P.; writing—original draft preparation, L.C.-P.; writing—review and editing, C.C.P., N.Ş.Ö., and C.P.; visualization, L.C.P.; supervision, C.C.P. and L.C.-P.; project administration, C.C.P.; funding acquisition, C.C.P. and L.C.-P. All authors have read and agreed to the published version of the manuscript.

Funding: This research was funded by Natural Sciences and Engineering Research Council of Canada (NSERC) grant number 105379 to C.C. Parrish, the Canada Foundation for Innovation (CFI) grant number 11231 to A. Mercier, and the Consejo Nacional de Ciencia y Tecnología CONACyT, grant number 37567. Part of the work was a postdoctoral study supported by the Scientific and Technological Research Council of Turkey (TUBITAK) by the 2219—Postdoctoral Fellowship Program—2014(2).

Acknowledgments: We thank D. Stansbury, K. Tipple, D. Pittman, and V.E. Wareham, from the Department of Fisheries and Oceans (DFO), for their support on board the vessel and/or with the species identification, as well as J. Wells for technical support and E. Montgomery for help with sample collection. We thank those responsible for the deep-water DFO project, Jean-François Hamel and Annie Mercier from the Department of Ocean Sciences at Memorial University of Newfoundland, and Horacio Pérez-España from University of Veracruz for the CONACyT project. Lastly, we thank the Consejo Nacional de Ciencia y Tecnología CONACyT for the sabbatical fellowship at Memorial University of Newfoundland granted to LCP (CVU 201104).

Conflicts of Interest: The authors declare no conflict of interest. The funders had no role in the design of the study; in the collection, analyses, or interpretation of data; in the writing of the manuscript, or in the decision to publish the results.

References

1. Thistle, D. The deep-sea floor: An overview. In *Ecosystems of the Deep Oceans*; Tyler, P.A., Ed.; Elsevier Science Publisher B.V.: Amsterdam, The Netherlands, 2003; pp. 5–38.
2. Campanyà-Llovet, N.; Snelgrove, P.V.; Parrish, C.C. Rethinking the importance of food quality in marine benthic food webs. *Prog. Oceanogr.* **2017**, *156*, 240–251. [CrossRef]
3. Drazen, J.C.; Phleger, C.F.; Guest, M.A.; Nichols, P.D. Lipid, sterols and fatty acid composition of abyssal holothurians and ophiuroids from the North-East Pacific Ocean: Food web implications. *Comp. Biochem. Physiol. B Biochem. Mol. Biol.* **2008**, *151*, 79–87. [CrossRef]
4. Govenar, B. Energy transfer through food webs at hydrothermal vents: Linking the lithosphere to the biosphere. *Oceanography* **2012**, *25*, 246–255. [CrossRef]
5. Boschker, H.T.S.; Middelburg, J.J. Stable isotopes and biomarkers in microbial ecology. *FEMS Microbiol. Ecol.* **2002**, *40*, 85–95. [CrossRef]
6. Nichols, D. Biological Markers in the Marine Environment. Ph.D. Thesis, University of Melbourne, Melbourne, Australia, 1983.
7. Sargent, J.R.; Parkes, R.J.; Mueller-Harvey, I.; Henderson, R.J. Lipid biomarkers in marine ecology. In *Microbes in the Sea*; Sleigh, M.A., Ed.; Ellis Horwood: Chichester, UK, 1987; pp. 119–138.
8. Parrish, C.C. Dissolved and particulate marine lipid classes: A review. *Mar. Chem.* **1988**, *23*, 17–40. [CrossRef]
9. Budge, S.M.; Iverson, S.J.; Koopman, H.N. Studying trophic ecology in marine ecosystems using fatty acids: A primer on analysis and interpretation. *Mar. Mamm. Sci.* **2006**, *22*, 759–801. [CrossRef]
10. Litzow, M.A.; Bailey, K.M.; Prahl, F.G.; Heintz, R. Climate regime shifts and reorganization of fish communities: The essential fatty acid limitation hypothesis. *Mar. Ecol. Prog. Ser.* **2006**, *315*, 1–11. [CrossRef]

11. Laureillard, J.; Saliot, A. Biomarkers in organic matter produced in estuaries: A case study of the Krka Estuary (adriatic Sea) using the sterol marker series. *Mar. Chem.* **1993**, *43*, 247–261. [CrossRef]
12. Li, W.; Dagaut, J.; Saliot, A. The application of sterol biomarkers to the study of the sources of particulate organic matter in the Solo River system and serayu River, Java, Indonesia. *Biochemistry* **1995**, *31*, 139–154. [CrossRef]
13. Crockett, E.L. Cholesterol function in plasma membranes from ectotherms: Membrane-specific roles in adaptation to temperature. *Amer. Zool.* **1998**, *38*, 291–304. [CrossRef]
14. Nes, W.R. Role of sterols in membranes. *Lipids* **1974**, *9*, 596–612. [CrossRef] [PubMed]
15. Morris, R.; Culkin, F. Fish. In *Marine Biogenic Lipids, Fats and Oils*; Ackman, R.G., Ed.; CRC Press, Inc.: Boca Raton, FL, USA, 1989; pp. 146–178.
16. Lehninger, A. Biosynthesis of Lipids. In *Biochemistry*; Worth Publishers Inc.: New York, NY, USA, 1975; pp. 583–614.
17. Napolitano, G.E.; Ackman, R.G.; Silva-Serra, M.A. Incorporation of dietary sterols by the sea scallop *Placopecten magellanicus* (Gmelin) fed on microalgae. *Mar. Biol.* **1993**, *117*, 647–654. [CrossRef]
18. Paibulkichakul, C.; Piyatiratitivorakul, S.; Kittakoop, P.; Viyakarn, V.; Fast, A.W.; Menasveta, P. Optimal dietary levels of lecithin and cholesterol for black tiger prawn *Penaeus monodon* larvae and postlarvae. *Aquaculture* **1998**, *167*, 273–281. [CrossRef]
19. Parrish, C.C. Lipids in marine ecosystems. *ISRN Oceanogr.* **2013**. [CrossRef]
20. Jones, G.J.; Nichols, P.D.; Shaw, P.M. Analysis of microbial sterols and hopanoids. In *Chemical Methods in Prokaryotic Systematic*; Goodfellow, M., O'Donnell, A.G., Eds.; John Wiley: Chichester, UK, 1994; pp. 163–195.
21. Wei, J.H.; Yin, X.; Welander, P.V. Sterol Synthesis in Diverse Bacteria. *Front. Microbiol.* **2016**, *7*, 990. [CrossRef] [PubMed]
22. Desmond, E.; Gribaldo, S. Diversity of a key eukaryotic feature genome. *Biol. Evol.* **2009**, 364–381. [CrossRef]
23. Shmoop University Inc. 2020. Available online: https://www.shmoop.com/study-guides/biology/animal-evolution-diversity/animal-family-tree (accessed on 11 April 2020).
24. Zhang, T.; Yuan, D.; Xie, J.; Lei, Y.; Li, J.; Fang, G.; Tian, L.; Liu, J.; Cui, Y.; Zhang, M.; et al. Evolution of the cholesterol biosynthesis pathway in animals. *Mol. Biol. Evol.* **2019**, *36*, 2548–2556. [CrossRef]
25. Ruess, L.; Müller-Navarra, D.C. Essential Biomolecules in Food Webs. *Front. Ecol. Evol.* **2019**, *7*, 269. [CrossRef]
26. Kanazawa, A. Sterols in marine invertebrates. *Fish. Sci.* **2001**, *67*, 997–1007. [CrossRef]
27. Martin-Creuzburg, D.; Oexle, S.; Wacker, A.J. Thresholds for sterol-limited growth of Daphnia magna: A comparative approach using 10 different sterols. *J. Chem. Ecol.* **2014**, *40*, 1039–1050. [CrossRef]
28. Carreón-Palau, L.; Parrish, C.C.; Del Angel-Rodríguez, J.A.; Pérez-España, H. Seasonal Shifts in Fatty Acids and Sterols in Sponges, Corals, and Bivalves, in a southern Gulf of Mexico coral reef under river influence. *Coral Reefs*, (accepted).
29. Del Angel-Rodríguez, J.A.; Carreón-Palau, L.; Parrish, C.C. Identification and quantification of sterols in coral reef food webs. In *Sterols: Types, Classification and Structure*, 1st ed.; Jimenez, S., Ed.; Nova Science Publishers Inc.: New York, NY, USA, 2020; pp. 1–42.
30. Parzanini, C.; Parrish, C.C.; Hamel, J.-F.; Mercier, A. Functional diversity and nutritional content in a deep-sea faunal assemblage through total lipid, lipid class, and fatty acid analyses. *PLoS ONE* **2018**, *13*, e0207395. [CrossRef] [PubMed]
31. Carreón-Palau, L.; Parrish, C.C.; Del Angel-Rodríguez, J.A.; Pérez-España, H.; Aguiñiga-García, S. Revealing organic carbon sources fueling a coral reef food web in the Gulf of Mexico using stable isotopes and fatty acids. *Limnol. Oceanogr.* **2013**, *58*, 593–612. [CrossRef]
32. Henrichs, S.M. Organic matter in coastal marine sediments. In *The Global Coastal Ocean: Multiscale Interdisciplinary Processes, The Sea*; Robinson, A.R., Brink, K.H., Eds.; Harvard University Press: Boston, MA, USA, 2005; Volume 13, pp. 129–162.
33. Reed, J.K. Deepest distribution of Atlantic hermatypic corals discovered in the Bahamas. In Proceedings of the Fifth International Coral Reef Symposium Congress, Tahiti, French Polynesia, 27 May–1 June 1985; Volume 6, pp. 249–254.
34. Fricke, H.W.; Vareschi, E.; Schlichter, D. Photoecology of the coral *Leptoseris fragilis* in the Red Sea twilight zone (an experimental study by submersible). *Oecologia* **1987**, *73*, 371–381. [CrossRef] [PubMed]

35. Maragos, J.E.; Jokiel, P. Reef corals of Johnston Atoll: One of the worlds's most isolated reefs. *Coral Reefs* **1986**, *4*, 141–150. [CrossRef]
36. Gold, D.A.; Grabenstatter, J.; Mendoza, A.; Riesgo, A.; Ruiz-Trillo, I.; Summons, R.E. Sponge sterol biomarker hypothesis. *Proc. Nat. Acad. Sci. Mar.* **2016**, *113*, 2684–2689. [CrossRef]
37. Weete, J.D.; Abril, M.; Blackwell, M. Phylogenetic Distribution of Fungal Sterols. *PLoS ONE* **2010**, *5*, e10899. [CrossRef]
38. Zakharenko, A.; Romanchenko, D.; Thinh, P.D.; Pikula, K.; Hang, C.T.T.; Yuan, W.; Xia, X.; Chaika, V.; Chernyshev, V.; Zakharenko, S.; et al. Features and Advantages of Supercritical CO_2 Extraction of Sea Cucumber *Cucumaria frondosa japonica* Semper, 1868. *Molecules* **2020**, *25*, 4088. [CrossRef]
39. Giraldo, C.; Mayzaud, P.; Tavernier, E.; Irisson, J.O.; Penot, F.; Becciu, J.; Chartier, A.; Boutoute, M.; Koubbi, P. Lipid components as a measure of nutritional condition in fish larvae (*Pleuragramma antarcticum*) in East Antarctica. *Mar. Biol.* **2013**, *160*, 877–887. [CrossRef]
40. Carreón-Palau, L.; Parrish, C.C.; Pérez-España, H.; Aguiñiga-García, S. Elemental ratios and lipid classes in a coral reef food web under river influence. *Prog. Oceanogr.* **2018**, *164*, 1–11. [CrossRef]
41. Maillet, G.; Casault, B.; Pepin, P.; Johnson, C.; Plourde, S.; Starr, M.; Caverhill, C.; Maass, H.; Spry, J.; Fraser, S.; et al. Ocean Productivity Trends in the Northwest Atlantic During 2013. *NAFO SCR Doc.* **2014**, *14*, 1–30.
42. Salas-Monreal, D.; Marin-Hernandez, M.; Salas-Perez, J.J.; Salas-de-Leon, D.A.; Monreal-Gomez, M.A.; Pérez-España, H. Coral reef connectivity within the Western Gulf of Mexico. *J. Mar. Syst.* **2018**, *179*, 88–99. [CrossRef]
43. The Geographical Location and Depth Profile of the Northwest Atlantic and Southwest Gulf of Mexico Sites. Available online: https://www.nafo.int/About-us/Maps (accessed on 30 September 2019).
44. Snelgrove, P.; Haedrich, R. Structure of the deep demersal fish fauna off Newfoundland. *Mar. Ecol. Prog. Ser.* **1985**, *27*, 99–107. [CrossRef]
45. Williams, R.G.; Follows, M.J. The Ekman transfer of nutrients and maintenance of new production over the North Atlantic. *Deep Sea Res. Part. I Oceanogr. Res. Pap.* **1998**, *45*, 461–489. [CrossRef]
46. Afanasyev, Y.D.; Nezlin, N.P.; Kostianoy, A.G. Patterns of seasonal dynamics of remotely sensed chlorophyll and physical environment in the Newfoundland region. *Remote Sens. Environ.* **2001**, *76*, 268–282. [CrossRef]
47. Okolodkov, Y.B.; Aké-Castillo, J.A.; Gutiérrez-Quevedo, M.G.; Pérez-España, H.; Salas-Monreal, D. Annual cycle of the plankton biomass in the National Park Sistema Arrecifal Veracruzano, southwestern Gulf of Mexico. In *Zooplankton and Phytoplankton*; Kattel, G., Ed.; Nova Science: New York, NY, USA, 2011; pp. 1–26.
48. Parrish, C.C. Separation of aquatic lipid classes by Chromarodthin-layer chromatography with measurement by Iatroscan flame ionization detection. *Can. J. Fish. Aquat. Sci.* **1987**, *44*, 722–731. [CrossRef]
49. Copeman, L.A.; Parrish, C.C. Lipids classes, fatty acids, and sterols in seafood from Gilbert Bay, southern Labrador. *J. Agric. Food Chem.* **2004**, *52*, 4872–4881. [CrossRef]
50. McLafferty, F.W.; Turecek, F. *Interpretation of Mass Spectra*, 4th ed.; University Sciences Books: Sausalito, CA, USA, 1993; p. 360. Available online: https://www.nafo.int/About-us/Maps (accessed on 30 September 2019).
51. Salas, S.; Chakraborty, K. First report of bioactive sterols from the muricid gastropod *Chicoreus ramosus*. *Steroids* **2018**, *137*, 57–63. [CrossRef]
52. Díaz de Vivar, M.E.D.; Zárate, E.V.; Rubilar, T.; Epherra, L.; Avaro, M.G.; Sewell, M.A. Lipid and fatty acid profiles of gametes and spawned gonads of *Arbacia dufresnii* (Echinodermata: Echinoidea): Sexual differences in the lipids of nutritive phagocytes. *Mar. Biol.* **2019**, *166*, 96. [CrossRef]
53. Pozharitskaya, O.N.; Alexander, N.; Shikov, A.N.; Laakso, I.; Seppänen-Laakso, T.; Makarenko, I.E.; Faustova, N.M.; Makarova, M.N.; Makarov, V.G. Bioactivity and chemical characterization of gonads of green sea urchin *Strongylocentrotus droebachiensis* from Barents Sea. *J. Funct. Foods* **2015**, *17*, 227–234. [CrossRef]

Publisher's Note: MDPI stays neutral with regard to jurisdictional claims in published maps and institutional affiliations.

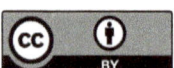

© 2020 by the authors. Licensee MDPI, Basel, Switzerland. This article is an open access article distributed under the terms and conditions of the Creative Commons Attribution (CC BY) license (http://creativecommons.org/licenses/by/4.0/).

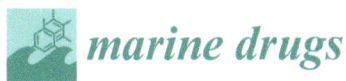

Article

Fucosylated Chondroitin Sulfates from the Sea Cucumbers *Paracaudina chilensis* and *Holothuria hilla*: Structures and Anticoagulant Activity

Nadezhda E. Ustyuzhanina [1,*], Maria I. Bilan [1], Andrey S. Dmitrenok [1], Alexandra S. Silchenko [2], Boris B. Grebnev [2], Valentin A. Stonik [2], Nikolay E. Nifantiev [1] and Anatolii I. Usov [1,*]

[1] N.D. Zelinsky Institute of Organic Chemistry, Russian Academy of Sciences, Leninsky Prospect 47, 119991 Moscow, Russia; bilan@ioc.ac.ru (M.I.B.); dmt@ioc.ac.ru (A.S.D.); nen@ioc.ac.ru (N.E.N.)
[2] G.B. Elyakov Pacific Institute of Bioorganic Chemistry, Far Eastern Branch of the Russian Academy of Sciences, Prospect 100 let Vladivostoku 159, 690022 Vladivostok, Russia; sialexandra@mail.ru (A.S.S.); grebnev_bor@mail.ru (B.B.G.); stonik@piboc.dvo.ru (V.A.S.)
* Correspondence: ustnad@gmail.com (N.E.U.); usov@ioc.ac.ru (A.I.U.); Tel.: +7-495-135-8784 (N.E.U.)

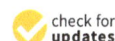

Received: 29 September 2020; Accepted: 26 October 2020; Published: 28 October 2020

Abstract: Fucosylated chondroitin sulfates (FCSs) **PC** and **HH** were isolated from the sea cucumbers *Paracaudina chilensis* and *Holothuria hilla*, respectively. The purification of the polysaccharides was carried out by anion-exchange chromatography on a DEAE-Sephacel column. The structural characterization of the polysaccharides was performed in terms of monosaccharide and sulfate content, as well as using a series of nondestructive NMR spectroscopic methods. Both polysaccharides were shown to contain a chondroitin core [→3)-β-D-GalNAc (N-acethyl galactosamine)-(1→4)-β-D-GlcA (glucuronic acid)-(1→]$_n$, bearing sulfated fucosyl branches at O-3 of every GlcA residue in the chain. These fucosyl residues were different in their pattern of sulfation: **PC** contained Fuc2S4S and Fuc4S in a ratio of 2:1, whereas **HH** included Fuc2S4S, Fuc3S4S, and Fuc4S in a ratio of 1.5:1:1. Moreover, some GalNAc residues in **HH** were found to contain an unusual disaccharide branch Fuc4S-(1→2)-Fuc3S4S-(1→ at O-6. Sulfated GalNAc4S6S and GalNAc4S units were found in a ratio of 3:2 in **PC** and 2:1 in **HH**. Both polysaccharides demonstrated significant anticoagulant activity in a clotting time assay, which is connected with the ability of these FCSs to potentiate the inhibition of thrombin and factor Xa in the presence of anti-thrombin III (ATIII) and with the direct inhibition of thrombin in the absence of any cofactors.

Keywords: sea cucumber; *Holothuria hilla*; *Paracaudina chilensis*; fucosylated chondroitin sulfate; anticoagulant activity

1. Introduction

Fucosylated chondroitin sulfates (FCSs) are the unique polysaccharides found exclusively in the body walls of sea cucumbers. These biopolymers are composed of D-glucuronic acid, N-acetyl-D-galactosamine, L-fucose, and sulfate residues [1–3]. A chondroitin core of FCSs [→3)-β-D-GalNAc-(1→4)-β-D-GlcA-(1→]$_n$ contains α-L-fucosyl branches attached to O-3 of GlcA or to O-6 of GalNAc [1–6]. Sulfate groups may occupy different positions of GalNAc, Fuc, and even GlcA residues. Depending on the species of sea cucumber, FCSs include GalNAc units sulfated at O-4 or at both O-4 and O-6; fucosyl branches Fuc2S4S, Fuc3S4S, and Fuc4S; as well as GlcA residues sulfated at O-3 or at both O-2 and O-3 [3–8]. In addition, difucosyl branches attached to O-3 of GlcA are known as very rare structural fragments of FCSs. Thus, FCS from *Holothuria* (*Ludwigothuria*) *grisea* was shown to contain the branch α-L-Fuc-(1→2)-α-L-Fuc3S-1→ [9]. The branch α-L-Fuc-(1→2)-α-L-Fuc3S4S-1→ was observed in FCS from *Eupentacta fraudatrix* [8]. FCS from *Holothuria lentiginosa* contains the fragment α-L-Fuc-(1→3)-α-L-Fuc4S-1→ linked also to O-3 of GlcA [10].

The fine structure of FCSs significantly influences biological activity, which is connected with the interaction of polysaccharides with different proteins. Thus, the intensively studied anticoagulant activity of FCSs was shown to be determined by their ability to potentiate the inhibition of thrombin and factor Xa in the presence of anti-thrombin III (ATIII) [1,3,5,6,11–14]. Other mechanisms mediated by heparin cofactor II and FXase were also considered [15–17]. The presence of fucosyl branches sulfated at O-4 in FCSs was found to be essential for the anticoagulant effect [13,18]. The anti-inflammatory activity of FCSs is connected with their binding to P- and L-selectins [19]. Recently, the anti-angiogenic effect of FCS from *Hemioedema spectabilis* was demonstrated in vitro [20], which is probably mediated by the interaction of the polysaccharide with growth factors [21].

In this communication, we describe the structural characterization of two FCSs (**PC** and **HH**) isolated from the sea cucumbers *Paracaudina chilensis* and *Holothuria hilla*, respectively. The anticoagulant activity of these polysaccharides was studied in vitro.

The sea cucumber *Holothuria hilla*, belonging to the order Holothuriida, is a widely distributed species in the South China Sea, especially near the shore of Fujian Province of China, Dongshan Island, and the Vietnamese seashore. The chemical composition of this sea cucumber was studied in 2006–2007 by Chinese researchers, who isolated and elucidated the structures of three novel triterpene glycosides, hillasides A–C [22,23], together with the previously known holothurins A and B. These glycosides are xylosides of holostane aglycones, differing in their structures of aglycones and carbohydrate side chains. It is interesting to mention that one of them, hillaside C, contained a disaccharide chain composed of two xylose residues, which was found in the triterpene glycosides of sea cucumbers for the first time. Hillasides were shown to exhibit significant cytotoxic activity (in vitro). The polysaccharides of *H. hilla* have not been previously studied.

Paracaudina chilensis belongs to the order Molpadiida, the representatives of which have been poorly studied in regard to their chemistry. A new triterpene glycoside, caudinoside A, was isolated from this sea cucumber (named *Paracaudina ransonetii*) in 1986. The structure of native aglycone, 3β-hydroxy-16-ketoholosta-9(11),25-diene, and the monosaccharide composition of the carbohydrate chain (xylose, quinovose, glucose, and 3-O-methylglucose in the ratio of 1:1:3:1) were established, but the whole chemical structure of caudinoside A remains unelucidated [24]. In addition, the amino acid sequence of the major globin isolated from coelomic cells of *P. chilensis* was determined [25], and gelatin hydrolysates were shown to possess antioxidant activity, demonstrating a reasonable radical scavenging effect and preventing the damage of rabbit liver and mitochondria (the species name was erroneously written as 'chinens' in this publication) [26]. As in the case of *H. hilla*, the polysaccharide composition of *P. chilensis* has not been investigated previously.

2. Results and Discussion

Crude extracts of sulfated polysaccharides were obtained from the body walls of sea cucumbers *Paracaudina chilensis* and *Holothuria hilla* by the conventional solubilization of biomass in the presence of papain [27] followed by the treatment of the extract with hexadecyl-trimethylammonium bromide to precipitate the sulfated components, which were then transformed into water-soluble sodium salts by stirring the components with NaI in ethanol. According to their composition, crude preparations contained sulfated fucans and FCS as the main components. Both crude extracts were subjected to anion-exchange chromatography on a DEAE-Sephacel column. The fractions eluted with 1.0 M NaCl were designated as **PC** for *P. chilensis* and **HH** for *H. hilla*. These preparations contained GlcA, GalNAc, Fuc, and sulfate in ratios (Table 1) typical for holothurian FCSs. The detection of minor Gal and GlcN in hydrolysates was explained by the possible presence of small amounts of other glycosaminoglycans, which could not be eliminated by anion-exchange chromatography. The molecular weights of the polysaccharides were estimated as 28.9 kDA for **PC** and 26.7 kDa for **HH** by gel-permeation chromatography [28].

Table 1. Percentages of crude polysaccharide preparations and composition of fucosylated chondroitin sulfates **PC** and **HH** (in *w/w* %).

Polysaccharide	Yield	Fuc	GlcA	SO₃Na	GlcN	GalN	Gal
HH	16.1	10.8	13.3	21.2	-	10.7	1.6
PC	20.9	10.9	11.4	21.3	1.2	8.8	4.3

The structures of polysaccharides **PC** and **HH** were characterized in more detail using NMR spectroscopic methods. The presence of Fuc, GalNAc, and GlcA units in both polysaccharides was confirmed by the characteristic values of chemical shifts of C-6 for Fuc (δ 17.2 ppm) and GlcA (δ 176.0 ppm), as well as of C-2 for GalNAc (δ 52.7 ppm) in ^{13}C NMR spectra (Figure 1). The anomeric regions in the ^{1}H NMR spectra of the polysaccharides were quite different, indicating the presence of different fucosyl branches (Figure 2).

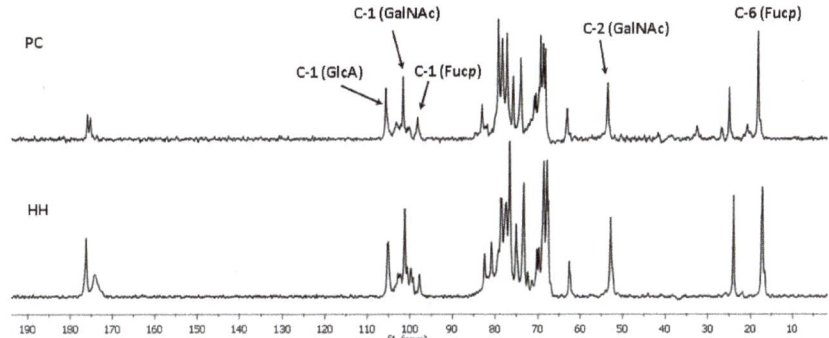

Figure 1. The ^{13}C NMR spectra of the fucosylated chondroitin sulfates **PC** and **HH**.

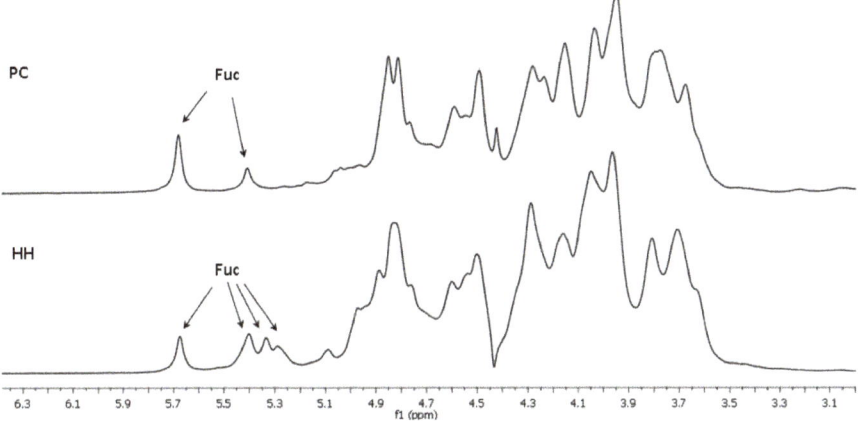

Figure 2. Fragments of ^{1}H NMR spectra of the fucosylated chondroitin sulfates **PC** and **HH**.

The application of 2D NMR experiments correlation spectroscopy (COSY), total correlation spectroscopy (TOCSY), heteronuclear single quantum coherence (HSQC), and rotating-frame nuclear Overhauser effect spectroscopy (ROESY) led to assigning all of the signals of the major components in the ^{1}H and ^{13}C NMR spectra of the polysaccharides (Figures 3 and 4 and Figures S1–S3, Table 2). Analysis of the spectra of **PC** revealed the similarity of its structure to those described previously for FCS from other species of sea cucumbers [4,19,29]. Thus, the signals of GlcA, GalNAc, and Fuc units were related to the core [→3)-β-D-GalNAc-(1→4)-β-D-GlcA-(1→]$_n$, bearing fucosyl branches at O-3 of every GlcA unit (see repeating unit **I** in Figure 3) [4,19]. There were two fucosyl units Fuc2S4S (**D**) and Fuc4S (**F**) that differed in pattern of sulfation, which was indicated by the downfield chemical shifts of the signals of respective protons in the ^{1}H NMR spectrum (Table 2). The ratio of units **D** and **F** was determined using the integral intensities of the respective H-1 signals and was found to be 2:1. The linkages between the fucosyl units and O-3 of GlcA were confirmed by the correlation H-1(Fuc)-H-3(GlcA) in the ROESY spectrum (Figure S2). Sulfated GalNAc4S6S (**B**) and GalNAc4S (**C**) units were found in an approximate ratio of 3:2 in **PC** by integration of the intensities of the cross-peaks related to H-6–C-6 interaction in units **B** and **C** in the HSQC spectrum.

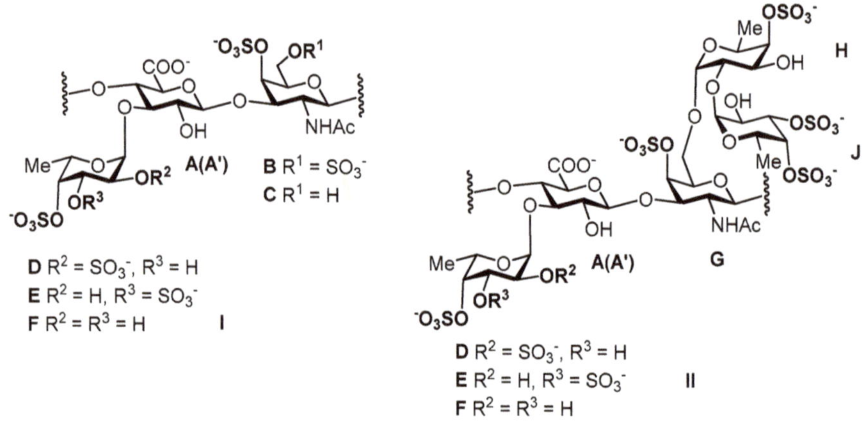

Figure 3. Repeating blocks of fucosylated chondroitin sulfates **PC** (units **A–D, F**) and **HH** (units **A–J**). Unit **A** bears Fuc2S4S (**D**), whereas unit **A'** bears Fuc3S4S (**E**) or Fuc4S (**F**).

The structure of polysaccharide **HH** was more complex than that of **PC**. Two branched repeating blocks **I** and **II** were determined in **HH** (Figure 3). The first one was typical for all FCSs and contained three different fucosyl branches Fuc2S4S (**D**), Fuc3S4S (**E**), and Fuc4S (**F**) in a ratio of ~1.5:1:1 (calculated using the integral intensities of the respective H-1 signals, Figure S4). Units GalNAc4S6S (**B**) and GalNAc4S (**C**) were found in a ratio of 2:1. The repeating block **II** along with the fucosyl residue at O-3 of GlcA contained the unusual difucosyl branch attached to O-6 of GalNAc(**G**) and formed by units **H** and **J**. The chemical shift of the H-1 signal of unit **H** (δ 5.28 ppm) differed from those of units **D, E,** and **F**. This led to the assessment of the signals of the spin system of unit **H** using the COSY, TOCSY, and ROESY experiments (Figures S1–S3) and allowed for the determination of the signals of the respective carbon atoms from the HSQC spectrum (Figure 4B). The attachment of unit **H** to O-6 of GalNAc (**G**) was confirmed by the presence of the cross-peak H1(**H**)-H6(**G**) in the ROESY spectrum. The downfield chemical shift of the C-2 signal of **H** (δ 72.8 ppm) indicated the position of glycosylation (compared with δ 69.8 ppm for Fuc4S **F**). Detailed analysis of the ROESY spectrum revealed one more fucosyl unit **J** (δ 5.41 ppm) linked to O-2 of residue **H**, as the cross-peak H1(**J**)-H2(**H**) was detected. The positions of sulfate groups in units **H** and **J** were determined by the downfield chemical shifts of signals of the respective protons. Therefore, the presence of the unusual branch Fuc4S-(1→2)-Fuc3S4S-(1→ linked to O-6 of GalNAc was confirmed. The ratio of units **H** and **E** was estimated to be about 1:1 (Figure S4). Previously, difucosyl branches in holothurian FCSs were found to be attached to O-3 of GlcA but not to O-6 of GalNAc [8–10].

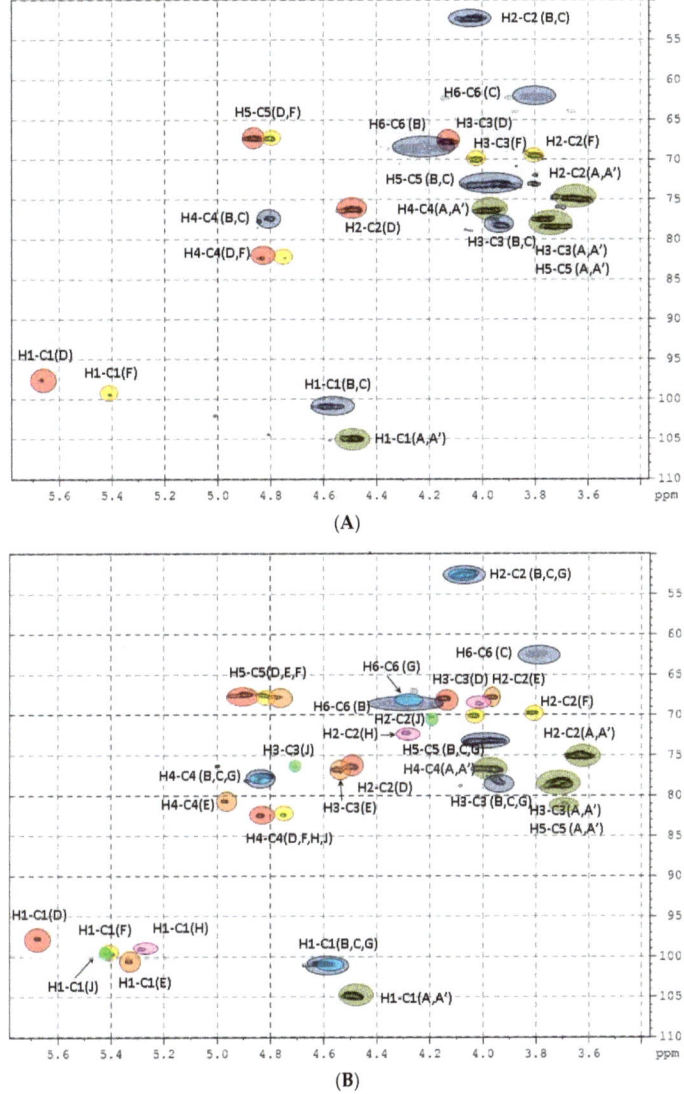

Figure 4. The HSQC NMR spectra of polysaccharides **PC** (**A**) and **HH** (**B**).

FCSs are known to demonstrate anticoagulant activity; therefore, we have studied two new polysaccharides **PC** and **HH** as anticoagulant agents in vitro. Heparin and low-molecular-weight heparin (enoxaparin) were used as standards. In addition, we have studied FCS **CD**, isolated previously from the sea cucumber *Cucumaria djakonovi* [30]. The latter polysaccharide includes the linear non-fucosylated disaccharide fragments →3)-β-D-GalNAc4S6S-(1→4)-β-D-GlcA-(1→, →3)-β-D-GalNAc4S-(1→4)-β-D-GlcA-(1→, and →3)-β-D-GalNAc6S-(1→4)-β-D-GlcA-(1→ along with the branched unit **I** (Figure 3). In the clotting time assay (activated partial thromboplastin time (APTT) test), the effects of **PC** and **HH** were higher than that of enoxaparin but lower than that of heparin, whereas polysaccharide **CD** was less active than enoxaparin (Figure 5A). The values of 2APTT (the concentration that led to a 2-fold increase of time of clot formation) were 0.8 ± 0.1 µg/mL for heparin, 2.5 ± 0.1 µg/mL for **HH**, 2.8 ± 0.1 µg/mL for **PC**, 3.7 ± 0.2 µg/mL for enoxaparin, and 5.0 ± 0.1 µg/mL for **CD**.

Table 2. Chemical shifts of the signals in the ^{1}H and ^{13}C NMR spectra of the fucosylated chondroitin sulfates **PC** and **HH** (the bold numerals indicate the positions of sulfate).

Residue	H1/C1	H2/C2	H3/C3	H4/C4	H5/C5	H6/C6
A→4)-β-D-GlcpA-(1→	4.48/ 105.0	3.64/ 75.0	3.72/ 77.8	3.96/ 76.6	3.70/ 78.1	- 176.0
A′→4)-β-D-GlcpA-(1→	4.48/ 105.0	3.60/ 75.0	3.68/ 80.7	4.00/ 76.6	3.71/ 78.1	- 176.0
B→3)-β-D-GalpNAc4S6S-(1→	4.58/ 100.9	4.07/ 52.7	3.95/ 77.9	**4.81**/ **77.2**	4.00/ 73.2	**4.33, 4.20** 68.5
C→3)-β-D-GalpNAc4S-(1→	4.58/ 100.9	4.07/ 52.7	3.95/ 77.9	**4.81**/ **77.2**	4.02/ 76.2	3.81/ 62.3
D α-L-Fucp2S4S-(1→	5.68/ 97.7	**4.47**/ **76.6**	4.17/ 67.8	**4.86**/ **82.5**	4.90/ 67.5	1.37/ 16.9
E α-L-Fucp3S4S-(1→	5.34/ 100.5	3.95/ 67.6	**4.53**/ **76.6**	**4.99**/ **80.6**	4.80/ 67.6	1.37/ 17.2
F α-L-Fucp4S-(1→	5.40/ 99.6	3.82/ 69.7	4.04/ 70.0	**4.77**/ **82.4**	4.80/ 67.6	1.37/ 17.2
G→3)-β-D-GalpNAc4S-(1→	4.47/ 105.1	3.38/ 73.9	3.59/ 75.2	**4.81**/ **77.2**	4.02/ 76.2	3.81/ 62.3
H→2)-α-L-Fucp4S-(1→	5.28/ 99.1	4.28/ 72.8	4.00/ 68.6	**4.84**/ **82.5**	NdNd	1.37/ 17.2
J α-L-Fucp3S4S-(1→	5.41/ 99.6	4.19/ 70.9	**4.69**/ **76.6**	**4.99**/ **80.6**	NdNd	1.37/ 17.2

Nd—not determined.

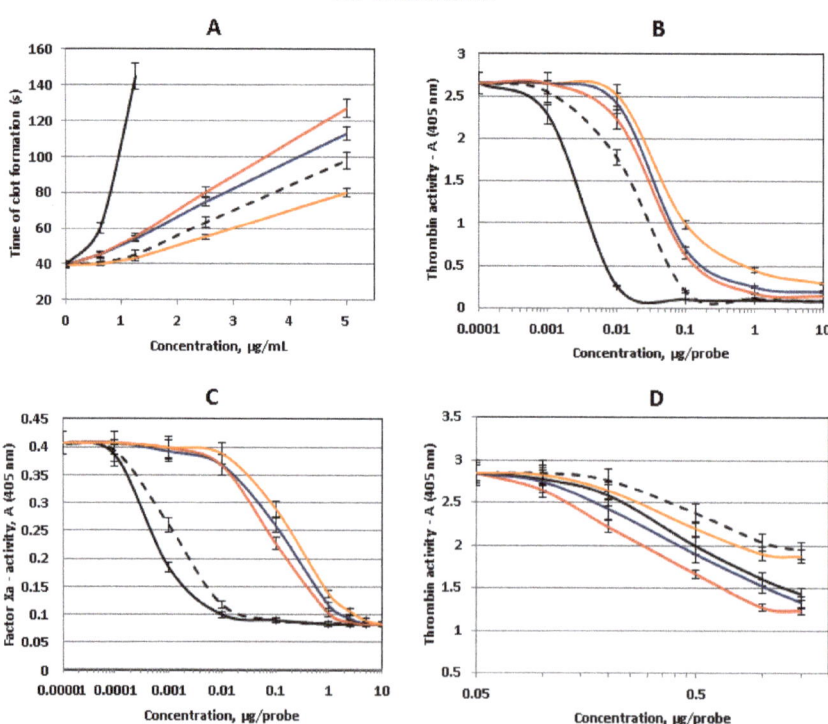

Figure 5. Anticoagulant activity of polysaccharides **PC** (blue), **HH** (red), **CD** (orange), heparin (black), and enoxaparin (dotted line). (**A**) Activate partial thromboplastin time (APTT) assay, (**B**) anti-IIa-activity in the presence of antithrombin III (ATIII), (**C**) anti-Xa-activity in the presence of ATIII, and (**D**) anti-IIa-activity without ATIII. $n = 4$, $p < 0.05$.

Thrombin and factor Xa are considered to be the main players in the coagulation cascade [1,6]. These serine proteases could be inhibited by ATIII, and this interaction is significantly increased in the presence of heparinoids. Therefore, we then studied the ability of the polysaccharides to potentiate the inhibition of thrombin and factor Xa in the presence of ATIII. In these experiments, all of the studied polysaccharides demonstrated the activity, but the values of the effects were lower than those of heparinoids (Figure 5B,C). Interesting results were obtained in the experiment with thrombin but without ATIII (Figure 5D). **HH** inhibited thrombin activity more effectively than **PC** and **CD**, and this phenomenon may be explained by the presence of disaccharide branches in **HH**. Notably, the activity of **HH** and **PC** was higher than that of heparin in this experiment. Previously, direct thrombin inhibition was described for fucoidans from brown seaweeds, the polysaccharides enriched in fucose content [31]. This mechanism might be taken into consideration, as it could impact the coagulation cascade.

3. Materials and Methods

3.1. General Methods

The procedures for the determination of neutral monosaccharides, sulfate, and uronic acids were described previously [32–34]. The molecular weights of polysaccharides were evaluated by chromatographic comparison with standard pullulans [28].

3.2. Isolation of Polysaccharides

The samples of sea cucumber *Holothuria hilla* were collected in the summer of 1990, on the seashore of D'Arros Island (Seyshelles) at a depth of 10 m by scuba divers. The taxonomic identification was made by Prof. V.S. Levin of the G.B. Elyakov Pacific Institute of Bioorganic Chemistry of the Far Eastern Branch of the Russian Academy of Sciences (PIBOC FEB RAS). The samples of *Paracaudina chilensis* were collected in the Trinity Bay, Peter the Great Gulf, the Sea of Japan in the summer of 2019 at a depth of 5–7 m. The taxonomic identification was carried out by Boris B. Grebnev (PIBOC FEB RAS). Both animals were fixed with ethanol. The sea cucumbers were cut into pieces, extracted twice with refluxed 70% EtOH, and the residue of animal material was air-dried.

According to the conventional procedure [27], dried and minced biomass of *H. hilla* (40 g) was suspended in 300 mL of 0.1 M sodium acetate buffer (pH 6.0), containing papain (1 g), ethylenediaminetetraacetic acid (EDTA) (0.4 g), and L-cysteine hydrochloride (0.2 g), and incubated at 45–50 °C for 24 h. After centrifugation, an aqueous hexadecyl-trimethylammonium bromide solution (10%, 30 mL) was added to the supernatant; the resulting precipitate was isolated by centrifugation and washed successively with water and ethanol. Then, it was stirred with a 20% ethanolic NaI solution (5 × 40 mL) for 2–3 days, washed with ethanol, dissolved in water, and lyophilized to obtain the crude polysaccharide preparation **HH-SP**, yield 1.9 g (4.7%), composition: Fuc 16.6%, uronic acids 3.0%, GlcN 2.1%, GalN 5.2%, Gal 2.1%, and SO_3Na 15.8%. An aqueous solution of **HH-SP** (249 mg in 50 mL) was placed on a column (3 × 10 cm) with DEAE (Diethylaminoethyl)-Sephacel in Cl$^-$ form and eluted with water, followed by a NaCl solution of increasing concentration (0.5, 0.75, 1.0, and 1.5 M), each time until the absence of a positive reaction of eluate for carbohydrates [35]. Fractions were desalted on a Sephadex G-15 (Sigma-Aldrich, St. Louis, MO, USA. Catalog number: G15120) column and lyophilized. According to composition (Table 1), the fraction eluted with 1.0 M NaCl was designated as **HH** and studied further as preparation of FCS. Similar treatment of *P. chilensis* biomass (45 g) gave rise to crude polysaccharide preparation **PC-SP**, yield 1.2 g (2.7%), and preparation of FCS eluted from the DEAE-Sephadex with 1.0 M NaCl was designated as **PC** (Table 1).

3.3. NMR Spectroscopy

The NMR spectra were recorded using Zelinsky Institute Shared Research Facilities Center. The sample preparation and the conditions of the experiments were described previously [7].

3.4. Clotting Time Assay

The APTT test was performed as described previously [14]. Heparin (Sigma-Aldrich, St. Louis, MO, USA. Catalog number: 51550), enoxaparin (Clexane®, Sanofi, Paris, France), and FCS **CD** were used as references.

3.5. Effect of Polysaccharides on Thrombin or Factor Xa Inactivation by Antithrombin III

Both experiments were carried out at 37 °C in 96-well plates using MultiscanGo (Thermo Fisher Scientific, Stockholm, Sweden). Tris-HCl buffer was used as a control.

A ReaChrom ATIII test kit (Renam, Moscow, Russia) was used for the measurement of thrombin activity. A solution of a polysaccharide sample (**PC**, **HH**, **CD**, heparin, or enoxaparin) (20 µL) with concentrations of 500, 50, 5, 0.5, and 0.05 µg/mL in Tris-HCl buffer was added to 50 µL of a solution of ATIII (0.2 U/mL) in Tris-HCl buffer (0.15 µM, pH 8.4). After a 3-min incubation, an aqueous solution of thrombin (50 µL, 20 U/mL) was added, and the mixture was incubated for 2 min. Then, a chromogenic substrate (50 µL, 2 mM) was added, and the mixture was kept for 2 min. Absorbance of p-nitroaniline (405 nm) was measured.

A ReaChrom Heparin kit (Renam, Moscow, Russia) was used for the measurement of factor Xa activity. A solution of a polysaccharide sample (**PC**, **HH**, **CD**, heparin, or enoxaparin) (20 µL) with concentrations of 500, 50, 5, 0.5, and 0.05 µg/mL in Tris-HCl buffer was added to 50 µL of a solution of ATIII (0.5 U/mL) in Tris-HCl buffer. After a 3-min incubation, an aqueous solution of factor Xa (50 µL, 2 U/mL) was added, and the mixture was incubated for 2 min. The mixture was worked up, treated with chromogenic substrate, and analyzed as described above.

3.6. Effect of Polysaccharides on Thrombin Inactivation without ATIII

A ReaChrom ATIII test kit (Renam, Moscow, Russia) was used for the experiments. An aqueous solution of thrombin (50 µL, 20 U/mL) and a solution of a polysaccharide sample (**PC**, **HH**, **CD**, heparin, or enoxaparin) (20 µL) with concentrations of 750, 500, 250, 100, and 50 µg/mL in Tris-HCl buffer were added to 50 µL of Tris-HCl buffer. The mixture was incubated for 3 min. Then, 50 µL of a chromogenic substrate (2 mM) was added, and the incubation was continued for 2 min. The absorbance of p-nitroaniline (405 nm) was measured. Tris-HCl buffer was used as a control.

3.7. Statistical Analysis

All biological experiments were performed in quadruplicate ($n = 4$). The results are presented as Mean ± SD. Statistical significance was determined with Student's t test. The p values less than 0.05 were considered significant.

4. Conclusions

Two new sulfated polysaccharides **PC** and **HH** were isolated from the sea cucumbers *Paracaudina chilensis* and *Holothuria hilla*, respectively. The main components of these biopolymers were GlcA, GalNAc, Fuc, and sulfate, indicating **PC** and **HH** as fucosylated chondroitin sulfates. Based on the data of the NMR spectra, both polysaccharides were shown to contain a chondroitin core [→3)-β-D-GalNAc-(1→4)-β-D-GlcA-(1→]$_n$, bearing sulfated fucosyl branches at O-3 of every GlcA residue in the chain. These fucosyl residues were different in their pattern of sulfation: **PC** contained Fuc2S4S and Fuc4S in a ratio of 2:1, while **HH** included Fuc2S4S, Fuc3S4S, and Fuc4S in a ratio of 1.5:1:1. Moreover, some GalNAc residues in **HH** were found to contain the unusual disaccharide branch Fuc4S-(1→2)-Fuc3S4S-(1→ at O-6. Sulfated GalNAc4S6S and GalNAc4S units were found in a ratio of 3:2 in **PC** and 2:1 in **HH**. Both polysaccharides demonstrated significant anticoagulant activity in the clotting time assay, which is connected with the ability of these FCSs to potentiate inhibition of thrombin and factor Xa in the presence of ATIII and with the direct inhibition of thrombin in the absence of any cofactors.

Supplementary Materials: The following are available online at http://www.mdpi.com/1660-3397/18/11/540/s1, Figure S1: The COSY NMR spectra of polysaccharides **PC (I)** and **HH (II)**, Figure S2: The ROESY NMR spectra of polysaccharides **PC (I)** and **HH (II)**, Figure S3: The TOCSY NMR spectra of polysaccharides **PC (I)** and **HH (II)**, and Figure S4: The calculation of the ratios of units H:E and D:E:F in polysaccharide **HH** using the integral intensities of the respective H-1 signals.

Author Contributions: Conceptualization, A.I.U., N.E.N., V.A.S., and N.E.U.; methodology, A.I.U., M.I.B., and N.E.U.; analysis, M.I.B., N.E.U., A.S.D, and A.S.S.; investigation, M.I.B., N.E.U., A.S.D., A.S.S., and A.I.U.; resources, B.B.G. and A.S.S.; original draft preparation, N.E.U. and A.I.U.; review and editing, all authors; supervision, A.I.U., N.E.N., and V.A.S. All authors have read and agreed to the published version of the manuscript.

Funding: This research was funded by the Russian Science Foundation, grant number 19-73-20240.

Conflicts of Interest: The authors declare no conflict of interest. The funders had no role in the design of the study; in the collection, analyses, or interpretation of data; in the writing of the manuscript; or in the decision to publish the results.

References

1. Pomin, V.H. Holothurian fucosylated chondroitin sulfates. *Mar. Drugs* **2014**, *12*, 232–254. [CrossRef] [PubMed]
2. Myron, P.; Siddiquee, S.; Azad, S.A. Fucosylated chondroitin sulfate diversity in sea cucumbers: A review. *Carbohydr. Polym.* **2014**, *112*, 173–178. [CrossRef]
3. Pomin, V.H.; Vignovich, W.P.; Gonzales, A.V.; Vasconcelos, A.A.; Mulloy, B. Galactosaminoglycans: Medical Applications and Drawbacks. *Molecules* **2019**, *24*, 2803. [CrossRef]
4. Ustyuzhanina, N.E.; Bilan, M.I.; Nifantiev, N.E.; Usov, A.I. New insight on the structural diversity of holothurian fucosylated chondroitin sulfates. *Pure Appl. Chem.* **2019**, *91*, 1065–1071. [CrossRef]
5. Chen, S.; Xue, C.; Yin, L.; Tang, Q.; Yu, G.; Chai, W. Comparison of structures and anticoagulant activities of fucosylated chondroitin sulfates from different sea cucumbers. *Carbohydr. Polym.* **2011**, *83*, 688–696. [CrossRef]
6. Mourão, P.A.S. Perspective on the use of sulfated polysaccharides from marine organisms as a source of new antithrombotic drugs. *Mar. Drugs* **2015**, *13*, 2770–2784. [CrossRef] [PubMed]
7. Ustyuzhanina, N.E.; Bilan, M.I.; Dmitrenok, A.S.; Tsvetkova, E.A.; Shashkov, A.S.; Stonik, V.A.; Nifantiev, N.E.; Usov, A.I. Structural characterization of fucosylated chondroitin sulfates from sea cucumbers *Apostichopus japonicus* and *Actinopyga mauritiana*. *Carbohydr. Polym.* **2016**, *153*, 399–405. [CrossRef]
8. Ustyuzhanina, N.E.; Bilan, M.I.; Dmitrenok, A.S.; Nifantiev, N.E.; Usov, A.I. Two fucosylated chondroitin sulfates from the sea cucumber *Eupentacta fraudatrix*. *Carbohydr. Polym.* **2017**, *164*, 8–12. [CrossRef]
9. Chen, S.; Li, G.; Wu, N.; Guo, X.; Liao, N.; Ye, X.; Liu, D.; Xue, C.; Chai, W. Sulfation pattern of the fucose branch is important for the anticoagulant and antithrombotic activities of fucosylated chondroitin sulfates. *Biochim. Biophys. Acta* **2013**, *1830*, 3054–3066. [CrossRef]
10. Soares, P.A.G.; Ribeiro, K.A.; Valente, A.P.; Capillé, N.V.; Oliveira, S.-N.M.C.G.; Tovar, A.M.F.; Pereira, M.S.; Vilanova, E.; Mourão, P.A.S. A unique fucosylated chondroitin sulfate type II with strikingly homogeneous and neatly distributed α-fucose branches. *Glycobiology* **2018**, *28*, 565–579. [CrossRef]
11. Carvalhal, F.; Cristelo, R.R.; Resende, D.I.S.P.; Pinto, M.M.M.; Sousa, E.; Correia-da-Silva, M. Antithrombotics from the Sea: Polysaccharides and Beyond. *Mar. Drugs* **2019**, *17*, 170. [CrossRef]
12. Mourão, P.A.S.; Boisson-Vidal, C.; Tapon-Bretaudiere, J.; Drouet, B.; Bros, A.; Fischer, A. Inactivation of thrombin by a fucosylated chondroitin sulfate from echinoderm. *Thromb. Res.* **2001**, *102*, 167–176.
13. Liu, X.; Hao, J.; Shan, X.; Zhang, X.; Zhao, X.; Li, Q.; Wang, X.; Cai, C.; Li, G.; Yu, G. Antithrombotic activities of fucosylated chondroitin sulfates and their depolymerized fragments from two sea cucumbers. *Carbohydr. Polym.* **2016**, *152*, 343–350. [CrossRef]
14. Ustyuzhanina, N.E.; Bilan, M.I.; Dmitrenok, A.S.; Borodina, E.Y.; Stonik, V.A.; Nifantiev, N.E.; Usov, A.I. A highly regular fucosylated chondroitin sulfate from the sea cucumber *Massinium magnum*: Structure and effects on coagulation. *Carbohydr. Polym.* **2017**, *167*, 20–26. [CrossRef]
15. Wu, M.; Wen, D.; Gao, N.; Xiao, C.; Yang, L.; Xu, L.; Lian, W.; Peng, W.; Jiang, J.; Zhao, J. Anticoagulant and antithrombotic evaluation of native fucosylated chondroitin sulfates and their derivatives as selective inhibitors of intrinsic factor Xase. *Eur. J. Med. Chem.* **2015**, *92*, 257–269. [CrossRef]
16. Yan, L.; Li, J.; Wang, D.; Ding, T.; Hu, Y.; Ye, X.; Linhardt, R.J.; Chen, S. Molecular size is important for the safety and selective inhibition of intrinsic factor Xase for fucosylated chondroitin sulfate. *Carbohydr. Polym.* **2017**, *178*, 180–189. [CrossRef]

17. Yan, L.; Wang, D.; Zhu, M.; Yu, Y.; Zhang, F.; Ye, X.; Linhardt, R.J.; Chen, S. Highly purified fucosylated chondroitin sulfate oligomers with selective intrinsic factor Xase complex inhibition. *Carbohydr. Polym.* **2019**, *222*, 115025. [CrossRef]
18. Pomin, V.H.; Mourão, P.A.S. Specific sulfation and glycosylation—A structural combination for the anticoagulation of marine carbohydrates. *Front. Cell. Infect. Microbiol.* **2014**, *4*, 33. [CrossRef]
19. Panagos, C.G.; Thomson, D.S.; Moss, C.; Hoghes, A.D.; Kelly, M.S.; Liu, Y.; Chai, W.; Venkatasamy, R.; Spina, D.; Page, C.P.; et al. Fucosylated chondroitin sulfates from the body wall of the sea cucumber *Holothuria forskali*. Conformation, selectin binding, and biological activity. *J. Biol. Chem.* **2014**, *289*, 28284–28298. [CrossRef]
20. Ustyuzhanina, N.E.; Bilan, M.I.; Dmitrenok, A.S.; Shashkov, A.S.; Ponce, N.M.A.; Stortz, C.A.; Nifantiev, N.E.; Usov, A.I. Fucosylated chondroitin sulfate from the sea cucumber *Hemioedema spectabilis*: Structure and influence on cell adhesion and tubulogenesis. *Carbohydr. Polym.* **2020**, *234*, 115895. [CrossRef]
21. Li, Q.; Cai, C.; Chang, Y.; Zhang, F.; Linhardt, R.J.; Xue, C.; Li, G.; Yu, G. A novel structural fucosylated chondroitin sulfate from *Holothuria mexicana* and its effects on growth factors binding and anticoagulation. *Carbohydr. Polym.* **2018**, *181*, 1160–1168. [CrossRef]
22. Wu, J.; Yi, Y.-H.; Tang, H.-F.; Wu, H.-M. Hillasides A and B, two new cytotoxic triterpene glycosides from the sea cucumber *Holothuria hilla* Lesson. *J. Asia Nat. Prod. Res.* **2007**, *9*, 609–615. [CrossRef]
23. Wu, J.; Yi, Y.-H.; Tang, H.F.; Zou, Z.-R.; Wu, H.-M. Structure and cytotoxicity of a new lanostan-type triterpene glycoside from the sea cucumber *Holothuria hilla*. *Chem. Biodivers.* **2006**, *3*, 1249–1254. [CrossRef]
24. Kalinin, V.I.; Malyutin, A.N.; Stonik, V.A. Caudinoside A—A new triterpene glycoside from the holothurian *Paracaudina ransonetii*. *Chem. Nat. Compd.* **1986**, *22*, 355–356. [CrossRef]
25. Suzuki, T. Amino acid sequence of a major globin from the sea cucumber Paracaudina chilensis. *Biochim. Biophys. Acta* **1989**, *998*, 292–296. [CrossRef]
26. Zeng, M.; Xiao, F.; Li, B.; Zhao, Y.; Liu, Z.; Dong, S. Study on free radical scavenging activity of sea cucumber (*Paracaudina chinens* var.) gelatin hydrolysate. *J. Ocean. Univ. China* **2007**, *6*, 255–258. [CrossRef]
27. Vieira, R.P.; Mulloy, B.; Mourão, P.A.S. Structure of a fucose-branched chondroitin sulfate from sea cucumber. Evidence for the presence of 3-O-sulfo-β-D-glucuronosyl residues. *J. Biol. Chem.* **1991**, *266*, 13530–13536.
28. Guo, X.; Condra, M.; Kimura, K.; Berth, G.; Dautzenberg, H.; Dubin, P.L. Determination of molecular weight of heparin by size exclusion chromatography with universal calibration. *Anal. Biochem.* **2003**, *312*, 33–39. [CrossRef]
29. Pomin, V.H. NMR structural determination of unique invertebrate glycosaminoglycans endowed with medical properties. *Carbohydr. Res.* **2015**, *413*, 41–50. [CrossRef]
30. Ustyuzhanina, N.E.; Bilan, M.I.; Panina, E.G.; Sanamyan, N.P.; Dmitrenok, A.S.; Tsvetkova, E.A.; Ushakova, N.A.; Shashkov, A.S.; Nifantiev, N.E.; Usov, A.I. Structure anf anti-inflammatory activity of a new unusual fucosylated chondroitin sulfate from *Cucumaria djakonovi*. *Mar. Drugs* **2018**, *16*, 389. [CrossRef]
31. Ustyuzhanina, N.E.; Ushakova, N.A.; Zyuzina, K.A.; Bilan, M.I.; Elizarova, A.L.; Somonova, O.V.; Madzhuga, A.V.; Krylov, V.B.; Preobrazhenskaya, M.E.; Usov, A.I.; et al. Influence of fucoidans on hemostatic system. *Mar. Drugs* **2013**, *11*, 2444–2458. [CrossRef]
32. Bilan, M.I.; Grachev, A.A.; Ustuzhanina, N.E.; Shashkov, A.S.; Nifantiev, N.E.; Usov, A.I. Structure of a fucoidan from the brown seaweed *Fucus evanescens* C.Ag. *Carbohydr. Res.* **2002**, *337*, 719–730. [CrossRef]
33. Bilan, M.I.; Zakharova, A.N.; Grachev, A.A.; Shashkov, A.S.; Nifantiev, N.E.; Usov, A.I. Polysaccharides of algae: 60. Fucoidan from the Pacific brown alga *Analipus japonicus* (Harv.) Winne (Ectocarpales, Scytosiphonaceae). *Russ. J. Bioorg. Chem.* **2007**, *33*, 38–46. [CrossRef]
34. Usov, A.I.; Bilan, M.I.; Klochkova, N.G. Polysaccharides of algae: 48. Polysaccharide composition of several calcareous red algae: Isolation of alginate from *Corallina pilulifera* P. et R. (Rhodophyta, Corallinaceae). *Bot. Mar.* **1995**, *38*, 43–51. [CrossRef]
35. Dubois, M.; Gilles, K.A.; Hamilton, J.K.; Rebers, P.A.; Smith, F. Colorimetric method for determination of sugars and related substances. *Anal. Chem.* **1956**, *28*, 350–356. [CrossRef]

Publisher's Note: MDPI stays neutral with regard to jurisdictional claims in published maps and institutional affiliations.

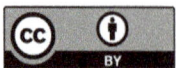

© 2020 by the authors. Licensee MDPI, Basel, Switzerland. This article is an open access article distributed under the terms and conditions of the Creative Commons Attribution (CC BY) license (http://creativecommons.org/licenses/by/4.0/).

MDPI\
St. Alban-Anlage 66\
4052 Basel\
Switzerland\
Tel. +41 61 683 77 34\
Fax +41 61 302 89 18\
www.mdpi.com

Marine Drugs Editorial Office\
E-mail: marinedrugs@mdpi.com\
www.mdpi.com/journal/marinedrugs

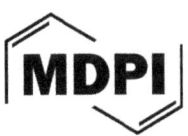

www.ingramcontent.com/pod-product-compliance
Lightning Source LLC
LaVergne TN
LVHW070717100526
838202LV00013B/1111